WHAT YOU MUST KNOW ABOUT

VITAMINS MINERALS HERBS AND SO MUCH MORE

SECOND EDITION

PAMELA WARTIAN SMITH, MD, MPH

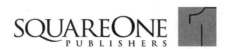

SQUAREONE
PUBLISHERS

EDITOR: Joanne Abrams
COVER DESIGNER: Jeannie Rosado
TYPESETTER: Gary A. Rosenberg

The information and advice contained in this book are based upon the research and the personal and professional experiences of the author. They are not intended as a substitute for consulting with a healthcare professional. The publisher and author are not responsible for any adverse effects or consequences resulting from the use of any of the suggestions, preparations, or procedures discussed in this book. All matters pertaining to your physical health should be supervised by a healthcare professional. It is a sign of wisdom, not cowardice, to seek a second or third opinion.

Square One Publishers
115 Herricks Road
Garden City Park, NY 11040
(516) 535-2010 • (877) 900-BOOK
www.squareonepublishers.com

Library of Congress Cataloging-in-Publication Data

Names: Smith, Pamela Wartian, author.
Title: What you must know about vitamins, minerals, herbs and so much more
  : choosing the nutrients that are right for you / Pamela Wartian Smith.
Description: Second edition. | Garden City Park : Square One Publishers,
  2020. | Includes index.
Identifiers: LCCN 2019024117 (print) | LCCN 2019024118 (ebook) | ISBN
  9780757004711 (paperback) | ISBN 9780757054716 (epub)
Subjects: LCSH: Naturopathy. | Dietary supplements. | Herbs—Therapeutic
  use. | Vitamins. | Nutrition. | Self-care, Health.
Classification: LCC RZ440 .S58 2020 (print) | LCC RZ440 (ebook) | DDC
  615.5/35—dc23
LC record available at https://lccn.loc.gov/2019024117
LC ebook record available at https://lccn.loc.gov/2019024118

Printed in the United States of America

10   9   8   7   6   5   4   3

Contents

PART 2: HEALTH CONDITIONS

In memory of Dr. Walter Crinnion. Every so often, we encounter a visionary who lights the torch of illumination so brightly, we cannot look away. Dr. Walter Crinnion is the man who enlightened us in the field of Environmental Medicine.

Acknowledgments

The wisdom of so many fine people has led me to this book. I cannot hope to name them all. In thanking a few, I extend my thanks to all.

To Roger Williams and Linus Pauling, who were the forerunners in the field of orthomolecular/functional medicine.

To my contemporaries, Drs. David Perlmutter, Steven Sinatra, Alan Gaby, Ronald Klatz, Robert Goldman, Shari Lieberman, Mark Houston, Patrick Quillin, Elizabeth Stuller, Todd LePine, Jill Carnahan, Lyn Patrick, and Filomena Trindade, who have taught me so much.

To Rudy Shur and Joanne Abrams at Square One Publishers, for their hard work and dedication to this project without which this book would never have been published. I am truly blessed to have the best publisher and editor that any author could have.

To my husband, Christopher Smith, for his enduring patience and support.

To God, for always lighting my path.

Introduction

Do you need to take vitamins and other nutrients? In what amounts should you take them? Which supplements are the most effective? What should you take for a specific illness or chronic problem? Answering these questions is a fundamental aspect of good health and longevity—but there are so many countering viewpoints regarding nutrients and nutrient supplementation that it can be hard to know what to do. This book will provide you with the critical information necessary to find the answers that are right for you.

Various health committees have attempted to provide nutritional guidelines. The Food and Nutrition Board of the National Academy of Science, for example, developed its recommended daily allowance (RDA) and its reference daily intake (RDI). However, these dietary suggestions, which are often strictly adhered to by well-meaning individuals, are designed to prevent disease. They are not designed to help people achieve optimal wellness—which should be the goal.

Furthermore, the RDA and RDI were developed without considering that each person requires a different amount of vitamins, minerals, and other nutrients. To fully promote your body's health, your nutritional intake must reflect such factors as soil depletion, the need for more antioxidants, the medications you're taking, vitamin interactions, stress, age, lifestyle, and genetics. Therefore, you cannot trust that your healthy friend's nutritional plan will necessarily work for you.

Proper determination of what your body needs is imperative. Almost 75 percent of your health and life expectancy is based on lifestyle, environment, and nutrition. Just as important, these factors also greatly influence the number of years you spend healthy. This statement has been proven by studies which show that "not only do persons with better health habits survive longer, but in such individuals, disability is postponed and compressed into fewer years at the end of life." An article in *The New England Journal of Medicine* illustrated

1

this point. After examining diet, lifestyle, and the risk of type 2 diabetes mellitus in women, the author concluded that the majority of type 2 diabetes cases are preventable with the adoption of a healthy lifestyle.

Similarly, researchers in the *Journal of the American Medical Association* stated, "Suboptimal vitamin states are associated with many chronic diseases including cardiovascular disease, cancer, and osteoporosis. It is important for physicians to identify patients with poor nutrition or other reasons for increased vitamin needs." They suggested that, "Most people do not consume an optimal amount of all vitamins by diet alone . . . it appears prudent for all adults to take vitamin supplements."

What You Must Know About Vitamins, Minerals, Herbs, and So Much More, Second Edition provides the information you need to know about nutrients—including signs of deficiencies, therapies for various diseases and disorders, and the dangers of certain interactions. Since the first edition of this book was published, patients have asked me many questions concerning supplements that have become known to the public only in the last few years—supplements such as cocoa and CBD oil. This second edition includes information about these substances so that you can learn if they might benefit you. It's important to recognize that in addition to research being performed on "new" nutrients, it continues to be conducted on supplements that have been studied and used for many years—supplements such as lutein, glucosamine, quercetin, and red yeast rice, to name just a few. Therefore, in this edition, I have also expanded and updated the information provided on many other nutrients. This revised material—always backed by rigorous scientific studies as well as my own experience working with patients—will allow you to make informed decisions, optimize your health, and live your life well.

The Purpose
of This Book

Many people claim that good health is their top priority. They may eat healthy foods, exercise vigorously, and visit their doctor on a regular basis. Unfortunately, in today's society, these good habits aren't enough to maintain optimal health. As you read on page 1, vitamin and minerals have a direct effect on both life span and quality of life—and modern-day food does not contain all the essential nutrients.

There are several reasons why you can't get all the nutrients you need from food. Most soil is now depleted of many important minerals, including zinc and magnesium. Selenium, a trace mineral that contributes to good health in small amounts but can be toxic in large amounts, is depleted in some areas while in overabundance in others. If the soil in which fruits and vegetables are grown is not rich in the proper minerals, these foods will not contain an adequate supply of nutrients.

Also, fruits and vegetables begin to lose their nutritional value immediately after they are picked. Cold storage continues this destruction of nutrients. Stored grapes, for example, lose up to 30 percent of their B vitamins by the time they arrive in most grocery stores. When tangerines are stored for eight weeks, they lose almost half of their vitamin C. Storing asparagus for one week can cause them to lose up to 90 percent of their vitamin C. The best and most effective time to eat fruits and vegetables is immediately after they are picked. Unfortunately, most of us are not in a position to do so.

Cooking, too, can destroy some of the nutrients found in produce. In fact, the longer you cook fruits and vegetables, the less nutrients remain. Therefore, you should try to eat these foods raw or lightly steamed, and, if possible, soon after they are picked.

Along with cooking, some of the ways in which food today is handled and prepared destroy some of the nutritional value it retained after being picked.

3

Many foods are blanched, sterilized, canned, and otherwise processed—all practices that decrease nutritional value. The milling of grains, for example, removes twenty-six essential nutrients and much of their fiber.

Because so much of the food we eat is depleted of essential vitamins and minerals, we must look elsewhere for these nutrients. In today's society, the consumption of supplements has become fundamental for good health. *What You Must Know About Vitamins, Minerals, Herbs, and So Much More* will assist you in choosing the nutrients required to keep your family healthy. It will also help you discover other nutrient-rich foods.

Unfortunately, even eating food that is rich in nutrients does not guarantee that you are receiving the nutrients you need. The nutrients may not be in a form that is *bioavailable*—able to be absorbed and utilized by the body. Despite the healthy perception of orange juice, for example, 40 percent of its vitamin C is biologically inactive. Yet most nutritional listings do not differentiate between nutrients that are biologically available and those that are biologically unavailable, leaving many health-conscious consumers in the dark.

There are also processes within your body that necessitate the constant refueling of nutrients. *Free radicals* are molecules created in the body by reactions that occur to produce energy and other substances. These molecules lack electrons, so they search the body for healthy cells and steal their electrons, modifying or killing the cells as a result. This process, called *oxidation,* causes *oxidative stress,* which can lead to tissue damage, disease, and aging. Free radical production requires more nutrients to avoid this harmful oxidative stress than in previous generations—further increasing the importance of good nutrition.

Yet free radicals also occur in the environment. In fact, they now occur in the environment more than ever before. Causes of free radical production outside the body include television screens; cell phones; computer screens; airplane trips; hair dryers; fluorescent lights; microwaves; toxic exposure to chemicals in food, water, and air; and excessive sunlight. This exposure to free radicals in the environment causes an extra load of oxidation that the body cannot handle. Oxidation in your body is like rust on your car. If extra free radicals are bombarding your body all day long, your system can "rust" on the inside. There may be physical results, such as cataract formation or sunburns. To stop the oxidative process, you can take *antioxidants,* which donate an electron to the free radical and help stop the destructive course.

There are different antioxidants that can be consumed to diminish oxidation. It is paramount that they be balanced. In certain conditions, too much of one antioxidant may hinder the protective effects of other antioxidants. Examples of antioxidants are vitamin A, vitamin C, vitamin E, selenium, coenzyme

Q_{10}, alpha lipoic acid, melatonin, garlic, and glutathione. I will describe these important antioxidants in further detail later in this book.

As you age, your body converts less vitamin D into the active form, and makes less alpha lipoic acid and coenzyme Q_{10}. This means that your body needs to find these nutrients elsewhere. As you will discover in later chapters, you can help your body age more comfortably by providing these nutrients in abundance.

Lifestyle is yet another factor that influences your need for nutrients. Stress, for example, depletes the body of certain vitamins and minerals, while drinking alcohol depletes the body of biotin, copper, zinc, and vitamins B_1, B_6, B_{12}, and C. Our eating habits can also cause major nutritional problems. As Dr. Michael Colgan states in his book *The New Nutrition*, "The American diet is a major cause of disease." The American diet is examined in the inset below.

The American Diet

According to most top nutritionists, the American diet is a serious cause for concern. As children develop, it is very important that they both receive necessary nutrients and learn healthy eating habits. Unfortunately, this is not the case for most American children. The following is an eye-opening list of the top three vegetables eaten by American children and teens.

- French fries—which account for 25 percent of all the vegetables they consume.

- Iceberg lettuce—which is 99 percent water with no nutritional value.

- Ketchup—which is one-half sugar.

Adults do not fare much better. The Second National Health and Nutrition Examination (NHANES II) conducted a survey that revealed the following.

- Less than 10 percent of Americans consume five servings of fruits and vegetables each day.

- 40 percent of Americans do not consume daily fruit or fruit juice.

- 50 percent of Americans do not consume daily garden vegetables.

- 70 percent of Americans do not consume daily fruit or vegetables rich in vitamin C.

- 80 percent of Americans do not consume daily fruit or vegetables rich in carotenoids.

Diet and nutrition play a major role in influencing how your genes express themselves. As Dr. Leo Galland pointed out, "It depends as much upon the milieu in which a gene functions as it does upon the DNA sequence of the genome." Therefore, even if you have inherited a gene for a particular illness such as Alzheimer's disease, whether the disease manifests itself depends on your environment, the food you eat, the toxins you are around, your stress level, and the nutrients your body receives. Dr. Roger Williams discusses this situation in his book *Biochemical Individuality: The Basis for the Genotropic Concept.* He states, "Nutrition applied with due concern for individual genetic variations, which may be large, offers the solution to many baffling health problems." Let's again compare your body to a car. If you feed it good fuel (nutritious food), it will run well, need little repair, and last a long time. If you put low octane fuel in your premium car (your body), it will not run well (develop disease and shorten life expectancy).

Some physicians say there is a lack of peer review studies or scientific evidence to show that vitamin and nutritional therapies work. Yet every year, there are thousands of studies on vitamins published, and thousands more on antioxidants. In fact, more research has been published on nutrients than on medications!

The therapeutic techniques described throughout this book are supported by thousands of literary references from respected, peer-reviewed scientific and medical publications. David Perlmutter, MD, a respected neurologist and author of BrainRecovery.com, said on his website, "It has been said that knowledge is power, but clearly in this context, knowledge is health." This knowledge is now available to you.

In Part 1, this book examines vitamins, minerals, fatty acids, amino acids, and other nutrients that help maintain health and aid in reducing disease. The suggested dosages are for people twelve years old or older and at least one hundred pounds in weight. Dosage is expressed in either milligrams or international units (a unit of measurement used in pharmacology) unless otherwise stated. Many of the nutrients, such as vitamins and minerals, can be consumed either in supplements or in foods, so you will also find lists of foods that contain high amounts of each relevant nutrient. It is important to note that in the numbered lists, the foods found at the top of the list contain more of the nutrient under discussion. Lists that are not numbered are in alphabetical order.

Part 2 of this book presents nutritional programs for various disorders and conditions, from acne to wounds. In each case, you will find an explanation of the problem, including possible symptoms and causes. This is followed by a table that lists supplements which can help you avoid, recover from, or manage the condition.

The information and recommendations provided in Parts 1 and 2 have been based on thousands of scientific studies and academic papers, along with clinical experience. Because this new edition covers so many more supplements than were discussed in the first edition, we were faced with the possibility of devoting 100 pages or more to a reference section. Since this would have made the book longer and far more costly, we decided to place the references on the publisher's website, which you can access at www.squareonepublishers.com, under the listing of my book.

As you read this book, keep in mind that, along with proper nutritional intake, choosing the right healthcare provider is important to overall health. I strongly suggest finding a specialist fellowship-trained in functional, anti-aging medicine, or personalized medicine. (See the Resources for contact information.)

Functional medicine is an integrative, science-based healthcare approach that treats illness and promotes wellness by tailoring individual therapies to restore physiological, psychological, and structural balance. This method of returning balance to your body in an effort to prevent and treat chronic disease—rather than simply treating the acute illness—can be quite effective. Functional medicine practitioners can also help you make informed nutritional decisions. *Anti-aging medicine* is a functional medicine approach that focuses on the biochemically unique aspects of each patient to prevent age-related decline. It seeks to prevent and treat age-related diseases, while also extending and improving quality of life for its patients. *Personalized medicine*—also called *individualized* or *precision medicine*—uses genomic (gene-based) information to determine an individual's susceptibility to various health problems, identifies appropriate preventive measures, and chooses targeted therapies that promote wellness. More information on the topics of functional, anti-aging, and personalized medicine can be found at www.faafm.com.

A number of factors, ranging from foods grown in nutrient-poor soil to cooking methods that destroy vitamins and minerals, can make it impossible to get all the nutrients your body requires from your diet. *What You Must Know About Vitamins, Minerals, Herbs, and So Much More* provides you with the up-to-date information you need to promote and maintain optimal health for yourself and your family.

Mixing Supplements, Drugs, and Food

The importance of consuming vitamins, minerals, and other nutrients cannot be overstated. At the same time, it is a process that must be monitored. The interaction of certain supplements, drugs, and food can be detrimental to your health rather than beneficial. Before starting any supplement regimen, therefore, you must be aware of possible side effects and contraindications. The following lists provide examples of problems that can occur from some fairly common interactions. These lists should not be viewed as being all-inclusive. Throughout Part 1, in the discussion of each supplement, you'll find specific cautions regarding its use as well as information on side effects and possible interactions with medications and other supplements. When you start putting together a supplement regimen—possibly based on a supplements table found in Part 2—it is important to read the relevant entries in Part 1 so that you fully understand each nutrient you take. It is also smart to work closely with your healthcare provider and pharmacist, as they understand the medications you're taking and can help ensure that your regimen is not only effective but also safe.

COMBINING NUTRITIONAL SUPPLEMENTS WITH MEDICATION

Some medications can deplete your body of specific nutrients, and some nutritional supplements can increase or decrease your body's absorption of some medications, changing their effect. Sometimes, these interactions can be quite serious, such as when a blood-thinning supplement increases the effect of a blood-thinning drug. The following list provides common examples of different supplement-medication interactions. If you are taking any medications—even drugs that don't appear on this list—it's crucial to discuss any nutritional changes with your healthcare provider or pharmacist. Your provider can guide you in replacing any depleted nutrients and alert you to supplements and medications that have the potential to interact.

- Antiarrhythmic medications, such as disopyramide and quinidine sulfate, can cause magnesium deficiency.

- Anticonvulsants (seizure medications) can deplete the body of carnitine.

- Birth control pills and other forms of estrogen replacement deplete the body of B vitamins.

- Calcium can inhibit the absorption of certain drugs, such as tetracycline and thyroid medications.

- Chamomile can increase the risk of bleeding when taking blood thinners like warfarin.

- Colchicine reduces the absorption of beta-carotene. It may also reduce the absorption of magnesium, potassium, and vitamin B_{12}.

- Digoxin (a medication usually prescribed for heart-related problems) can increase the rate of calcium excretion from the body.

- Diuretics (water pills) can decrease levels of magnesium, potassium, sodium, and zinc.

- Estrogen replacement increases calcium absorption.

- Fiber can decrease the absorption of digoxin.

- Ginkgo biloba can interact with a wide range of medications, including blood thinners, MAO inhibitors, and blood pressure drugs.

- Histamine-2 receptor antagonists (H2-blockers), such as cimetidine, can prevent or block the production of stomach acid and decrease vitamin D activity.

- HMG-CoA reductase inhibitors (statin drugs), used to lower cholesterol, can decrease your body's ability to make adequate coenzyme Q_{10}.

- Long-term use of antacids can lead to decreased folic acid absorption.

- Medications used to lower blood sugar—such as glyburide, acetohexamide, and tolazamide—can lead to coenzyme Q_{10} deficiency.

- Methotrexate, used to treat cancer and autoimmune disorders, can decrease beta-carotene, folic acid, and vitamin B_{12}.

Combining Grapefruit with Medication

Grapefruit is a highly nutritious food. It is packed with vitamin C, potassium, glutathione, and lycopene; is rich in antioxidants; and is high in fiber. In fact, you'll see it in some of the Food Sources lists in Part 1. Unfortunately, grapefruit is also unique in that it can interact with a number of medications in different ways, delaying the absorption of the drug, increasing the level of the drug, or causing side effects ranging from hives to insomnia. When taken with certain medications, grapefruit juice can even cause kidney and liver toxicity.

How does grapefruit cause these effects? Many drugs are metabolized (broken down) in the small intestine with the help of an isoenzyme called CYP3A4. Grapefruit juice can block the action of this isoenzyme so that instead of being metabolized, the medication enters the blood and stays in the body longer. The result, quite simply, is too much of that drug in the body.

In a few cases, grapefruit has a very different effect. Some drugs are moved by transporters into the body's cells, and grapefruit juice can impede the action of the transporters, decreasing the amount of the drug in your body so that it is not able to work as well as it should. In other words, there is too little of the drug in the body.

The printed information that accompanies your prescription or OTC medication will tell you if you have to avoid grapefruit juice. Nevertheless, it makes sense to check with your healthcare provider or pharmacist to see if you have to avoid grapefruit juice altogether or simply cut down on the amount consumed. The side effects listed below will give you some idea of the potential problems that can be caused by this food.

- Grapefruit can cause flushing, headaches, and increased heart rate if eaten while taking calcium-channel blockers, which are taken to decrease blood pressure.

- Grapefruit increases quinidine levels.

- Grapefruit can cause irregular heart rhythms if eaten while taking the antihistamine terfenadine.

- Grapefruit can increase levels of benzodiazepines.

- Grapefruit can cause kidney and liver toxicity if it is eaten while taking cyclosporine.

- Grapefruit increases caffeine levels and can cause nervousness and insomnia.

- Grapefruit can decrease the absorption of macrolide antibiotics such as clarithromycin.

- Grapefruit can decrease the absorption of the antihistamine fexofenadine.

- Grapefruit can increase the medication level of HMG-CoA reductase inhibitors (statin drugs).

- Grapefruit can increase the level of warfarin, a medication that affects blood clotting.

- Grapefruit can delay the absorption of sildenafil, a male impotence medication.

- Grapefruit can cause hives if taken with the pain reliever naproxen.

- Grapefruit can increase the amount of carbamazepine absorbed by the body, leading to nausea, tremors, drowsiness, dizziness, or agitation.

- Grapefruit can elevate blood levels of amiodarone, causing nausea, drowsiness, tremors, or agitation.

- Grapefruit can increase estrogen levels in both men and women. No interaction with medication is necessary for this to occur.

- Potassium-sparing diuretics deplete your body of folic acid, calcium, and zinc.

- Regular use of aspirin decreases folate levels.

- Too much vitamin B_6 can decrease the effectiveness of levodopa, a treatment for Parkinson's disease.

COMBINING SUPPLEMENTS

Vitamins, minerals, and other nutritional supplements can interact with one another, as well as with medications. These relationships and interrelationships can have various effects—some good, and some bad. The following examples show how certain supplements interact. (For more information on supplement interactions and absorption, see the inset on page 65.)

- A certain amount of vitamin C is necessary for your body to use selenium effectively.

- Vitamin C can enhance the availability of vitamin A.

- Too much zinc can decrease calcium absorption.

- Vitamin D increases the absorption of calcium and magnesium.

- Vitamin D helps your body use zinc effectively.

- Too much copper can decrease the uptake of manganese in your system.

- A vitamin A deficiency can decrease iron utilization.

- Too much iron can lower your manganese and copper levels.

- Too much vitamin B_2 (riboflavin) can cause a magnesium deficiency.

- Vitamin B_6 (pyridoxine) can cause a decrease in copper absorption.

- A vitamin E deficiency can decrease absorption of vitamin A.

- A vitamin B_6 (pyridoxine) deficiency can lead to a decreased use of selenium.

- Adequate phosphorus intake is needed to maintain vitamin D.

- High doses of fish oil (omega-3 fatty acids) combined with blood-thinning herbs such as ginkgo biloba can cause bleeding.

- The herb fenugreek can inhibit the absorption of iron supplements.

- Taking melatonin with other supplements that have sedative effects, such as valerian and St. John's wort, can increase both the intended effects and the side effects of the melatonin.

PART 1

Nutrients

1

Vitamins

Vitamins are substances that occur naturally in both plants and animals and are essential—in small amounts—for normal growth and nutrition. They are divided into two categories: fat-soluble vitamins and water-soluble vitamins.

Fat-soluble vitamins include vitamins A, D, E, and K. With the exception of vitamin K, these nutrients are stored in the body for long periods of time. For that reason, vitamins A, D, and E generally pose a risk for toxicity if they are taken in excess.

Water-soluble vitamins, such as the B-complex vitamins and vitamin C, are not stored in the body, but are eliminated via the urine on the same day they are ingested. Because these nutrients are so quickly flushed out, the body requires a daily supply. In fact, B vitamins should be taken twice a day for optimal health.

In this chapter, you will first read about fat-soluble vitamins. Then, you will turn your attention to water-soluble vitamins.

Although it has long been the topic of much debate, we now know that the quality of the vitamins—as well as other supplements—that you take *does* make a difference. Whether or not the substance will work for you depends on factors such as form, purity, and bioavailability. Supplements are divided into four grades, or quality categories, that take these factors into account. To learn more about this, turn to the inset on page 18.

As you become familiar with the different vitamins discussed in this chapter, be sure to give careful consideration to each one's potential side effects and contraindications. As you read in the section "Mixing Supplements, Drugs, and Food," which begins on page 9, there are various reactions that can occur when different substances are taken together. Similarly, taking too much of a certain vitamin can result in either the deficit of another vitamin or an unpleasant or even dangerous health issue. Yet, as you will see, nutritional deficiencies can

Determining the Quality of Nutritional Supplements

An important part of any supplement plan is choosing good-quality products. This guarantees that the vitamins, minerals, herbs, and other nutrients you take will provide the benefits your body needs.

Nutritional supplements are divided into four categories. To be considered a better grade, a supplement must be tested by an outside (third-party) source that can verify its quality. Below, you will find a brief description of each of these categories.

- **Pharmaceutical grade:** Supplements of this grade meet the highest regulatory requirements for purity, dissolution (ability to be dissolved), and absorption as verified by an outside party. In terms of purity, these supplements must be 99-percent pure, with no binders, fillers, dyes, or other unknown substances. These are the supplements most often sold by licensed healthcare practitioners.

- **Medical grade:** These supplements are of a high grade although they may not conform to the standards of pharmaceutical grade products. Prenatal vitamins are usually in this category.

- **Cosmetic or nutritional grade:** These supplements are often not tested for purity, dissolution, or absorption. They may not have a high concentration of their listed active ingredient. This is the grade of supplement most often sold in health food stores.

- **Feed or agricultural grade:** Supplements of this grade are used for veterinary purposes. Never use supplements of this grade.

result in equally serious problems. Visit your healthcare professional if you have any questions as you develop your optimal vitamin regimen.

Every year, over 75 percent of your body is reconstructed from the nutrients you consume either in food or in supplement form. The quality of these nutrients determines the quality of your cells, how well they function, and if they are able to prevent disease. Nutrients even affect your DNA.

To maximize your supplements' shelf life and potency, store them in a cool, dry place, away from heat, moisture, and direct light. Avoid keeping them in the refrigerator, where the humidity can cause the nutrients to degrade.

In addition to aiming for the highest grade of supplement, be aware that the form of the nutrient used is very important. For instance, calcium citrate is a more *bioavailable* form than calcium carbonate, which means that a greater proportion of the nutrient is utilized for body functions. Whenever possible, choose natural forms of nutrients. Natural vitamin E, for example, is better absorbed and more active than the synthetic version. Why are less effective forms of nutrients sometimes used? In most cases, it is more cost effective for the manufacturer to use the lower-quality form. Throughout the book, whenever pertinent, I guide you to the best available form of the nutrient.

When choosing herbal supplements—and other supplements, as well—you'll want a product that has been screened for purity. An adulteration screen can tell you if the supplements contain any toxic metals, such as arsenic, lead, mercury, or cadmium. Supplements should also be screened for other contaminants, including other pharmaceuticals, pesticides, fungicides, insecticides, and other toxic ingredients. (To learn more about choosing the best herbal supplements, see page 186.)

Although you can (and should) check supplement labels to make sure that the products you buy contain no unwanted ingredients, the fact is that laboratory testing is necessary to determine a supplement's contents and bioavailability. That's why the best way to insure a supplement's quality is to buy pharmaceutical grade products. A good first step would be to seek out a healthcare provider who is trained in integrative medicine and can guide you to high-quality supplements. Also see page 485 for a list of pharmaceutical grade companies from which you can order products.

Always take supplements with a full glass of water, as this will help them work properly. If possible, take them with food (as long as the food does not contain a lot of fiber), which will enhance your body's absorption of the nutrients. Fat-soluble vitamins should be taken once a day. Water-soluble vitamins, on the other hand, leave the body more quickly, so they should be taken twice daily. Therefore, if the daily dose of a water-soluble vitamin is 100 milligrams, you should take 50 milligrams twice a day. As you read through this chapter, you will find more specific information that will allow you to design a safe and effective vitamin regimen.

FAT-SOLUBLE VITAMINS

VITAMIN A AND THE CAROTENOIDS

Vitamin A is a fat-soluble vitamin that can be divided into two groups: retinoids (or aldehydes) and carotenoids. *Retinoids,* which come from animal sources, provide active vitamin A—vitamin A that is ready for use by the body. *Carotenoids,* which come from plant sources, include some substances that the body converts to vitamin A, as well as some substances that are not transformed into vitamin A but have other functions in the body. In our discussion below, we first look at active vitamin A and the provitamin A carotenoids that the body converts to vitamin A. We then separately examine three carotenoids that are *not* converted to vitamin A.

VITAMIN A AND THE PROVITAMIN A CAROTENOIDS

As you learned above, foods from animal sources—meat and poultry (especially liver), fish, and dairy products—provide the body with active vitamin A, which is also referred to as preformed vitamin A. But you also get this important nutrient from provitamin A carotenoids, which the body converts into active vitamin A. The best known and most thoroughly studied provitamin is beta-carotene, but this group also includes alpha-carotene and beta-cryptoxanthin.

It's worth noting that there is an important difference between preformed vitamin A and provitamin A. If taken in high doses, preformed vitamin A can be toxic. (Remember that as a fat-soluble vitamin, it is stored in the body rather than being regularly flushed out.) But your body converts only as much vitamin A from the provitamin A carotenoids as it needs, so use of the provitamins—beta-carotene, for instance—is not associated with toxicity.

■ Functions of Vitamin A in Your Body

- Assists immune function by improving white blood cells, natural killer cells, macrophages, and T and B lymphocytes

- Helps protect the retina from oxidative stress, reducing the risk of macular degeneration

- Involved in cellular communication

- Necessary for the growth and development of bones and teeth
- Needed for the growth and support of the skin
- Needed to detoxify certain highly toxic compounds
- Reduces the risk of cancer, including cervical, esophageal, bladder, stomach, skin, leukemia, and lymphoma
- Responsible for healthy mucous membranes
- Regulates gene expression

■ Symptoms of Vitamin A Deficiency

- ☐ Decreased steroid synthesis
- ☐ Dry eyes
- ☐ Fatigue
- ☐ Hypothyroidism (underactive thyroid)
- ☐ Increased susceptibility to infections, including vaginal yeast infections
- ☐ Infertility in males (negatively affects sperm development)
- ☐ Iron deficiency anemia
- ☐ Night blindness
- ☐ Poor tooth and bone formation
- ☐ Poor wound healing
- ☐ Rough, scaly skin
- ☐ Vision loss due to retinal damage

■ Causes of Vitamin A Deficiency

- Celiac disease
- Chronic high alcohol intake
- Crohn's disease
- Cystic fibrosis
- Decreased pancreatic or biliary secretion
- Diabetes
- Duodenal bypass surgery
- Giardiasis
- Inadequate intake of foods rich in vitamin A and carotenoids
- Malabsorption
- Malnutrition
- Some medications, from antibiotics to cholesterol-lowering medicine, can lower vitamin A levels. Ask your healthcare provider or pharmacist if any of your medications, including over-the-counter products, have the potential to cause a vitamin A deficiency.
- Ulcerative colitis
- Vitamin E deficiency, which can decrease the absorption of vitamin A

Food Sources of Vitamin A

The following foods are numbered so that the foods which contain the most vitamin A are at the top of the list. As the list proceeds, the foods contain progressively less vitamin A. As explained in the vitamin A discussion, animal foods provide preformed vitamin A while certain plant foods provide provitamin A carotenoids, which the body converts to vitamin A. To highlight this distinction, all foods that provide the provitamin form have been marked with an asterisk (*).

1. Lamb liver
2. Beef liver
3. Calf liver
4. Red chili peppers*
5. Dandelion greens*
6. Chicken liver
7. Carrots*
8. Dried apricots*
9. Collard greens*
10. Kale*
11. Sweet potatoes*
12. Parsley*
13. Spinach*
14. Turnip greens*
15. Mustard greens*
16. Swiss chard*
17. Beet greens*
18. Chives*
19. Butternut squash*
20. Watercress*
21. Mangos*
22. Sweet red peppers*
23. Hubbard squash*
24. Cantaloupe*
25. Butter
26. Endive*
27. Apricots*
28. Broccoli spears*
29. Whitefish
30. Green onions*
31. Romaine lettuce*
32. Papayas*
33. Nectarines*
34. Prunes*
35. Pumpkin*
36. Swordfish*
37. Whipped cream
38. Peaches*
39. Acorn squash*
40. Egg yolks
41. Chicken
42. Sour red cherries*
43. Butterhead lettuce*
44. Asparagus*
45. Tomatoes*
46. Green chili peppers*
47. Green peas*
48. Elderberries*
49. Watermelon*
50. Rutabagas*
51. Brussels sprouts*
52. Okra*
53. Yellow cornmeal*
54. Yellow squash*

■ Conditions That Can Benefit from Vitamin A

- Acne
- Acute promyelocytic leukemia
- Age-related macular degeneration
- Alcoholism
- Asthma
- Cancer (prevention)
- Cataracts
- Celiac disease

- Crohn's disease
- Cystic fibrosis
- Diabetes
- Dry-eye syndrome
- Duodenal bypass surgery
- Giardiasis
- Hepatitis C
- Hypothyroidism (underactive thyroid)
- Ichthyosis (a skin disorder)
- Iron deficiency anemia*
- Lichen planus (an inflammatory condition)
- Measles
- Menorrhagia (abnormally heavy menstrual bleeding)
- Predisposition to coronary artery disease
- Predisposition to glaucoma and cataracts
- Premenstrual syndrome (PMS)
- Psoriasis
- Retinitis pigmentosa
- Seborrhea
- Sinusitis and rhinitis
- Susceptibility to infection
- Ulcerative colitis
- Wrinkles (use topically)

*Used in conjunction with iron, vitamin A has been shown to improve iron deficiency anemia more effectively than either nutrient alone. Vitamin A deficiency often occurs with iron deficiency.

■ Recommended Dosage

5,000 to 10,000 international units (IU) daily. If you are a smoker, do not take more than 8,000 IU a day, because larger doses of this vitamin are associated with an increased risk of lung cancer in smokers. Note that vitamin C can enhance the availability of vitamin A.

Because large doses of preformed vitamin A can cause problems (see the discussions below), it is recommended that you take a supplement that includes vitamin A and mixed carotenoids. Your body will convert the provitamin A carotenoids into active vitamin A only as needed. When choosing a supplement, look for these provitamin A amounts:

alpha-carotene: 1 to 2 milligrams daily.

beta-carotene: 3 to 6 milligrams daily.

beta-cryptoxanthin: 4 milligrams daily.

■ Substances That Increase Vitamin A Levels

- Oral contraceptives

■ Side Effects and Contraindications

Excessive vitamin A consumption can cause liver damage, bone loss, and even death. If you are taking a high dose (more than 20,000 IU a day), you need to have your calcium and liver enzymes measured on a regular basis. If you have liver disease, are a smoker, are exposed to asbestos, or are pregnant, you should not consume more than 8,000 IU of vitamin A each day.

An intake of large doses of vitamin A can decrease the absorption of vitamin K and may also interfere with the ability of vitamin D to help maintain calcium balance in the body. In addition, vitamin A supplements may interact poorly with certain medications, such as tetracycline and birth control pills. Speak to your healthcare provider or pharmacist to see if it is safe to take this nutrient with your medications and if any cautions should be exercised. To be completely safe, have your healthcare provider measure your vitamin A levels.

Note that the provitamin A carotenoids—alpha-carotene, beta-carotene, and beta-cryptoxanthin—have not been shown to have side effects in general, most likely because they are converted into vitamin A only as needed. However, supplements of beta-carotene have been shown to increase the risk of lung cancer in smokers.

■ Symptoms of Vitamin A Toxicity

☐ Appetite loss	☐ Dizziness	☐ Irritability
☐ Bone pain	☐ Dry, itchy skin	☐ Joint pain
☐ Cerebral edema	☐ Enlarged liver or spleen	☐ Loss of eyebrows
☐ Coarse hair		☐ Malaise
☐ Cracked lips	☐ Fatigue	☐ Nausea and vomiting
☐ Depression	☐ Hair loss	
☐ Diplopia (double vision)	☐ Headache	☐ Weight loss

LYCOPENE

The carotenoid lycopene gives a number of fruits and vegetables their red color and is found in particularly high amounts in tomatoes and tomato products. In fact, in North America, 85 percent of dietary lycopene comes from tomato products. Cooking tomatoes and tomato products, as you do when you prepare a tomato-based pasta sauce, makes lycopene easier for the body to use.

This carotenoid is a powerful antioxidant that is believed to protect the body's cells from damage by free radicals. (See the inset below.) For this reason, there has been a good deal of research into its possible use to prevent cancer and other disorders that are linked to free radicals and oxidative stress.

What Are Carotenoids and How Do They Protect Our Health?

Carotenoids are a class of *phytonutrients* (literally, *plant chemicals*). There are over 700 carotenoids on Earth, and 60 of them are found in food, where they lend bright red, yellow, and orange hues to many fruits and vegetables.

Despite the large number of carotenoids present in food sources, the typical American diet includes only six carotenoids: alpha-carotene, beta-carotene, beta-cryptoxanthin, lycopene, lutein, and zeaxanthin. As explained in the discussion of vitamin A (see page 20), alpha-carotene, beta-carotene, and beta-cryptoxanthin are provitamin A carotenoids, which means that they are converted into vitamin A in the intestine or liver. Lutein, lycopene, and zeaxanthin are not converted into vitamin A.

Whether or not they can be transformed into vitamin A, all carotenoids are known for their health benefits. Most likely, these benefits are due to the carotenoids' role as *antioxidants*—powerful substances that help protect us from disease by neutralizing health-damaging free radicals. Because each carotenoid is unique, each is best known for the specific benefits it provides. For instance, lutein is well known for protecting the eye from macular degeneration, and lycopene is best recognized for providing protection from prostate cancer.

We cannot manufacture carotenoids; we have to get them from our diet. To reap the many benefits offered by these amazing substances, be sure to eat lots of brightly colored fruits and veggies. Carotenoids are plant pigments, so the more vividly colored your produce, the more likely you are to get the carotenoids you need. Sweet potatoes, dark leafy greens like spinach and kale, watermelons, tomatoes, and butternut squash are not only delicious but also packed with health-promoting plant chemicals. Just be aware that a good diet sometimes isn't enough. That's why it's smart to also take supplements that supply mixed carotenoids. The dosage information provided in this chapter will guide you in getting all the carotenoids your body requires.

■ Functions of Lycopene in Your Body

- Decreases LDL (bad) cholesterol

- Helps prevent prostate cancer

- May help prevent bladder, breast, colon, lung, ovarian, and pancreatic cancer

■ Symptoms of Lycopene Deficiency

While there are no known symptoms of lycopene deficiency, the lack of lycopene—like the lack of other carotenoids—can increase the risk of chronic disorders such as heart disease and cancer.

■ Causes of Lycopene Deficiency

- Low dietary intake of foods containing this nutrient

Food Sources of Lycopene

- Apricots
- Dark green leafy vegetables
- Guavas
- Pink grapefruit
- Tomatoes
- Watermelon

■ Conditions That Can Benefit from Lycopene

- Asthma

- Cataracts

- Human papillomavirus (HPV)

- Predisposition to prostate cancer and possibly other cancers, including bladder, breast, colon, lung, ovarian, and pancreatic cancer

■ Recommended Dosage

5 to 20 milligrams daily.

■ Side Effects and Contraindications

In general, lycopene supplements are well tolerated. Some people have experienced GI complaints such as diarrhea, gas, nausea, and vomiting.

LUTEIN AND ZEAXANTHIN

In nature, the carotenoids lutein and zeaxanthin appear to absorb excess light as a means of preventing sunlight—especially high-energy blue light—from damaging plants. Similarly, in humans, these nutrients increase the density of macular pigment, enabling the eyes to better filter out blue wavelengths of light that can cause the damage associated with macular degeneration. Like all carotenoids, lutein and zeaxanthin are also powerful antioxidants that help protect the body from free radicals. (See the inset on page 25.)

■ Functions of Lutein and Zeaxanthin in Your Body

- Helps prevent cataracts
- Improves the function of the retina
- Increases the density of the protective pigmented cells in the retina
- Increases the electrical activity in the retina in response to light stimulus
- Protects against and treats macular degeneration

■ Symptoms of Lutein and Zeaxanthin Deficiency

While there are no known symptoms of lutein and zeaxanthin deficiency, the lack of these nutrients can increase the risk of cataracts and macular degeneration.

■ Causes of Lutein and Zeaxanthin Deficiency

- Low dietary intake of foods containing these nutrients

Food Sources of Lutein and Zeaxanthin

- Avocados
- Broccoli
- Brussels sprouts
- Carrots
- Collard greens
- Dandelion greens
- Egg yolks
- Kale
- Mustard greens
- Peas
- Spinach
- Summer and winter squash
- Turnip greens
- Yellow corn

Conditions That Can Benefit from Lutein and Zeaxanthin

- Cataracts
- Decline of cognitive function
- Macular degeneration

Recommended Dosage

6 to 12 milligrams daily of lutein and 2 milligrams daily of zeaxanthin. It should be noted that most supplements designed to prevent or treat macular degeneration provide 10 milligrams of lutein.

Side Effects and Contraindications

There are no reported side effects of lutein or zeaxanthin supplementation.

VITAMIN D

Vitamin D is provided by just a few foods, most of which come from animal sources. Although some vitamin D is found in plants, the plant form, vitamin D_2, is not readily used by the body. The body also produces vitamin D when sunshine strikes the skin, but with the current emphasis on minimizing sun exposure to lower the risk of skin cancer, many Americans avoid the sun or use sunscreen. Considering these factors, it is not surprising that 75 percent of the United States population is deficient in this important vitamin. Because vitamin D has so many vital functions in the body, supplementation is often necessary to make sure you get what you need for good health.

Functions of Vitamin D in Your Body

- Aids in the absorption of calcium from the intestinal tract
- Aids in the prevention and treatment of insulin resistance
- Helps the body assimilate phosphorus
- Helps the pancreas release insulin
- Important for thyroid function
- Is anti-inflammatory
- Necessary for blood clotting
- Necessary for growth and development of bones and teeth
- Regulates gene expression

- Stimulates bone cell mineralization

■ Symptoms of Vitamin D Deficiency

☐ Cognitive decline

☐ Increased risk of bone loss

☐ Low calcium levels

☐ Low phosphate levels

☐ Muscle spasms

☐ Softening of the bones (rickets in children and osteomalacia in adults)

Food Sources of Vitamin D

The following foods are numbered so that the foods that contain the most vitamin D are at the top of the list. As the list proceeds, the foods contain progressively less vitamin D.

1. Canned sardines
2. Salmon
3. Tuna
4. Shrimp

5. Butter
6. Sunflower seeds
7. Liver
8. Eggs

9. Fortified milk
10. Mushrooms
11. Natural cheese

■ Causes of Vitamin D Deficiency

- Aging process
- Decreased fat absorption (as a result of short bowel syndrome, sprue, or certain medications)
- Inadequate exposure to the sun
- Some drugs—such as prednisone, phenobarbital, and fat-blocking medications—can cause a vitamin D deficiency. Speak to your healthcare provider or pharmacist to learn if any of the drugs you're taking might cause vitamin D loss.
- Sunscreen use

■ Conditions That Can Benefit from Vitamin D

- Autoimmune diseases
- Cancer prevention and treatment

- Cardiovascular disease
- Cognitive decline

- Congestive heart failure
- Depression
- Diabetes
- Epilepsy
- Fibromyalgia
- Hypertension (high blood pressure)
- Hypothyroidism (underactive thyroid)
- Inflammatory conditions
- Migraine headaches
- Multiple sclerosis
- Musculoskeletal pain
- Osteoarthritis
- Osteoporosis/osteopenia (bone loss)
- Polycystic ovary syndrome
- Uterine fibroids

■ Recommended Dosage

Before using vitamin D supplements, consult your healthcare provider, who should order blood tests to determine how much vitamin D you need to consume. Studies have shown that the preferred form of vitamin D supplements is vitamin D_3.

To get enough vitamin D from the sun's rays, expose your face and arms for ten to fifteen minutes at least three times a week without sunscreen. Do not overdo sun exposure, though, and be careful to avoid sunburn. The use of sunscreen decreases the absorption of vitamin D into the skin. If you are very fair and need to wear sunscreen, you may have to take additional vitamin D.

■ Side Effects and Contraindications

The optimal blood level of vitamin D is 55 to 80 ng/mL (nanomoles per liter). Some people may not be able to supplement to an optimal level of vitamin D because a hypersensitivity to this nutrient may cause them to develop high calcium blood levels (hypercalcemia). People are most likely to be hypersensitive to vitamin D supplementation if they have one of the following conditions: cancer, Crohn's disease, granulomatous diseases, hyperparathyroidism, sarcoidosis, or tuberculosis.

■ Symptoms of Vitamin D Toxicity

Although Vitamin D is stored in the body, vitamin D toxicity is rare. It can occur, though, if you take overly high doses of the supplement. This is why it's so important to consult with your healthcare provider before using vitamin D.

The following are possible symptoms of vitamin D toxicity.

- Heart arrhythmias (irregular heartbeat)
- Hypercalcemia (elevated calcium levels in the blood)
- Hypercalciuria (elevated calcium levels in the urine)
- Joint pain
- Loss of appetite
- Muscle weakness
- Nausea
- Polyuria (large amounts of dilute urine)
- Weight loss

VITAMIN E

Vitamin E—sometimes referred to as the "master antioxidant"—includes two classes of fat-soluble compounds, the tocopherols and the tocotrienols. Each of these classes contains four compounds. The tocopherols are made up of alpha-tocopherol, beta-tocopherol, gamma-tocopherol, and delta-tocopherol. The tocotrienols are made up of alpha-tocotrienol, beta-tocotrienol, gamma-tocotrienol, and delta-tocotrienol.

The eight vitamin E compounds come in both natural and synthetic forms. Natural vitamin E is called d-alpha (or d-beta, d-gamma, or d-delta), and synthetic vitamin E is noted as dl-alpha (or dl-beta, dl-gamma, or dl-delta). Vitamin E is better absorbed by the body and better metabolized by the liver when a natural form of the nutrient is used.

Of all the vitamin E compounds, alpha-tocopherol is the most biologically active, followed by beta-tocopherol, gamma-tocopherol, and delta-tocopherol. The tocotrienols—alpha-tocotrienol, beta-tocotrienol, gamma-tocotrienol, and delta-tocotrienol—are less active than the tocopherol forms of vitamin E, but still perform important functions in the body.

Below, you will learn the functions of tocopherols followed by the functions of tocotrienols. You will then find more general information about Vitamin E as a whole—what the deficiency symptoms are, what the food sources are, and more. The "Recommended Dosage" section gives you the proper doses for both tocopherols, which are most commonly used to treat the conditions discussed in Part 2 of this book, and tocotrienols, which are less often suggested in Part 2.

■ Functions of Tocopherols in Your Body

- Can stop cholesterol-like substances from damaging blood vessels
- Enhance the immune system

- Help prevent Alzheimer's disease
- Help prevent lung, esophageal, and colorectal cancer
- Help relieve atrophic vaginitis
- Improve the action of insulin

- Inhibit platelet adhesion
- Needed by the ovaries to function properly
- Protect vitamin A and increase its storage
- Relieve hot flashes

■ Functions of Tocotrienols in Your Body

- Fight inflammation
- Lower cholesterol

- Reduce risk of cancer
- Reverse plaque build-up

■ Symptoms of Vitamin E Deficiency

☐ Ataxia (loss of control over body movements)

☐ Hemolytic anemia (premature destruction of red blood cells)

☐ Immunological abnormalities

☐ Increase in the enzymes creatine kinase and pyruvate kinase

☐ Peripheral neuropathy (damage to peripheral nerves)

☐ Platelet dysfunction

☐ Retinopathy (a disease of the retina)

☐ Skeletal myopathy (a disease of the muscles)

■ Causes of Vitamin E Deficiency

- Excessive alcohol
- Excessive vitamin A

- Pectin (a natural substance used to thicken jams and jellies)
- Smoking

■ Conditions That Can Benefit from Vitamin E

- Arthritis
- Asthma
- Cancer prevention
- Cardiovascular disease
- Cataracts

- Chronic fatigue syndrome
- Claudication (cramping pain in legs)
- Cystic fibrosis
- Fibrocystic breast disease

- Hepatitis
- Hot flashes
- Huntington's chorea
- Hypercholesterolemia (high cholesterol)
- Hypertension (high blood pressure)
- Hypertriglyceridemia (high triglycerides)
- Impotence

- Infertility
- Osteoporosis
- Painful menstrual cycles
- Parkinson's disease
- Premenstrual syndrome (PMS)
- Restless leg syndrome
- Scleroderma and other autoimmune diseases
- Skin aging
- Sunburn protection

Food Sources of Vitamin E

The following foods are numbered so that those which contain the most Vitamin E are at the top of the list. As the list proceeds, the foods contain progressively less Vitamin E. Note that these foods largely contain the vitamin E compounds known as tocopherols. Tocotrienols—the other class of vitamin E compounds—are not found in many common foods.

1. Wheat germ
2. Sunflower seeds
3. Sunflower seed oil
4. Safflower oil
5. Almonds
6. Sesame oil
7. Peanut oil
8. Corn oil
9. Wheat germ
10. Peanuts
11. Olive oil
12. Soybean oil
13. Roasted peanuts
14. Peanut butter
15. Butter
16. Spinach
17. Oatmeal
18. Bran
19. Asparagus
20. Salmon
21. Brown rice
22. Whole rye bread
23. Dark rye bread
24. Pecans
25. Wheat germ
26. Rye and wheat crackers
27. Whole wheat bread
28. Carrots
29. Peas
30. Walnuts
31. Bananas
32. Eggs
33. Tomatoes
34. Lamb

Recommended Dosage

For general wellness and the treatment of most health disorders, I recommend mixed tocopherols. When treating high cholesterol and high triglycerides, I recommend mixed tocotrienols. Be aware that most vitamin E supplements provide only alpha-tocopherol, but products containing only mixed tocopherols or only mixed tocotrienols are available.

Tocopherols: 100 to 400 international units (IU) of mixed tocopherols daily.

Tocotrienols: 400 international units (IU) of mixed tocotrienols daily.

■ Side Effects and Contraindications

Ferrous sulfate, used to treat iron deficiency, destroys vitamin E and should not be taken with it. Other forms of iron, such as ferrous gluconate and ferrous fumarate, do not have this negative effect.

Vitamin E is a blood thinner, so if you are taking blood thinners (Plavix, for instance), consult your healthcare provider about the amount of vitamin E that is right for you.

Some people experience diarrhea, flatulence, nausea, and/or heart palpitations when taking large doses of vitamin E. If you experience these symptoms, reduce your dose.

VITAMIN K

Vitamin K is a unique nutrient. Only about 25 percent of this vitamin comes from dietary sources, while about 75 percent is produced in the intestinal tract by friendly bacteria. The vitamin occurs in two major forms: K_1 (phylloquinone) and K_2 (menaquinone). In general, K_1 is the form derived from dietary sources, while K_2 is produced by intestinal bacteria.

Like other fat-soluble vitamins, this nutrient depends on a healthy liver and gallbladder to be properly absorbed, but unlike the other vitamins in this category, vitamin K is not stored by the body. This can make it difficult to get all of the vitamin K required for good health. In fact, studies have shown that more vitamin K is needed than previously thought, especially as people age. You can develop a deficiency of vitamin K in as little as seven days if your diet does not provide enough of this nutrient. You then may need to take supplemental vitamin K, but it is always best to get as much of this nutrient as possible in your diet and to have a healthy gut that is able to make the vitamin K that you need.

Vitamin K was originally identified because of its important role in blood clot formation. We now know that it plays a role in many vital processes.

■ Functions of Vitamin K in Your Body

- Helps prevent and treat osteoporosis

- Helps prevent brain cell death in older individuals

- Important for normal cell growth and proliferation

- Inhibits the growth and invasiveness of some forms of cancer

- Plays an important role in the formation of strong bones

- Reduces cardiovascular disease by enhancing vascular health and elasticity

- Regulates blood coagulation (clotting) due to laceration or other injury

■ Symptoms of Vitamin K Deficiency

- ☐ Bleeding from the gums
- ☐ Bloody stools
- ☐ Bruising easily
- ☐ Excessive bleeding from wounds or surgical sites
- ☐ Excessive menstrual bleeding

- ☐ Hematomas (a collection of blood caused by a break in blood vessels)
- ☐ Loss of bone density
- ☐ Nosebleeds
- ☐ Petechiae (red or purple spots on the skin caused by broken capillaries)

■ Causes of Vitamin K Deficiency

- Certain medications, from anticoagulants to broad-spectrum antibiotics, can cause a vitamin K deficiency. Speak to your healthcare provider or pharmacist to learn if any drugs you're taking might be causing low vitamin K production or absorption.

- Consumption of foods made with hydrogenated fats

- Excessive supplementation of vitamins A and E

- Fat malabsorption due to disorders such as celiac disease, removal of part of intestine, or other causes

- Gallstones

- Insufficient consumption of vitamin K-rich foods, such as leafy greens
- Lack of adequate beneficial bacteria in the intestine

Food Sources of Vitamin K

The following foods are numbered so that the foods which contain the most vitamin K are at the top of the list. As the list proceeds, the foods contain progressively less vitamin K.

1. Turnip greens	10. Butter	18. Corn oil
2. Broccoli	11. Pork liver	19. Peaches
3. Lettuce	12. Oats	20. Beef
4. Cabbage	13. Green peas	21. Chicken liver
5. Beef liver	14. Whole wheat	22. Raisins
6. Spinach	15. Green beans	23. Tomato
7. Watercress	16. Pork	24. Milk
8. Asparagus	17. Eggs	25. Potato
9. Cheese		

■ Conditions That Can Benefit from Vitamin K

- Cardiovascular disease
- Osteopenia and osteoporosis
- Cancer (prevention)
- Memory loss (prevention)
- Problems with bleeding and blood clotting

■ Recommended Dosage

If you eat a sound diet and have a healthy gastrointestinal tract, you may not need to supplement with vitamin K. However, since many people do not eat as well as they should and have a gastrointestinal tract that is not operating optimally, you might benefit from vitamin K supplements. If you do need additional vitamin K, choose K_2 and take 50 to 100 micrograms a day. If you have heart disease or osteoporosis, you may want to supplement with MK-7, which is better absorbed and stays in the body longer.

■ Side Effects and Contraindications

For most people, vitamin K_1 and vitamin K_2 are safe and do not cause any side effects. Synthetic vitamin K may cause toxicity, so always look for the natural form. Also, supplementation of vitamin K can alter the effectiveness of anticoagulant medications such as Coumadin. If you are using a blood thinner, be sure to speak to your healthcare provider before taking vitamin K.

WATER-SOLUBLE VITAMINS

VITAMIN B COMPLEX

Vitamin B was once thought to be a single nutrient, but researchers later found that the original "soup" which showed vitamin activity actually contained not one vitamin but eleven of them, each with a unique structure and unique functions. Although many of these nutrients work together to help you achieve optimal health, they are not actually related to one another despite their names.

One characteristic that B vitamins *do* share is that they are all water-soluble, which means they are eliminated from the body the same day they are ingested. Because it is vital to have an adequate amount of B vitamins in your body, you should consume them at least twice a day. For instance, if you are taking 100 milligrams of B_1, or thiamine, you should take 50 milligrams of thiamine twice a day.

High-dose supplementation of a single B vitamin can cause imbalances of other B vitamins. Therefore, you should take a multivitamin that contains these vitamins rather than taking each B vitamin individually unless you are instructed to by your doctor.

Members of the Vitamin B Complex

All of the following vitamins except for vitamin B_{10} are described in detail in the pages that follow. No section has been included on B_{10} (para-aminobenzoic acid) because very little is known about this nutrient at this time. What happened to the "missing" B vitamins: B_4, B_8, and B_{11}? They are no longer considered vitamins.

- Vitamin B_1 (Thiamine)
- Vitamin B_2 (Riboflavin)
- Vitamin B_3 (Niacin and Niacinamide)

- Vitamin B_5 (Pantothenic acid)
- Vitamin B_6 (Pyridoxine)
- Vitamin B_7 (Biotin)
- Vitamin B_9 (Folic acid)
- Vitamin B_{10} (Para-aminobenzoic acid)
- Vitamin B_{12} (Cobalamin)
- Inositol

B_1 (THIAMINE)

The first B vitamin discovered was thiamine (or thiamin). Thiamine is involved in many of the body's activities, including the burning of carbohydrates for energy. This nutrient is found in a large number of foods, as well as in both individual supplements and supplements that contain all of the B vitamins.

■ Functions of B_1 in Your Body

- Helps the body adapt to stress and avoid adrenal burnout
- Needed for proper metabolism of thyroid hormones
- Needed for synthesis of nucleic acids and certain coenzymes
- Needed for the making of aldosterone, a steroid hormone
- Required for energy production
- Required for proper nerve function
- Used for the activation of enzymes in the adrenal glands
- Used in the synthesis of the neurotransmitter acetylcholine (the main neurotransmitter of memory)

■ Symptoms of B_1 Deficiency

- ☐ Beriberi (only in late-stage B_1 deficiency)
- ☐ Confusion
- ☐ Fatigue
- ☐ Forgetfulness
- ☐ Gastrointestinal disturbances
- ☐ General weakness
- ☐ Headache
- ☐ Irritability
- ☐ Loss of appetite
- ☐ Mild depression
- ☐ Nervousness
- ☐ Poor memory
- ☐ Racing heart
- ☐ Sleep disturbance
- ☐ Vision problems

Food Sources of B₁

The following foods are numbered so that the foods which contain the most vitamin B_1 are at the top of the list. As the list proceeds, the foods contain progressively less vitamin B_1. Note that grains lose up to 100 percent of their thiamine content when processed. Also, marinating your meat in wine, soy sauce, or vinegar depletes its level of thiamine by 50 to 75 percent.

1. Brewer's yeast
2. Wheat germ
3. Sunflower seeds
4. Rice polishings
5. Pine nuts
6. Peanuts (with skins)
7. Brazil nuts
8. Pork
9. Pecans
10. Soybean flour
11. Pinto and red beans
12. Split peas
13. Millet
14. Wheat bran
15. Pistachio nuts

16. Navy beans
17. Buckwheat
18. Oatmeal
19. Whole wheat flour
20. Whole wheat grain
21. Lima beans
22. Hazelnuts
23. Lamb heart
24. Wild rice
25. Whole grain rye
26. Cashews
27. Lamb liver
28. Mung beans
29. Whole ground cornmeal
30. Lentils

31. Beef kidneys
32. Green peas
33. Macadamia nuts
34. Brown rice
35. Walnuts
36. Garbanzo beans
37. Garlic
38. Beef liver
39. Almonds
40. Lima beans
41. Pumpkin and squash seeds
42. Fresh chestnuts
43. Soybean sprouts
44. Red chili peppers
45. Hulled sesame seeds

■ Causes of B₁ Deficiency

- Alcohol
- Blueberries
- Brussels sprouts

- Certain medications, from diuretics to oral contraceptives, can cause a thiamine deficiency. Speak to your healthcare provider or pharmacist to learn if any drugs you're taking might be causing thiamine loss.

- Coffee
- Horseradish
- Pickled foods
- Red beet root
- Seafood such as fish, shrimp, clams, and mussels
- Sugar
- Sulfites (a food additive)
- Tea

■ Conditions That Can Benefit from B₁

- Alcoholism
- Confusion
- Dementia
- Depression
- Fatigue
- Memory loss
- Neuropathy
- Pain

■ Recommended Dosage

10 to 100 milligrams daily. B vitamins are water-soluble and leave the body quickly, so they should be taken twice a day. Therefore, you should take 5 to 50 milligrams of B_1 twice a day as part of a B-complex supplement. High doses of B_1 may deplete your body of vitamin B_6 or magnesium, so do not exceed the recommended amount except under a doctor's orders.

■ Side Effects and Contraindications

Do not take the herb horsetail if you are taking thiamine, since it may destroy thiamine in the stomach. Iron decreases the body's absorption of thiamine, so take these two supplements at least two hours apart.

The possible side effects of thiamine supplementation include the following:

- Mild rash
- Nausea
- Restlessness
- Sweating

B₂ (RIBOFLAVIN)

Vitamin B_2, or riboflavin, is very much involved in your body's energy processes, as well as in many other processes. For example, it is vital for healthy thyroid function and for healthy eyes. Fortunately, this important nutrient is found in many foods, including meats, vegetables, beans, and grains.

Food Sources of B$_2$

The following foods are numbered so that the foods which contain the most vitamin B$_2$ are at the top of the list. As the list proceeds, the foods contain progressively less vitamin B$_2$. Be aware that processing food decreases its riboflavin content by up to 80 percent, so opt for whole foods whenever possible.

1. Brewer's yeast	16. Soy flour	31. Pine nuts
2. Lamb liver	17. Wheat bran	32. Sunflower seeds
3. Beef liver	18. Mackerel	33. Pork
4. Calf liver	19. Collards	34. Navy beans
5. Beef kidneys	20. Soybeans	35. Beet and mustard greens
6. Chicken liver	21. Eggs	
7. Lamb kidneys	22. Split peas	36. Lentils
8. Chicken giblets	23. Beef tongue	37. Prunes
9. Almonds	24. Kale	38. Rye
10. Wheat germ	25. Parsley	39. Whole grains
11. Wild rice	26. Cashews	40. Mung beans
12. Mushrooms	27. Rice bran	41. Pinto and red beans
13. Egg yolks	28. Veal	
14. Millet	29. Salmon	42. Black-eyed peas
15. Hot red peppers	30. Broccoli	43. Okra

■ Functions of B$_2$ in Your Body

- Acts as a catalyst in several reactions that process carbohydrates, fats, and proteins
- Involved in the metabolism of drugs and environmental toxins
- Involved in the metabolism of vitamin K
- Needed for energy metabolism
- Needed to convert vitamin B$_6$, folic acid, vitamin A, and niacin into their active forms

- Protects glutathione, an antioxidant required for eye health
- Required for proper thyroid function
- Used in lipid metabolism
- Used in the formation of aldosterone, a steroid hormone

■ Symptoms of B₂ Deficiency

- ☐ Depression
- ☐ Dry, cracking skin
- ☐ Exhaustion
- ☐ Eyes that are light-sensitive and easily fatigued

■ Substances That Reduce the Bioavailability of B₂

- Alcohol
- Caffeine
- Certain medications, from antibiotics to antacids, can decrease the bioavailability of this nutrient. Speak to your healthcare provider or pharmacist to learn if any of the drugs you're taking might be making your riboflavin supplements less effective.
- Saccharin
- Vitamin B₃
- Vitamin C
- Zinc

■ Conditions That Can Benefit from B₂

- Acne
- Alcoholism
- Arthritis
- Athlete's foot
- Baldness
- Cataracts
- Depression
- Diabetes mellitus
- Diarrhea
- Failure to detoxify effectively
- Hysteria
- Indigestion
- Light sensitivity
- Migraines
- Nerve damage
- Reddening of the eyes
- Scrotal skin changes
- Seborrheic dermatitis
- Skin changes around the mouth
- Stress
- Visual changes

■ Recommended Dosage

10 to 100 milligrams daily. You need more B₂ during illness or athletic train-ing. B vitamins are water-soluble and leave the body quickly, so they should

be taken twice a day. Therefore, you should take 5 to 50 milligrams of B_2 twice a day as part of a B-complex supplement.

■ Side Effects and Contraindications

Usually, B_2 does not cause any side effects. However, high dose supplementation of a single B vitamin can cause imbalances of other B vitamins.

B₃ (NIACIN AND NIACINAMIDE)

Vitamin B_3 is used in at least forty chemical reactions in your body. One of this vitamin's best-known benefits is its ability to reduce elevated cholesterol levels. However, as stated under "Side Effects and Contraindications" (see page 45), taking this vitamin without the rest of the B complex can actually raise the risk of heart disease.

As a supplement, vitamin B_3 is available as both niacin (also called nicotinic acid) and niacinamide (also called nicotinamide). These supplements cannot be used interchangeably. For instance, niacin can be used to treat high cholesterol levels thanks to its role in fat metabolism, but niacinamide does not work for this purpose. Niacin is also effective in the treatment of circulatory disorders. Either niacin or niacinamide can be used to treat mental health disorders such as depression and anxiety.

■ Functions of B₃

- Can decrease lipoprotein A, high amounts of which are markers for an increased risk of heart disease
- Can lower LDL (bad) cholesterol and raise HDL (good) cholesterol
- Decreases fibrinogen levels, high amounts of which are related to heart disease
- Lowers triglycerides
- May improve diabetes
- Needed for the breakdown of carbohydrates, proteins, and fats into usable energy
- Needed for the proper function of the adrenal glands
- Provides energy to convert cholesterol to pregnenolone, a hormone needed to prevent memory loss
- Used in the metabolism of tryptophan and serotonin

Symptoms of B₃ Deficiency

☐ Anorexia

☐ Confusion

☐ Depression

☐ Dermatitis

☐ Fatigue

☐ Headaches

☐ Inability to detoxify

☐ Indigestion

☐ Insomnia

☐ Irritability

☐ Mouth ulcers

☐ Muscle weakness

☐ Nausea

☐ Pellagra (only in late-stage niacin deficiency)

☐ Skin changes around the mouth

Food Sources of B₃

The following foods are numbered so that the foods which contain the most B₃ are at the top of the list. As the list proceeds, the foods contain progressively less B₃.

1. Brewer's yeast
2. Rice bran
3. Rice polishings
4. Wheat bran
5. Peanuts with skin
6. Lamb liver
7. Pork liver
8. Peanuts without skin
9. Beef liver
10. Calf liver
11. Light meat turkey
12. Chicken liver
13. Light meat chicken
14. Trout
15. Halibut
16. Mackerel
17. Swordfish
18. Goose
19. Beef heart
20. Salmon
21. Veal
22. Beef kidneys
23. Wild rice
24. Chicken giblets
25. Lamb
26. Sesame seeds
27. Sunflower seeds
28. Beef
29. Pork
30. Brown rice
31. Pine nuts
32. Whole grain buckwheat
33. Red chili peppers
34. Whole wheat grain and flour
35. Wheat germ
36. Barley
37. Herring
38. Almonds
39. Shrimp
40. Split peas
41. Haddock

■ Conditions That Can Benefit from B₃

- Acne
- Depression
- Diabetes mellitus
- High cholesterol
- High triglycerides
- Intermittent claudication (cramping pain in legs due to poor circulation)

- Low HDL (good) cholesterol
- Memory loss
- Osteoarthritis
- Painful menstrual cycles
- Parkinson's disease
- Rheumatoid arthritis

■ Recommended Dosage

50 to 100 milligrams daily as part of a B-complex supplement. B vitamins are water-soluble and leave the body quickly, so they should be taken twice a day. To successfully lower cholesterol and triglycerides and be effective for mood swings, you may need larger doses of B₃. See your healthcare provider before supplementing with doses greater than 100 milligrams a day.

■ Side Effects and Contraindications

When you are first beginning niacin supplementation, it is fairly common to experience skin flushing, sensations of heat, stomach problems, or dry skin. However, these reactions typically subside within several weeks. For some conditions, instead of niacin, you can use niacinamide, which does not result in a niacin flush.

Doses of niacin or niacianamide above 100 milligrams a day can cause liver damage, peptic ulcers, high uric acid levels, or glucose intolerance. Furthermore, doses above 100 milligrams a day taken with a statin drug to lower cholesterol can lead to rhabdomyolysis, a potentially fatal breakdown of skeletal muscle. Never take this supplement without the other B-complex vitamins because doing so can cause your homocysteine levels to elevate, increasing your risk of heart disease and memory loss.

B₅ (PANTOTHENIC ACID)

Like many other elements of the vitamin B complex, B₅—also known as pantothenic acid—is involved in the body's metabolism of carbohydrates, fats, and proteins. Because this vitamin can be found in many different foods, it is named *pantothenic*, which is derived from the Greek word meaning *everywhere*.

■ Functions of B₅ in Your Body

- Aids in the formation of antibodies
- Aids in wound healing
- Helps with fatty acid manufacture and transport
- Helps your body use other vitamins
- Needed for the breakdown of carbohydrates, proteins, and fats into usable energy
- Needed for the synthesis of coenzyme A
- Stimulates adrenal gland
- Used in red cell production
- Used in the synthesis of several amino acids
- Used to make vitamin D

■ Symptoms of B₅ Deficiency

- ☐ Adrenal exhaustion
- ☐ Allergies
- ☐ Arthritis
- ☐ Burning sensation in feet
- ☐ Constipation
- ☐ Decreased immunity, making the body susceptible to frequent infections
- ☐ Decreased production of hydrochloric acid, which can lead to decreased absorption of minerals, along with skin problems and digestive issues
- ☐ Depression
- ☐ Duodenal ulcers
- ☐ Eczema
- ☐ Enlarged, chunky, furrowed tongue
- ☐ Fatigue
- ☐ Gout
- ☐ Graying hair
- ☐ Headache
- ☐ Hypertension (high blood pressure)
- ☐ Insomnia
- ☐ Intestinal inflammation
- ☐ Muscle cramps
- ☐ Nerve degeneration
- ☐ Restlessness
- ☐ Upper respiratory tract infections
- ☐ Vomiting

Food Sources of B₅

The following foods are numbered so that the foods which contain the most vitamin B₅ are at the top of the list. As the list proceeds, the foods contain progressively less vitamin B₅.

1. Brewer's yeast
2. Calf liver
3. Chicken liver
4. Beef kidneys
5. Peanuts
6. Mushrooms
7. Soybean flour
8. Split peas
9. Beef tongue
10. Perch
11. Blue cheese
12. Pecans
13. Soybeans
14. Eggs
15. Lobster
16. Oatmeal
17. Buckwheat flour
18. Sunflower seeds
19. Lentils
20. Whole grain rye flour
21. Cashews
22. Salmon
23. Camembert cheese
24. Garbanzo beans
25. Toasted wheat germ
26. Broccoli
27. Hazelnuts
28. Dark meat turkey
29. Brown rice
30. Whole wheat flour
31. Sardines
32. Red chili peppers
33. Avocados
34. Veal
35. Black-eyed peas
36. Wild rice
37. Cauliflower
38. Dark meat chicken
39. Kale

■ Causes of B₅ Deficiency

- Caffeine

- Certain medications, from estrogen supplements to sleeping pills, can cause a B₅ deficiency. Speak to your healthcare provider or pharmacist to learn if any drugs you're taking might be causing loss of this nutrient.

■ Conditions That Can Benefit from B₅

- Acne
- Adrenal dysfunction
- Allergies
- Anemia
- Cold sores
- Elevated triglycerides
- Fatigue
- Genital herpes
- Infection
- Osteoarthritis
- Problems with detoxification
- Rheumatoid arthritis

- Shingles
- Ulcerative colitis

■ Recommended Dosage

50 to 100 milligrams a day as part of a B-complex supplement. B vitamins are water-soluble and leave the body quickly, so they should be taken twice a day. Higher doses may need to be used as a therapy for a disease process. Use larger doses only under the direction of your healthcare provider.

■ Side Effects and Contraindications

High-dose supplementation of a single B vitamin can cause imbalances of other B vitamins. In the case of pantothenic acid, this can lead to the following side effects:

- Dizziness
- Joint pain
- Nausea
- Headache
- Muscle pain
- Sore throat

B₆ (PYRIDOXINE)

Pyridoxine acts as a partner (coenzyme) for more than one hundred different enzymes, assisting in enzyme activity. As you get older, the efficiency with which you utilize B_6 decreases, so it may be necessary to increase your intake of this nutrient as you age.

■ Functions of B₆ in Your Body

- Increases immune system response
- Involved in strengthening connective tissue
- Key to the synthesis of several neurotransmitters (chemical messengers in the brain), including serotonin, norepinephrine, dopamine, and GABA
- Lowers homocysteine levels, decreasing the risk of heart disease and memory loss
- Needed for REM sleep
- Needed for the absorption of fats and proteins
- Needed for the production of hydrochloric acid
- Needed to detoxify chemicals
- Used in the synthesis of amino acids

Food Sources of B$_6$

The following foods are numbered so that the foods which contain the most B$_6$ are at the top of the list. As the list proceeds, the foods contain progressively less B$_6$.

1. Brewer's yeast
2. Sunflower seeds
3. Toasted wheat germ
4. Fresh tuna
5. Beef liver
6. Soybeans
7. Chicken liver
8. Walnuts
9. Fresh salmon
10. Fresh trout
11. Calf liver
12. Mackerel
13. Pork liver
14. Soybean flour
15. Lentils
16. Lima beans
17. Buckwheat flour
18. Black-eyed peas
19. Navy beans
20. Brown rice
21. Hazelnuts
22. Garbanzo beans
23. Pinto beans
24. Bananas
25. Pork
26. Fresh halibut
27. Beef kidneys
28. Avocados
29. Veal kidneys
30. Whole wheat flour
31. Chestnuts
32. Egg yolks
33. Kale
34. Rye flour
35. Spinach
36. Turnip greens
37. Sweet peppers
38. Potatoes
39. Prunes
40. Raisins
41. Sardines
42. Brussels sprouts
43. Elderberries
44. Fresh perch
45. Fresh cod
46. Barley
47. Camembert cheese
48. Sweet potatoes
49. Cauliflower
50. Popped popcorn
51. Red cabbage
52. Leeks

■ Symptoms of B$_6$ Deficiency

- ☐ Depression
- ☐ Fatigue
- ☐ Hyperactivity
- ☐ Insomnia
- ☐ Irritability
- ☐ Mental confusion
- ☐ Mouth ulcers
- ☐ Nervousness
- ☐ Numbness
- ☐ Skin lesions around the mouth
- ☐ Weakness

Understanding Methylated B Vitamins

Although the word may not be familiar to you, *methylation* is a simple process that occurs in every cell and tissue of the body when a "methyl group"—three hydrogen atoms and one carbon atom—becomes linked to another molecule. Methylation is vitally important to your well-being because it is critical to biochemical reactions that regulate DNA production, neurotransmitter production, estrogen metabolism, fat metabolism, eye health, cellular energy, liver health, and more.

The body relies on *methyl donors*—substances that can transfer a methyl group to another substance—to enable methylation to take place. While a number of substances can play this role, three of the most important donors are vitamins B_6, B_9, and B_{12}. Unfortunately, the modern diet is a poor source of B vitamins. Moreover, approximately 50 percent of the U.S. population has a genetic mutation (a variant of the gene MTHFR) that makes it difficult for the methylation process to occur. Considering the importance of this process to the proper function of body systems, it's easy to understand that this can lead to a variety of health problems. Poor methylation can even prevent you from utilizing the common forms of these B vitamins, which are not methylated.

Fortunately, if you have an MTHFR gene mutation, you can improve your body's methylation by taking active forms of vitamins B_6, B_9, and B_{12}. Also called methylated forms, they are, respectively, pyridoxal 5-phosphate, the active form of B_6; L-5-methyltetrahydrofolate, the active form of B_9; and methylcobalamin, the active form of B_{12}. These supplements can both help fuel the methylation process and ensure that your body is supplied with B vitamins that it can readily use.

Should you take methylated B vitamins just to make sure that you're getting active vitamins that can facilitate the methylation process? While this may seem like a reasonable course of action, it is important to understand that 50 percent of the population does *not* need methylated B vitamins. Even worse, if you take methylated B vitamins and do not need them, they will increase your risk of developing cancer even if you do not have a family history of cancer.

Fortunately, your healthcare provider can measure your body's ability to methylate by performing a genetic test to see if you have a variant of the MTHFR gene. Your provider can also test for levels of the amino acid homocysteine, which tend to be elevated when methylation is not occurring properly; or can order a test that evaluates the methylation cycle. It is vital to seek medical evaluation and advice before choosing B vitamins that are in the methylated form.

■ Causes of B₆ Deficiency

- Certain medications, from antibiotics to antidepressants to oral contraceptives, can cause a vitamin B_6 deficiency. Speak to your healthcare provider or pharmacist to learn if any drugs you're taking might be causing vitamin B_6 loss.
- Cigarette smoking
- Excessive exercise
- Food additives (FDC yellow #5)
- Pesticides

■ Conditions That Can Benefit from Vitamin B₆

- Asthma
- Atherosclerosis
- Autism
- Calcium oxalate kidney stones (prevention)
- Carpal tunnel syndrome
- Depression
- Diabetes mellitus
- Eczema
- Epilepsy
- Infertility
- Irritability
- Macular degeneration
- Monosodium glutamate (MSG) sensitivity or intolerance
- Nausea and vomiting related to pregnancy
- Nervous system dysfunction
- Osteoporosis
- Premenstrual syndrome (PMS)
- Schizophrenia
- Seborrheic dermatitis
- Sickle cell disease

■ Recommended Dosage

30 to 100 milligrams daily. B vitamins are water-soluble and leave the body quickly, so they should be taken twice a day as part of a B-complex supplement.

When an individual has a mutation of the gene MTHFR, it is necessary to take a methylated from of B_6 known as pyridoxal 5-phosphate. To learn more about this, see the inset on page 50.

■ Side Effects and Contraindications

At too high a dose (more than 100 milligrams a day), pyridoxine can cause a neuropathy (nerve disorder). If you are taking L-dopa for Parkinson's disease, do not take B_6 without first consulting your doctor.

B₇ (BIOTIN)

Most diets supply a good amount of biotin, as it is present in many foods. Moreover, this is one of the few vitamins that can be manufactured by the bacteria that live in the small intestines. Prolonged antibiotic use can lower the amount of biotin in the body by killing off beneficial bacteria, and poor gastrointestinal tract health can also cause a deficiency. Fortunately, supplements can help make up any shortfall.

Like many of the B vitamins, biotin converts food into energy, but it has other functions as well.

■ Functions of B₇ in Your Body

- Increases insulin sensitivity
- Needed for fatty acid synthesis
- Strengthens hair
- Strengthens nails
- Needed for the breakdown of carbohydrates, proteins, and fats into usable energy

■ Symptoms of B₇ Deficiency

- ☐ Brittle nails
- ☐ Cradle cap (infantile seborrheic dermatitis)
- ☐ Dandruff
- ☐ Depression
- ☐ Dry skin
- ☐ Fatigue
- ☐ Hair loss
- ☐ Hallucinations
- ☐ Localized numbness and tingling
- ☐ Muscle pain
- ☐ Nausea
- ☐ Reduced appetite
- ☐ Scaly dermatitis

■ Causes of B₇ Deficiency

- Certain medications, such as anticonvulsants, can cause a biotin deficiency. Speak to your healthcare provider or pharmacist to learn if any drugs you're taking might be causing biotin loss.
- Excess consumption of alcohol
- Long-term consumption of raw egg whites
- Poor gastrointestinal tract health

■ Conditions That Can Benefit from B₇

- Brittle nails
- Diabetes mellitus
- Diabetic neuropathy

- Hair loss
- Multiple sclerosis (MS)
- Seborrheic dermatitis

Food Sources of B7

The following foods are numbered so that the foods which contain the most vitamin B7 are at the top of the list. As the list proceeds, the foods contain progressively less vitamin B7.

1. Brewer's yeast
2. Lamb liver
3. Pork liver
4. Beef liver
5. Soy flour
6. Soybeans
7. Rice bran
8. Rice germ
9. Rice polishings
10. Egg yolk
11. Peanut butter
12. Walnuts
13. Roasted peanuts
14. Barley
15. Pecans
16. Oatmeal
17. Canned sardines
18. Whole eggs
19. Black-eyed peas
20. Split peas
21. Almonds
22. Cauliflower
23. Mushrooms
24. Whole wheat cereal
25. Canned salmon
26. Textured vegetable protein
27. Bran
28. Lentils
29. Brown rice

■ Recommended Dosage

300 to 600 micrograms daily as part of a B-complex supplement. B vitamins are water-soluble and leave the body quickly, so they should be taken twice a day. As a therapy for hair loss or multiple sclerosis, take 5 milligrams a day in addition to the B complex.

■ Side Effects and Contraindications

Usually, biotin does not cause any side effects. However, high-dose supplementation of a single B vitamin can cause imbalances of other B vitamins, which is why you should always take a B-complex supplement. Furthermore, high-dose biotin can result in false thyroid measurements. If you are taking high doses of this vitamin, stop taking biotin for at least five days before testing thyroid hormone levels.

B_9 (FOLIC ACID AND FOLATE)

Vitamin B_9 has many functions in the body but is especially important for the synthesis and repair of DNA and RNA, the formation of red blood cells, and the prevention of certain deformities in the developing fetus.

Folate levels in your body can become low in just a few weeks if you don't eat enough foods that are rich in this B vitamin, so supplementation can be important. The natural form of B_9 found in foods is folate; the synthetic form is folic acid. Since about half of the population has an impaired ability to convert supplemental folic acid to its active form, 5-methyltetrahydrofolate, supplemental folate is the best choice.

■ Functions of B_9 in Your Body

- Detoxifies hormones such as estrogen

- Detoxifies phenols (by-products of manufacturing) from the environment

- Essential for central nervous system function

- Essential for DNA and RNA synthesis

- Facilitates the synthesis of serotonin, dopamine, and norepinephrine (neurotransmitters involved in mood regulation)

- Lowers homocysteine levels, decreasing the risk of heart disease, bone loss, depression, and memory loss

- Needed for the proper health of all tissues, especially the mucous membrane tissues of the digestive tract, vagina, and cervix

- Needed for the synthesis of hemoglobin

- Produces complex phospholipids for neurological function

- Produces S-adenosylmethionine (SAMe), an important compound found in all living cells

- Protects the developing fetus from neural tube defects, such as spina bifida

■ Symptoms of B_9 Deficiency

- ☐ Birth defects affecting the neural tube
- ☐ Decreased resistance to infection
- ☐ Depression
- ☐ Diarrhea
- ☐ Drowsiness
- ☐ Graying hair
- ☐ Impaired wound healing

☐ Indigestion

☐ Inflamed and sore tongue with smooth and shiny appearance

☐ Insomnia

☐ Irritability

☐ Mental illness

☐ Numbness or tingling in hands and feet

☐ Slow, weakened pulse

☐ Toxemia

☐ Weakness

Food Sources of B₉

The following foods are numbered so that the foods which contain the most vitamin B₉ are at the beginning of the list. As the list proceeds, the foods contain progressively less B₉.

1. Brewer's yeast
2. Black-eyed peas
3. Rice germ
4. Soy flour
5. Wheat germ
6. Beef liver
7. Lamb liver
8. Soy beans
9. Pork liver
10. Bran
11. Kidney beans
12. Mung beans
13. Lima beans
14. Navy beans
15. Garbanzo beans
16. Asparagus

17. Lentils
18. Walnuts
19. Fresh spinach
20. Kale
21. Hazelnuts
22. Beet and mustard greens
23. Textured vegetable protein
24. Roasted peanuts
25. Peanut butter
26. Broccoli
27. Barley
28. Split peas
29. Whole wheat cereal
30. Brussels sprouts

31. Almonds
32. Whole wheat flour
33. Oatmeal
34. Cabbage
35. Dried figs
36. Avocados
37. Green beans
38. Corn
39. Fresh coconut
40. Pecans
41. Mushrooms
42. Dates
43. Blackberries
44. Ground beef
45. Oranges

■ Causes of B₉ Deficiency

● Alcohol

- Certain medications, from aspirin to valproic acid, can cause a vitamin B_9 deficiency. Speak to your healthcare provider or pharmacist to learn if any drugs you're taking might be causing B_9 loss.

- Diet low in folate-rich foods

- Genetic defects

- Inflammatory bowel disease (IBD)

- Malabsorption syndromes such as celiac disease

- Tobacco

■ Conditions That Can Benefit from B_9

- Birth defects such as neural tube and cleft palate (prevention)

- Cancer (prevention)

- Cervical dysplasia

- Depression

- Folate deficiency anemia

- Gingivitis

- Gout

- Hyperhomocysteinemia (high homocysteine levels)

- Macular degeneration

- Psoriasis

- Restless leg syndrome

■ Recommended Dosage

400 to 800 micrograms daily, preferably of active folate. B vitamins are water-soluble and leave the body quickly, so they should be taken twice a day. Doses above 400 micrograms should be taken only under the direction of your healthcare provider.

When an individual has a mutation of the gene MTHFR, it is necessary to take a methylated from of B_9 known as L-5-methyltetrahydrofolate. To learn more about this, see the inset on page 50.

After consuming digestive enzymes, wait at least two hours before taking B_9, or your absorption of the vitamin may be negatively affected.

■ Side Effects and Contraindications

Folic acid supplementation can mask the symptoms of B_{12} deficiency. For that reason, dosage should not exceed 400 micrograms per day without having your healthcare provider evaluate your B_{12} level.

Large doses of folic acid can cause insomnia, irritability, and gastrointestinal problems. If you are taking phenytoin (an anticonvulsant), do not take high doses of folic acid. Folic acid also interferes with seizure medications such as valproic acid, carbamazepine, and primidone. Consult your healthcare provider or pharmacist before taking this vitamin to see if any of the medications you are using may make it unwise to use B_9 supplements.

B_{12} (COBALAMIN)

Vitamin B_{12}—also referred to as cobalamin or, in its synthetic form, cyanocobalamin—is made by bacteria in the gastrointestinal tract and is also present in foods, most of animal origin. Hydrochloric acid releases B_{12} from food, at which point the vitamin can be absorbed by the body. This vitamin plays a crucial role in many important body functions, from the formation of red blood cells to energy production.

■ Functions of B_{12} in Your Body

- Essential for DNA synthesis
- Facilitates the metabolism of folic acid
- Helps synthesize proteins
- Involved in the formation and maturation of red blood cells
- Involved in the production of neurotransmitters (chemical messengers in the brain)
- Lowers homocysteine levels, decreasing the risk of heart disease, bone loss, depression, and memory loss
- Plays a key role in the release of energy into the cells
- Replenishes the protective covering of nerve and brain cells
- Required for proper digestion

■ Symptoms of B_{12} Deficiency

☐ Anemia

☐ Confusion

☐ Constipation

☐ Decreased levels of estrogen and progesterone in women

☐ Depression

☐ Diarrhea

☐ Dizziness

☐ Drowsiness

☐ Elevated levels of the amino acid homocysteine

☐ Fatigue

☐ Hallucinations

☐ Increased levels of the hormone cortisol

☐ Insomnia

☐ Irritability

☐ Memory loss

☐ Moodiness

☐ Numbness and tingling of extremities

☐ Poor appetite

☐ Sore tongue

☐ Stiffness

☐ Tinnitus (ringing in the ears)

☐ Weakness

Food Sources of B₁₂

The following foods are numbered so that the foods which contain the most vitamin B_{12} are at the beginning of the list. As the list proceeds, the foods contain progressively less B_{12}.

1. Lamb liver
2. Clams
3. Beef liver
4. Lamb kidneys
5. Calf liver
6. Beef kidneys
7. Chicken liver
8. Oysters
9. Sardines
10. Beef heart
11. Egg yolks
12. Lamb heart
13. Trout
14. Fresh salmon
15. Fresh tuna
16. Lamb
17. Thymus sweetbreads
18. Eggs
19. Dried whey
20. Beef
21. Edam cheese
22. Swiss cheese
23. Brie cheese
24. Gruyere cheese
25. Blue cheese
26. Fresh haddock
27. Fresh flounder
28. Scallops
29. Cheddar cheese
30. Cottage cheese
31. Mozzarella cheese
32. Halibut
33. Perch fillets
34. Fresh swordfish

■ Causes of B₁₂ Deficiency

- AIDS

- Alcoholism

- Certain medications, from antacids to oral hypoglycemic agents, can cause a B_{12} deficiency. Speak to your healthcare provider or pharmacist to learn if any drugs you're taking might be causing a loss of this vitamin.

- Digestive disorders and malabsorption syndromes, including celiac disease, Crohn's disease, and irritable bowel syndrome (IBS).

- *H. pylori* infection
- Inherited disorders
- Low levels of the protein called *intrinsic factor* due to penicious anemia or the aging process
- Nitrous oxide
- Strict vegan diet

■ Conditions That Can Benefit from B$_{12}$

- AIDS
- Anemia
- Anxiety
- Asthma
- Ataxia
- Bell's palsy
- Dementia
- Depression
- Epilepsy
- Fatigue
- Hepatitis
- Infertility

- Insomnia
- Irritability
- Leg cramps at night
- Macular degeneration
- Multiple sclerosis
- Neuropathy
- Numbness
- Psychosis
- Retinopathy (damage to the blood vessels of the retina)
- Sciatica

- Seborrheic dermatitis
- Tingling
- Tinnitus (ringing in the ears)
- Trigeminal neuralgia (chronic pain disorder affecting the trigeminal nerve)
- Vitiligo
- Xanthelasma (yellowish deposit of cholesterol under the skin, on or around the eyelids)

■ Recommended Dosage

400 to 1,000 micrograms daily. The B vitamins are water-soluble and leave the body quickly, so B$_{12}$ should be taken twice a day as part of a B-complex supplement. Your healthcare provider may suggest higher doses to you for some disease processes.

When an individual has a mutation of the gene MTHFR, it is necessary to take a methylated from of B$_{12}$ known as methylcobalamin. To learn more about this, see the inset on page 50.

■ Side Effects and Contraindications

There are no reported side effects of B$_{12}$ use.

INOSITOL

Considered part of the vitamin B complex, inositol is essential to both physical and mental function. It is available in certain foods as well as in supplements.

■ Functions of Inositol in Your Body

- Augments the effects of neurotransmitter release
- Can improve the quality of sleep
- Can reduce LDL (bad) cholesterol
- Has a significant impact on mood and cognition
- Helps form lecithin, which has many important functions
- Helps keep arteries from hardening
- Involved with metabolizing fats and cholesterol in the arteries and liver
- Is a component of every cell membrane
- Used to treat depression and panic disorders

■ Symptoms of Inositol Deficiency

☐ Anxiety

☐ Depression

☐ Difficulty falling asleep

☐ Fibroid tumors

☐ Premenstrual syndrome (PMS) symptoms

■ Causes of Inositol Deficiency

- High caffeine intake
- Long-term use of antibiotics

- Low dietary intake of foods containing inositol

Food Sources of Inositol

- Beans
- Brewer's yeast
- Fruits, especially citrus
- Grains
- Green leafy vegetables

- Meat
- Milk
- Nuts
- Raisins
- Wheat germ

■ Conditions That Can Benefit from Inositol

- Depression
- Fibroids
- Insomnia
- Liver disease
- Neuropathy
- Panic attacks
- Premenstrual syndrome (PMS)

■ Recommended Dosage

200 milligrams to 12 grams daily. B vitamins are water-soluble and leave the body quickly, so they should be taken twice a day. Dosages larger than 200 milligrams should be taken only under the supervision of a physician. Large doses of inositol used for insomnia are taken once a day, one hour before bedtime.

■ Side Effects and Contraindications

Do not take inositol if you have kidney failure. Inositol may stimulate uterine contractions, so women who wish to become pregnant should consult their doctor regarding its use.

VITAMIN C

Vitamin C cannot be made by the body and therefore must be consumed in food or supplements. Many people know that this water-soluble vitamin is needed to support immune function, but vitamin C is actually required for a large number of essential body functions. That's why it's so important that you get ample amounts of this nutrient.

■ Functions of Vitamin C in Your Body

- Acts as a diuretic
- Aids in the healing of wounds
- Aids in the synthesis of collagen
- Benefits the immune system by increasing the number of white blood cells and interferons
- Decreases adrenal steroid production
- Decreases the production of inflammatory leukotrienes
- Decreases the rate of gum disease

- Decreases the rate of stomach cancer
- Decreases the risk of heart disease
- Enhances the body's absorption of iron
- Helps regenerate vitamin E, glutathione, and uric acid
- Helps the metabolism of the amino acid tyrosine
- Helps the synthesis of the amino acid carnitine
- Increases fertility
- Increases HDL (good) cholesterol
- Increases nitric oxide
- Involved in catecholamine synthesis
- Involved in the production of the neurotransmitter serotonin
- Is a powerful antioxidant
- Lowers blood pressure
- Lowers levels of sorbitol, a substance that can damage the body
- Lowers the incidence of cataracts
- Lowers triglycerides
- Needed for the production of the hormone progesterone
- Needed to maintain levels of glutathione, an antioxidant
- Prevents free radical damage of LDL (bad) cholesterol
- Prevents some forms of lung disease
- Prevents the formation of nitrosamines, which can be carcinogenic
- Reduces bruising
- Reduces damage due to glycation
- Supports the energy-producing capacity of the mitochondria

■ Symptoms of Vitamin C Deficiency

- ☐ Anemia
- ☐ Bleeding gums
- ☐ Cardiovascular disease
- ☐ Dry hair
- ☐ Dry, rough, scaling skin
- ☐ Easy bruising
- ☐ Fatigue
- ☐ Frequent infections
- ☐ Impaired wound healing
- ☐ Joint pain
- ☐ Loose teeth
- ☐ Swollen and painful joints
- ☐ Weight loss

Food Sources of Vitamin C

The following foods are numbered so that the foods that contain the most vitamin C are at the top of the list. As the list proceeds, the foods contain progressively less vitamin C.

Be aware that the vitamin C content of foods is easily destroyed by light, heat, and chemicals. Fresh-cut lettuce, for example, loses half of its vitamin C in forty-eight hours unless it is stored in a dark refrigerator.

1. Red chili peppers
2. Guavas
3. Red sweet peppers
4. Kale leaves
5. Parsley
6. Collard leaves
7. Turnip greens
8. Green sweet peppers
9. Broccoli
10. Brussels sprouts
11. Mustard greens
12. Watercress
13. Cauliflower
14. Persimmons
15. Red cabbage
16. Strawberries
17. Papayas
18. Spinach
19. Oranges
20. Orange juice
21. Cabbage
22. Lemon juice
23. Grapefruit
24. Grapefruit juice
25. Elderberries
26. Calf liver
27. Turnips
28. Mangos
29. Asparagus
30. Cantaloupes
31. Swiss chard
32. Green onions
33. Beef liver
34. Okra
35. Tangerines
36. New Zealand spinach
37. Oysters
38. Young lima beans
39. Black-eyed peas
40. Soybeans
41. Green peas
42. Radishes
43. Raspberries
44. Chinese cabbage
45. Yellow summer squash
46. Loganberries
47. Honeydew melon
48. Tomatoes

■ Causes of Vitamin C Deficiency

- Aging
- Certain medications, from antibiotics to oral contraceptives, can cause a vitamin C deficiency.

Speak to your healthcare provider or pharmacist to learn if any drugs you're taking might be causing vitamin C loss.

- Diabetes mellitus
- High fever
- Smoking
- Stress

■ Conditions That Can Benefit from Vitamin C

- Adrenal dysfunction
- Cancer (prevention)
- Cardiovascular disease
- Cataract (prevention)
- Diabetes
- Fatigue
- Female hormone imbalance
- Fertility problems
- Hypertension
- Hypertriglyceridemia (high triglyceride levels)
- Poor wound healing
- Weak immune system

■ Recommended Dosage

1,000 to 5,000 milligrams daily. Vitamin C is water-soluble and leaves the body quickly, so it should be taken twice a day in divided doses.

■ Side Effects and Contraindications

Doses of vitamin C higher than 5,000 milligrams can be ingested, but may cause diarrhea. Buffered vitamin C, which is buffered with minerals, can often be taken without stomach upset. Do not take high doses if you are prone to kidney stones or gout.

Hemochromatosis occurs when the body accumulates excess iron. Vitamin C can increase this accumulation, so if you have this condition, avoid taking supplemental vitamin C.

If you have glucose-6-phosphate dehydrogenase (G6PD) deficiency, avoid IV vitamin C.

■ Symptoms of Vitamin C Toxicity

- ☐ Diarrhea
- ☐ Difficulty sleeping
- ☐ Fatigue
- ☐ Flushing of face
- ☐ Headache
- ☐ Nausea and vomiting

Increasing the Absorption of Your Vitamin and Mineral Supplements

No matter how beneficial a vitamin or mineral supplement may be, it will not help you unless your body is able to absorb and use it. The term *bioavailability* is used to describe the degree to which a supplement is absorbed by the body so that it can be used.

For every supplement, there are factors that influence its bioavailability. These factors include:

- **The chemical form of the supplement.** Some forms are more easily absorbed than others. Also, pharmaceutical grade supplements are more absorbable than lower grades. (For more about supplement quality, see the inset on page 18.)

- **The amount that's taken at one time.** Sometimes, it's better to take a nutrient in divided doses rather than a single dose because the body can't absorb a large amount at one time.

- **The other supplements with which it's taken.** While some nutrients can enhance the absorption of a particular supplement, others can decrease its absorption.

- **Food.** Generally, it's better to take supplements at mealtime, because when you eat, the digestive processes help you absorb nutrients. But while some foods can enhance the absorption of a particular supplement, others can decrease its absorption.

The following table will guide you in maximizing the absorption of certain vitamins and minerals.

Supplement	What You Can Do to Increase Absorption
Vitamin A and Carotenoids	Take with high-quality fats, such as olive oil, flax seeds, or avocado. Because Vitamin A is fat-soluble, it needs fat to be absorbed. Take with vitamin C, which enhances the absorption of vitamin A.
B Complex Vitamins	Take in divided (two) doses instead of one large dose.
Vitamin B_9 (folic acid and folate)	When taking B_9 and digestive enzymes, wait two hour after taking enzymes before taking B_9.
Vitamin B_{12} (cobalamin)	Take with vitamin C, which enhances the absorption of B_{12}. Vitamin C can be taken as a supplement or as an acidic food such as lemon juice.
Vitamin C	Take in divided (two) doses instead of one large dose.

Vitamin D	Take in the form of vitamin D_3. Take with high-quality fats, such as olive oil, flax seeds, or avocado. Because Vitamin D is fat-soluble, it needs fat to be absorbed.
Vitamin E	Unless otherwise directed, take in the form of mixed tocopherols, the more active type of vitamin E. Do not take with ferrous sulfate, which destroys vitamin E. Take with high-quality fats, such as olive oil, flax seeds, or avocado. Because Vitamin E is fat-soluble, it needs fat to be absorbed.
Vitamin K	Take in the form of vitamin $K_{,2}$. Take with high-quality fats, such as olive oil, flax seeds, or avocado. Because Vitamin K is fat-soluble, it needs fat to be absorbed. Avoid large doses of vitamin A, which can decrease the absorption of K.
Calcium	Take in divided (two) doses instead of one large dose. Take in the form of calcium citrate or hydroxyapatite. Do not take calcium carbonate, which is less absorbable. Take with vitamin D_3, which helps the body absorb, transport, and deposit calcium in the bones. Vitamin C and lysine can also increase calcium absorption. When taking calcium and iron, do not take at the same time of day. Calcium and iron compete with each other for absorption.
Chromium	Take in the form of chromium picolinate.
Copper	Take in the form of copper sulfate, copper gluconate, cupric acetate, or copper carbonate. Do not take cupric oxide, which is less absorbable. Wait two hours after eating fiber-rich foods before taking copper. When taking copper and zinc, take one in the morning and the other in the evening. Copper and zinc compete with each other for absorption.
Iron	Take ferrous supplements, such as ferrous sulfate, ferrous fumarate, and ferrous gluconate. Do not take ferric supplements, which are less absorbable. Take with vitamin C, cysteine, folic acid, or zinc. When taking iron and calcium, do not take at the same time of day. Iron and calcium compete with each other for absorption. When taking iron and zinc, take one in the morning and the other in the evening. Iron and zinc compete with each other for absorption. Do not take iron with fenugreek or bilberry, which can inhibit absorption.
Magnesium	Take in the form of magnesium citrate, magnesium glycinate, magnesium gluconate, or magnesium lactate. Do not take magnesium oxide, which is less absorbable. Take with vitamin D, which increases the absorption of magnesium.
Selenium	Take with vitamin C, which enhances the absorption of selenium.
Silicon	Take in the form of orthosilicic acid.
Zinc	Take in the form of zinc picolinate or zinc citrate. Do not take zinc sulfate, which is less absorbable. Take with vitamin D, which helps your body use zinc. When taking zinc and copper, take one in the morning and the other in the evening. Zinc and copper compete with each other for absorption. When taking zinc and iron, take one in the morning and the other in the evening. Zinc and iron compete with each other for absorption.

2

Minerals

Many important bodily functions require certain minerals in order to operate correctly. Yet minerals, unlike vitamins, cannot be produced by your body. Therefore, adequate consumption of minerals is very important for optimal health.

At the same time, you cannot simply load up on these nutrients. Every mineral is required by your body in a specific amount. This precise amount depends on many factors, including diet, medications, health, and the interaction of the mineral with other substances. (See page 9 for more on nutritional interactions.)

Minerals are divided into two groups: macro (or major) and micro (or minor). *Macrominerals* are required by your body in relatively high quantities. Generally, people need more than 200 milligrams of these nutrients a day. Calcium, chloride, magnesium, phosphorus, potassium, and sodium are all macrominerals.

Microminerals, on the other hand, are required by your body in trace amounts. Boron, chromium, cobalt, copper, iodine, iron, manganese, molybdenum, nickel, selenium, silicon, tin, vanadium, and zinc are microminerals.

In this chapter, macrominerals are discussed first, while the second half of the chapter describes microminerals. The nutrients are arranged alphabetically within these two sections. You will read important information about each mineral, including its functions, food sources, and recommended dosage. All dosages include what is consumed in both food and supplements. Furthermore, the dosages are for adults with normal kidney and liver function. You will also read about the symptoms that can occur if your body's storage of that mineral becomes deficient. This will allow you to plan your daily mineral intake and promote your optimal health.

The microminerals cobalt, nickel, and tin are not elaborated on because these minerals are sufficiently consumed through diet. There is, however, the possibility of ingesting too much of these nutrients. A toxic metal screen test can determine whether you are getting too much of these minerals. See "Resources" for the names and contact information of several laboratories that perform this test.

MACROMINERALS

CALCIUM

Calcium is the most abundant mineral in the body, and an essential component of a healthy diet. The body can absorb only about 500 milligrams of calcium at a time, so the daily intake should be divided into separate doses.

■ Functions of Calcium in Your Body

- Activates numerous enzymes
- Helps cholesterol make sex hormones
- Important for release of neurotransmitters (chemical "messengers" in the brain)
- Needed for the absorption of vitamin B_{12}
- Plays a crucial role in nerve impulse transmission
- Regulates ion transport in your cells
- Required (along with vitamin K) for blood to clot
- Used by muscles in energy production
- Vital for development of bones and teeth

■ Symptoms of Calcium Deficiency

☐ Hypertension (high blood pressure)

☐ Muscle spasms and twitching

☐ Osteoporosis/osteopenia (bone loss)

■ Causes of Calcium Deficiency (Hypocalcemia)

- Acidic foods
- Alcohol
- Aspartame
- Aspirin
- Caffeine
- Chocolate

Food Sources of Calcium

The following list is reprinted with permission from Jeffrey Bland's *Clinical Nutrition: A Functional Approach.* Foods that contain the most calcium are listed first, followed by foods that contain progressively less calcium. The number to the left of each food describes how many milligrams of calcium are in 100 grams (3.5 ounces) of that food.

1093	Kelp	73	Cooked soybeans
925	Swiss cheese	73	Pecans
750	Cheddar cheese	72	Wheat germ
352	Carob flour	69	Peanuts
296	Dulse	68	Miso
250	Collard leaves	68	Romaine lettuce
246	Turnip greens	67	Dried apricots
245	Barbados molasses	66	Rutabaga
234	Almonds	62	Raisins
210	Brewer's yeast	60	Black currant
203	Parsley	59	Dates
200	Corn tortillas with lime	56	Green snap beans
187	Dandelion greens	51	Globe artichoke
186	Brazil nuts	51	Prunes
151	Watercress	51	Pumpkin and squash seeds
129	Goat's milk		
128	Tofu	50	Beans
126	Dried figs	49	Common cabbage
121	Buttermilk	48	Soybean sprouts
120	Yogurt	46	Hard winter wheat
119	Beet greens	41	Orange
119	Wheat bran	39	Celery
118	Whole milk*	38	Cashews
114	Buckwheat, raw	38	Rye grain
110	Sesame seeds, hulled	37	Carrot
106	Ripe olives	34	Barley
103	Broccoli	32	Sweet potato
99	English walnut	32	Brown rice
94	Cottage cheese	29	Garlic
93	Spinach	28	Summer squash

27	Onion	16	Grapes
26	Lemon	16	Beets
26	Fresh green peas	14	Cantaloupe
25	Cauliflower	14	Jerusalem artichoke
25	Lentils	13	Tomato
22	Sweet cherry	12	Eggplant
22	Asparagus	12	Chicken
22	Winter squash	11	Orange juice
21	Strawberries	10	Beef
20	Millet	8	Bananas
19	Mung bean sprouts	7	Apples
17	Pineapple	3	Sweet corn

* Milk is not the best source of calcium because pasteurization destroys up to 32 percent of the available calcium.

- Cholestyramine
- Diet high in oxalate (found in spinach, almonds and cashews, baked potatoes with skin, sweet potatoes, miso soup, beets, cocoa powder, bran cereals, and raspberries)
- Diet high in phosphorus (found in soft drinks and white flour)
- Excessive protein consumption
- Excessive thyroid replacement
- Heavy exercise
- Heparin
- High-fiber foods consumed at the same time as mineral supplements
- Increased fat in diet
- Increased zinc consumption
- Low vitamin D
- Methotrexate
- Phenobarbital
- Phenytoin
- Steroids
- Sugar
- Tetracyclines
- Whole wheat

■ Conditions That Can Benefit from Calcium

- Colon cancer
- Elevated triglycerides
- High blood pressure
- Increased cholesterol
- Leg cramps

- Osteoporosis/osteopenia (bone loss)
- Preeclampsia
- Premenstrual syndrome (PMS)

Acid-Creating Foods

The average American diet includes many foods that, once eaten, create acid in your body. If you eat a majority of acidic foods and not enough alkaline foods, your body has to find alkalizing minerals elsewhere to neutralize its pH levels. It often has to resort to using the calcium and protein in your bones. As a result, your bones can become weakened, possibly irrevocably, and your body systems can age at an accelerated pace, resulting in a slew of related problems. The following foods create particularly high acidity levels in your body.

- Chocolate
- Dairy products, such as butter, cheese, ice cream, milk, and yogurt
- Sugar
- Honey
- Beverages such as beer, black tea, coffee, and soft drinks
- All fish and seafood
- All meats, such as beef, chicken, ham, turkey, and veal
- Grains and grain products, such as barley, oats, rice, wheat, and bread
- Nuts, except for almonds, cashews, chestnuts, and macadamia nuts
- A few fruits, including cranberries and dried fruit (Most fruits are alkalizing.)
- A few vegetables, including peas, spinach, rhubarb, and tomatoes (Most vegetables are alkalizing.)
- Processed soybeans
- White vinegar

■ Recommended Dosage

The body can absorb only 500 milligrams of calcium at a time. Therefore, to fully utilize the calcium you ingest, the following suggestions for daily calcium consumption should be split into doses. These amounts refer to your entire daily calcium intake, including what you eat and what you take in supplement form.

- Adult males: 500 milligrams daily.
- Menopausal women: 1,200 milligrams daily.
- Perimenopausal women: 800 milligrams daily.
- Pregnant or lactating women: 1,200 milligrams daily.

Always make sure you use only pharmaceutical-grade supplements. Lower-grade products may be contaminated with lead, mercury, arsenic, aluminum, or cadmium. Calcium carbonate is not as bioavailable as other forms of calcium. Instead, choose calcium citrate or hydroxyapatite, which are both good sources of calcium. The bioavailability of calcium citrate is 2.5 times that of calcium carbonate. If you have calcium-related kidney stones, use only the calcium citrate form. Finally, when you eat fiber-rich foods, wait two hours before taking a calcium supplement.

■ Substances That Increase Calcium Absorption

- Ascorbic acid (vitamin C)
- Citric acid
- Glycine
- Hydrochloric acid
- Lysine
- Vitamin D

■ Side Effects and Contraindications

- Decreases absorption of ciprofloxacin and most fluoroquinolone antibiotics
- Decreases aluminum absorption
- Increases the toxicity of digoxin
- Inhibits the absorption of tetracycline
- Interferes with the absorption of thyroid medication
- May interfere with the absorption of magnesium, zinc, iron, manganese, and phosphorus

■ Symptoms of Calcium Toxicity (Hypercalcemia)

Since the body is limited in its ability to absorb calcium, there are a few short-term effects (namely, constipation and kidney stones) of ingesting too much. However, long-term consumption of too much calcium can result in *hypercalcemia*—high levels of calcium in the blood. Additionally, combining excess calcium with excess vitamin D, which helps the body absorb calcium, can be very dangerous. There are also several diseases—certain cancers, granulomatous diseases, sarcoidosis, Crohn's disease, and hyperparathyroidism, for instance—that may make it unwise to take vitamin D since the combination can raise your calcium to above-normal levels. That's why it's so important to speak to your healthcare provider about your calcium needs. The following are symptoms of hypercalcemia.

☐ Clogged arteries

☐ Constipation

☐ Decreased iron absorption

☐ Decreased magnesium absorption

☐ Decreased uptake of manganese

☐ Decreased vitamin K production

☐ Decreased zinc absorption

☐ Kidney stones

☐ Thyroid dysfunction

CHLORIDE

Electrolytes are molecules in your plasma—the liquid portion of your blood—that maintain either a positive or negative charge. These charges allow them to respond to messages from your nervous system by conducting electrical currents through your body, enabling and regulating many bodily functions and systems. Chloride is one of the body's most important electrolytes. Along with sodium, chloride maintains membrane potential, which is the difference in electrical potential between the inside and outside of a cell. Also, chloride, in the form of hydrochloric acid (HCL), is a component of gastric acid, which aids in the absorption and digestion of nutrients in the stomach.

Food Sources of Chloride

Most people get a majority of their chloride from table or sea salt (sodium chloride), a substance that also contains potassium. People who use a salt substitute that contains potassium chloride get chloride from that product. Chloride can also be found in the following foods.

- Celery
- Lettuce
- Olives
- Tomatoes

■ Functions of Chloride in Your Body

- Generates and conducts electrical signals that play roles in many bodily functions

- Helps balance the fluid inside and outside cells

- Is a component of stomach acid

- Maintains pH balance

Electrolyte Imbalance and Chloride

It is very important that your body's electrolytes—such as chloride, sodium, and potassium—remain at their proper levels. *Electrolyte imbalance* (which is also called electrolyte disturbance) can occur if any of these substances has a sudden, abnormal change. The change can be an elevation or depletion of the electrolyte, and may be due to renal (kidney) failure or water loss, such as from long-time laxative abuse or excessive vomiting, diarrhea, or sweating. Therefore, sufferers of anorexia and bulimia are at particularly high risk. Electrolyte imbalance is usually the result of an underlying problem, such as dehydration or dysfunction of the endocrine system or kidneys, and is usually corrected by treating the initial problem. If an electrolyte imbalance is left untreated, it can cause heart-related issues such as irregular heart rhythms, organ failure, problems with the nervous system, or death. An abnormal level of chloride can take one of the forms described below.

Chloride Deficiency (Hypochloremia)

Chloride can exit the body through urine, sweat, or vomit, or can be lost as the result of kidney or adrenal gland disease. When too much of this mineral exits the body, *hypochloremia*, an abnormally low level of chloride, occurs. Some people experience headaches, nausea, or even cardiac arrest. Others experience water loss and dehydration.

Chloride Elevation (Hyperchloremia)

Any excess of chloride is usually removed from the body in urine, but sometimes elevated levels of chloride—*hyperchloremia*—do occur. Some people experience dehydration, diarrhea, muscle tension, or kidney disease. Diabetics with elevated chloride levels have a very difficult time maintaining healthy blood sugar levels. Treatment should involve pinpointing and treating the underlying problem.

■ Recommended Dosage

Because salt is so common in most of our diets, it is usually not necessary to take supplements or eat more salt-containing foods. In fact, most people consume too much salt. However, some people do need to add salt to their diets, particularly if they experience a good deal of stress. People with adrenal failure, for example, need to increase their salt intake. Your healthcare provider can help determine whether you need more or less salt in your diet.

Cautions When Using Potassium Chloride

As mentioned on page 73, some people use a salt substitute that contains potassium chloride. Although potassium chloride is usually safe to ingest, a number of drugs can interact with this substance. Before you use a product that contains potassium chloride, speak to your healthcare provider or pharmacist to see if it can be used safely along with your medications.

MAGNESIUM

Magnesium is a *cofactor*—a molecule that binds to and stimulates an enzyme—and is involved in the activation of over 300 enzymes in the body. It is a required component in the production of adenosine triphosphate (ATP), one of the body's main energy sources. Half of the body's magnesium is found in the bones and helps prevent bone loss. Moreover, one study showed that mildly low magnesium levels, caused by low dietary intake, predispose the body to the chronic inflammatory stress that can lead to the development of disease.

■ Functions of Magnesium in Your Body

- Acts as a natural anticonvulsant
- Acts as a natural tranquilizer
- Assists with nerve function
- Assists with skeletal muscle function
- Can help induce sleep
- Decreases blood vessel constriction
- Decreases risk of tooth decay
- Enhances the function of various brain antioxidants
- Essential to the life of all cells
- Helps heal wounds

- Helps prevent labor complications
- Helps synthesize and oxidize fatty acids
- Important for functions of the immune system
- Improves glucose uptake by insulin
- Improves muscle strength and endurance
- Increases HDL cholesterol
- Maintains normal heart rhythm
- Maximizes heart health
- May reduce risk of arrhythmia (irregular heart rhythm) after bypass surgery
- Metabolizes fats and carbohydrates for energy production
- Necessary for bone formation
- Necessary for steroid hormone production
- Necessary for teeth formation
- Necessary for protein synthesis
- Prevents production of inflammation-increasing chemicals
- Relaxes electrical impulses and encourages calmness
- Relaxes muscles to prevent cramping
- Removes excess ammonia
- Important for the metabolism of other nutrients, including calcium, copper, iron, phosphorus, potassium, sodium, and zinc

■ Symptoms of Magnesium Deficiency

☐ Aggressive behavior
☐ Anorexia nervosa/ weight loss
☐ Anxiety
☐ Back pain or spasm
☐ Carbohydrate cravings
☐ Chest tightness
☐ Cognitive decline
☐ Cold hands and feet
☐ Confusion
☐ Constipation

☐ Decreased appetite
☐ Delirium
☐ Depression
☐ Difficulty swallowing
☐ Fatigue
☐ Hyperexcitability
☐ Hyperventilation
☐ Insomnia
☐ Irritability
☐ Memory loss

☐ Muscle cramps, soreness, or twitches
☐ Nausea and vomiting
☐ Neck pain or spasm
☐ Numbness
☐ Palpitations
☐ Poor wound healing
☐ Salt cravings
☐ Sensitivity to light
☐ Sensitivity to noise

☐ Spontaneous carpopedal spasm (involuntary muscle contractions in hands and feet)

☐ Tingling

☐ TMJ pain (pain in jaw joint)

☐ Tremors

☐ Urinary spasm

☐ Vertigo

☐ Weakness

■ Causes of Magnesium Deficiency

- Alcoholism
- Diarrhea
- Diet high in oxalate (found in spinach, almonds and cashews, baked potatoes with skin, sweet potatoes, miso soup, beets, cocoa powder, bran cereals, and raspberries)
- Excessive caffeine intake
- Excessive sugar intake
- Extreme athletic competition
- Fiber excess
- Gastrointestinal disorders, including biliary and intestinal fistulas, celiac disease, infection, inflammatory bowel disease, malabsorption syndromes, pancreatitis, and partial bowel obstruction
- Heavy bleeding during menstrual cycle
- Certain medications. Some drugs, from antibiotics to steroids, can cause a magnesium deficiency. Speak to your healthcare provider or pharmacist to learn if any drugs you're taking might be causing magnesium loss.
- Parasitic infection
- Phosphates in soft drinks
- Pregnancy
- Stress
- Surgery
- Total parental nutrition (TPN)
- Trans fatty acids
- Trauma
- Vomiting

■ Conditions That Can Benefit from Magnesium

- Abnormal calcium deposits
- Agoraphobia
- Alcoholism
- Angina (chest pain)
- Anxiety disorder
- Asthma
- Attention deficit disorder (ADD)
- Autism
- Calcium-oxalate kidney stones
- Cardiac arrhythmias
- Cardiomyopathy
- Cardiovascular disease

Food Sources of Magnesium

The following list is reprinted with permission from *Clinical Nutrition: A Functional Approach* by Jeffrey Bland. Foods that contain the most magnesium are listed first, followed by foods that contain progressively less magnesium. The number to the left of each food describes how many milligrams of magnesium are in 100 grams (3.5 ounces) of that food.

760	Kelp	38	Sunflower seeds
490	Wheat bran	37	Barley
336	Wheat germ	37	Beans
270	Almonds	36	Dandelion greens
267	Cashews	36	Garlic
258	Blackstrap molasses	35	Raisins
231	Brewer's yeast	35	Fresh green peas
229	Buckwheat	34	Potato with skin
225	Brazil nuts	34	Crab
220	Dulse	33	Bananas
184	Hazelnuts	31	Sweet potatoes
175	Peanuts	30	Blackberries
162	Millet	25	Beets
160	Wheat grain	24	Cauliflower
142	Pecans	23	Carrots
131	English walnuts	22	Celery
115	Tofu	21	Beef
106	Beet greens	20	Asparagus
90	Coconut meat, dry	19	Chicken
88	Cooked soybeans	18	Green pepper
88	Spinach	17	Winter squash
88	Brown rice	16	Cantaloupe
71	Dried figs	16	Eggplant
65	Swiss chard	14	Tomatoes
62	Dried apricots	13	Cabbage
58	Dates	13	Grapes
57	Collard leaves	13	Milk
51	Shrimp	13	Mushrooms
48	Sweet corn	12	Onions
45	Avocado	11	Oranges
45	Cheddar cheese	11	Iceberg lettuce
41	Parsley	9	Plums
40	Prunes	8	Apples

- Chronic fatigue syndrome
- Chronic obstructive pulmonary disease (COPD)
- Claudication (type of cramping pain in leg)
- Congestive heart failure
- Dementia
- Depression
- Diabetes mellitus
- Endometriosis
- Fibromyalgia
- Heart attack
- High blood pressure
- Hypertention (high blood pressure)
- Hypoglycemia (low blood sugar)
- Insomnia
- Learning disabilities
- Low HDL (good) cholesterol
- Lupus
- Migraine headaches
- Mitral valve prolapse
- Muscle spasms
- Osteopenia/osteoporosis (bone loss)
- Pregnancy complications
- Premenstrual syndrome (PMS)
- Psychosis
- Restless leg syndrome
- Schizophrenia
- Sickle cell anemia
- Urinary problems

■ Recommended Dosage

400 to 800 milligrams daily. Some people have diarrhea if they take over 600 milligrams a day. In that case, the dose should be reduced. Magnesium citrate, magnesium glycinate, magnesium gluconate, and magnesium lactate are more easily absorbed than magnesium oxide.

■ Side Effects and Contraindications

Chronic kidney disease can cause magnesium to accumulate in the body, making it necessary to avoid magnesium supplements or to use them with caution. In addition, many medications, from calcium channel blockers to diuretics, can cause problems when taken with this nutrient. Speak to your healthcare provider or pharmacist to see if it is safe to take this nutrient with your medications and if any cautions should be exercised.

■ Symptoms of Magnesium Toxicity

☐ Drowsiness   ☐ Lethargy   ☐ Weakness

PHOSPHORUS

Phosphorus is essential to many life processes in all living organisms. The second most abundant mineral in the body, phosphorus is chiefly stored in the bones. There are also phosphate-containing molecules called phospholipids, which are a major component of cell membranes. In fact, this mineral has many vital functions.

■ Functions of Phosphorus in Your Body

- Assists with growth and healing of bones and teeth
- Develops and repairs body tissue
- Helps regulate enzymes
- Involved in many biochemical reactions
- Major component of bones and teeth
- Necessary for lipid metabolism
- Needed for energy production
- Used in the buffering system that maintains acid-alkaline balance

■ Symptoms of Phosphorus Deficiency (Hypophosphatemia)

☐ Anorexia nervosa/loss of appetite   ☐ Irregular breathing

☐ Anxiety   ☐ Joint stiffness

☐ Bone pain   ☐ Weakness

☐ Fragile bones

■ Causes of Phosphorus Deficiency

Most Americans are not deficient in phosphorus because it is found in most foods, including unhealthy but popular fare such as soft drinks and fast foods. The following conditions and substances, however, can lower phosphorus levels.

- Alcoholism
- Certain medications, from antacids to ace inhibitors, can lower phosphorus levels. Ask your healthcare provider or pharmacist if any of your medications, including over-the-counter products, have the potential to cause a phosphorus deficiency.

- Salt substitutes that contain high levels of potassium.
- Vitamin D deficiency

■ Conditions That Can Benefit from Phosphorus

- Calcium-based kidney stones
- Osteoporosis/osteopenia (bone loss)
- Hypercalcemia (elevated levels of calcium)

■ Recommended Dosage

Although most people in the United States are not deficient in phosphorus (particularly because soft drinks contain this mineral), it is suggested that if you have normal kidney function, you ingest the following amounts in the form of foods. Only rarely is a phosphorus supplement needed, so speak to your healthcare provider before taking one.

- Adults 19 to 24 years of age: 2,400 milligrams daily.
- Adults 25 years of age and older: 800 milligrams daily.
- Pregnant women: 1,200 milligrams daily.

■ Side Effects and Contraindications

People with severe kidney disease, which can cause phosphorus to accumulate in the body, or with problems regulating their calcium levels should not take a phosphorus supplement.

■ Symptoms of Phosphorus Toxicity (Hyperphosphatemia)

Several studies suggest that higher intakes of phosphorus are associated with an increased risk of cardiovascular disease. Using phosphorus supplements along with potassium supplements or potassium-sparing diuretics may result in hyperkalemia (high potassium level). Other possible side effects of high phosphorus levels include the following:

- Decreased levels of iron, calcium, magnesium, and/or zinc
- Diarrhea
- Fatigue
- Irritability
- Numbness

Food Sources of Phosphorus

The following list is reprinted with permission from Jeffrey Bland's *Clinical Nutrition: A Functional Approach.* Foods that contain the most phosphorus are listed first, followed by foods that contain progressively less phosphorus. The number to the left of each food describes how many milligrams of phosphorus are in 100 grams (3.5 ounces) of that food.

1753	Brewer's yeast	150	Lamb
1276	Wheat bran	119	Lentils
1144	Pumpkin and squash seeds	116	Mushrooms
		116	Fresh peas
1118	Wheat germ	111	Sweet corn
837	Sunflower seeds	101	Raisins
693	Brazil nuts	93	Whole milk
592	Sesame seeds, hulled	88	Globe artichoke
554	Soybeans	87	Yogurt
504	Almonds	80	Brussels sprouts
478	Cheddar cheese	79	Prunes
457	Pinto beans	78	Broccoli
409	Peanuts	77	Dried figs
400	Wheat	69	Yams
380	English walnuts	67	Soybean sprouts
376	Rye grain	64	Mung bean sprouts
373	Cashews	63	Dates
353	Beef liver	63	Parsley
338	Scallops	62	Asparagus
311	Millet	59	Bamboo shoots
290	Pearled barley	56	Cauliflower
289	Pecans	53	Potato with skin
267	Dulse	51	Okra
240	Kelp	51	Spinach
239	Chicken	44	Green beans
221	Brown rice	44	Pumpkin
205	Eggs	42	Avocados
202	Garlic	40	Beet greens
175	Crab	39	Swiss chard
152	Cottage cheese	38	Winter squash
150	Beef	36	Carrots

36	Onions	26	Eggplant
35	Red cabbage	26	Lettuce
33	Beets	24	Nectarines
31	Radish	22	Raspberries
29	Summer squash	20	Grapes
28	Celery	20	Oranges
27	Cucumbers	17	Olives
27	Tomatoes	16	Cantaloupe
26	Bananas	10	Apples
26	Persimmon	8	Pineapples

POTASSIUM

Electrolytes are molecules that serve to conduct electricity through the body. Every electrolyte has either a positive or negative charge that reacts to messages sent through the body by the nervous system. They react to these messages by conducting electric currents that regulate many functions and bodily systems. The electrolyte potassium is primarily intracellular (inside the cells) while the electrolytes sodium and chloride are primarily extracellular (outside the cells). Together, these three macrominerals maintain balance between the intra- and extracellular compartments in order to regulate many functions, including nerve transmission and muscle contractions. (To learn about electrolyte imbalance, see the inset on page 74.)

■ Functions of Potassium in Your Body

- Aids in maintaining cellular integrity (keeps the cells together)
- Needed for muscle contraction
- Preserves the acid-base balance
- Regulates fluid balance
- Transmits electrical signals between cells and nerves
- Used in glucose and glycogen metabolism

■ Symptoms of Potassium Deficiency (Hypokalemia)

- ☐ Arrhythmia (irregular heartbeat)
- ☐ Cardiac weakness
- ☐ Central nervous system changes
- ☐ Fragile bones

☐ Muscle weakness or pain   ☐ Slow heart rate

■ Causes of Potassium Deficiency (Hypokalemia)

- Aging
- Alcoholism
- Anorexia nervosa
- Bulimia
- Burns
- Diarrhea
- Excessive water loss
- Kidney disease
- Low levels of magnesium (magnesium is necessary for the body to process potassium)

- Low-potassium diet
- Some medications, from aspirin to penicillin, can cause potassium deficiency. Speak to your healthcare provider or pharmacist to see if any of the medications you are taking might be contributing to potassium deficiency.
- Starvation
- Vomiting

■ Symptoms of Elevated Potassium Levels (Hyperkalemia)

- ☐ Arrhythmia
- ☐ Chest pain
- ☐ Diarrhea
- ☐ General malaise

- ☐ Increased urination
- ☐ Muscle pain
- ☐ Paralysis

■ Causes of Elevated Potassium Levels (Hyperkalemia)

- Adrenal dysfunction
- Breakdown of cell function
- Congestive heart failure
- Endocrine problems
- Hormone problems
- Ineffective elimination from body
- Kidney disease
- Laxative abuse

- Many medications, from ACE inhibitors to NSAIDS, can cause elevated potassium levels. Speak to your healthcare provider or pharmacist to see if any of the medications you are taking might be contributing to high potassium levels.
- Severe dehydration

Food Sources of Potassium

The following list is reprinted with permission from Jeffrey Bland's *Clinical Nutrition: A Functional Approach.* Foods that contain the most potassium are listed first, followed by foods that contain progressively less potassium. The number to the left of each food describes how many milligrams of potassuim are in 100 grams (3.5 ounces) of that food.

8060	Dulse	322	Radishes
5273	Kelp	295	Cauliflower
920	Sunflower seeds	282	Watercress
827	Wheat germ	278	Asparagus
773	Almonds	268	Red cabbage
763	Raisins	264	Lettuce
727	Parsley	251	Cantaloupe
715	Brazil nuts	249	Lentils
674	Peanuts	244	Tomatoes
648	Dates	243	Sweet potatoes
640	Dried figs	234	Papaya
604	Avocados	214	Eggplant
603	Pecans	213	Green peppers
600	Yams	208	Beets
550	Swiss chard	202	Summer squash
540	Cooked soybeans	200	Oranges
529	Garlic	199	Raspberries
470	Spinach	191	Cherries
450	English walnuts	164	Strawberries
430	Millet	162	Grapefruit juice
416	Beans	158	Grapes
414	Mushrooms	157	Onions
407	Potatoes with skin	146	Pineapples
382	Broccoli	144	Milk, whole
370	Bananas	141	Lemon juice
370	Meats	130	Pears
369	Winter squash	129	Eggs
366	Chicken	110	Apples
341	Carrots	100	Watermelon
341	Celery	70	Brown rice, cooked

■ Conditions That Can Benefit from Potassium

- Arrhythmias
- Cardiovascular disease
- Diabetes mellitus
- Fatigue
- High blood pressure

- Postural low blood pressure (occurs when you stand from a sitting or lying position)
- Predisposition to kidney stones
- Predisposition to osteopenia/ osteoporosis (bone loss)
- Predisposition to stroke

■ Recommended Dosage

500 milligrams daily. Potassium supplements should be taken with water because they can damage the esophagus if they get caught in the throat.

■ Side Effects and Contraindications

Potassium supplements should be avoided if you have renal (kidney) failure. They should also be avoided if you are taking certain drugs, such as ACE inhibitors. Speak to your healthcare provider or pharmacist to see if it is safe to take potassium with your medications and if any cautions should be exercised.

SODIUM

Sodium, an electrolyte, plays several vital roles in the body. Perhaps most important, it helps control blood pressure and regulates the function of muscles and nerves. For sodium to do its job and keep the body functioning normally, the concentration of this nutrient must be carefully controlled and kept in balance with concentrations of two other important electrolytes, potassium and chloride. Too much sodium in the diet can disrupt this balance and lead to potentially deadly problems like high blood pressure, but abnormally low levels of sodium are also dangerous. (For more information on electrolyte imbalance, see the inset on page 74.) It is important to note that while low sodium levels can be harmful, most Americans should *reduce* their sodium intake.

■ Functions of Sodium in Your Body

- Generates and conducts electricity, which is involved in many functions
- Helps control blood pressure
- Helps transport carbon dioxide

- Needed for muscle contraction

- Required for amino acid transport

- Required for proper function of nervous system

- Responsible for nerve transmission

■ Symptoms of Sodium Deficiency (Hyponatremia)

- ☐ Change in body's acid-base balance

- ☐ Confusion

- ☐ Decreased elasticity of subcutaneous tissue (the tissue beneath the skin)

- ☐ Diminished reflexes

- ☐ General malaise

- ☐ Headache

- ☐ Impaired adrenal function

- ☐ Increased hematocrit (portion of blood that contains red blood cells)

- ☐ Low blood pressure

- ☐ Neurological disorders

- ☐ Tiredness

- ☐ Vomiting

■ Causes of Sodium Deficiency (Hyponatremia)

- Certain medications, from diuretics to NSAIDS, can cause a sodium deficiency. Speak to your healthcare provider or pharmacist to see if any of your medications has the potential to lead to this condition.

- Dehydration

- Disorders and conditions such as diarrhea, hyperglycemia, and malaria

- Excessive and persistent sweating, such as that associated with vigorous exercise

- Heart failure

- Some forms of kidney disease

■ Recommended Intake

Most people consume too much salt, often in the form of processed foods that are high in sodium. The average daily intake for Americans is 3,400 milligrams per day, while the recommended daily *limit* is 2,400 mg daily. Less commonly, some individuals that have low levels of the hormone cortisol may require an additional intake of sodium. Speak to your healthcare provider to determine what your daily intake of sodium should be.

Food Sources of Sodium

The following list is reprinted with permission from Jeffrey Bland's *Clinical Nutrition: A Functional Approach.* Foods that contain the most sodium are listed first, followed by foods that contain progressively less sodium. The number to the left of each food describes how many milligrams of sodium are in 100 grams (3.5 ounces) of that food, unless another measurement is given.

3007	Kelp	52	Watercress
2400	Green olives	50	Whole cow's milk
2132	Salt (one teaspoon)	49	Turnips
1428	Dill pickles	47	Carrots
1319	Soy sauce (one tablespoon)	47	Yogurt
		45	Parsley
828	Ripe olives	43	Artichokes
747	Sauerkraut	34	Dried figs
700	Cheddar cheese	30	Lentils
265	Scallops	30	Sunflower seeds
229	Cottage cheese	27	Raisins
210	Lobster	26	Red cabbage
147	Swiss chard	19	Garlic
130	Beet greens	19	White beans
130	Buttermilk	15	Broccoli
126	Celery	15	Mushrooms
122	Eggs	13	Cauliflower
110	Cod	10	Onions
71	Spinach	10	Sweet potatoes
70	Lamb	9	Lettuce
65	Pork	6	Cucumbers
64	Chicken	5	Peanuts
60	Beef	4	Avocados
60	Beets	3	Tomatoes
60	Sesame seeds	2	Eggplant

■ Symptoms of High Sodium Levels (Hypernatremia)

☐ Bone loss   ☐ Coma   ☐ Confusion

☐ Edema (swelling of tissues)   ☐ Irritability   ☐ Thirst

☐ High blood pressure   ☐ Lethargy   ☐ Weakness

☐ Seizures

■ Causes of High Sodium Levels (Hypernatremia)

- Burns
- Dehydration
- Diabetes insipidus (impaired thirst mechanism)
- Diarrhea
- Fever
- Kidney disease
- Some medications, such as steroids, can affect sodium levels. Check with your healthcare provider or pharmacist to learn if any medications you are taking can elevate sodium levels.
- Vomiting

■ Conditions That Can Benefit From Sodium

- Hypoadrenalism (low levels of the hormone cortisol)
- Hyponatremia (low sodium levels)
- Sunstroke
- Muscle cramps

MICROMINERALS

BORON

Boron, a micromineral, is required by the body in trace amounts. As an activating agent, it is responsible for triggering many important body functions, such as helping the body respond to various hormone activities. It also manages the balance of other essential minerals. Because this hormone is responsible for so many processes in the body, a boron deficiency can be serious.

■ Functions of Boron in Your Body

- Aids vitamin D in increasing mineral content of your bones
- Decreases inflammation
- Enhances cartilage formation

- Fights tooth decay

- Helps maintain memory and improve other brain functions

- Improves levels of HDL cholesterol, LDL cholesterol, and triglycerides

- Increases absorption of and regulates levels of calcium, magnesium, copper, and phosphorus

- Increases estrogen production in women

- Increases testosterone production in both men and women

- Is a cofactor in enzymatic reactions

- Promotes immune function in its role as an antioxidant

- Reduces risk of prostate cancer

Food Sources of Boron

The following list provides the boron content of a number of foods. Foods that contain the most boron are listed first, followed by foods that contain progressively less boron. The number to the left of each food describes how many milligrams of boron are in 100 grams (3.5 ounces) of that food

4.51	Raisins	0.71	Chickpeas
2.82	Almonds	0.7	Bananas
2.77	Hazelnuts	0.52	Peaches
2.11	Dried apricots	0.5	Red grapes
1.72	Brazil nuts	0.5	Celery
1.63	Walnuts	0.32	Pears
1.4	Red kidney beans	0.32	Red apples
1.18	Prunes	0.31	Broccoli
1.15	Raw cashews	0.3	Carrots
1.08	Dates	0.3	Oranges
0.74	Lentils	0.2	Onions

■ Symptoms of Boron Deficiency

☐ Arthritis

☐ Carpal tunnel syndrome

☐ Decreased focus and memory

☐ Depression

☐ Hormonal imbalance

☐ Impaired levels of HDL cholesterol, LDL cholesterol, and triglycerides

☐ Muscle pain or weakness

☐ Osteopenia/osteoporosis (bone loss)

☐ Receding gumlines

☐ Tooth decay

☐ Weak or brittle bones

■ Causes of Boron Deficiency

• Dietary insufficiency

• Disturbed calcium-magnesium balance

• Eating disorders (anorexia nervosa or bulimia)

• Malabsorption disorders

• Persistent vomiting

• Renal (kidney) disease

• Severe diarrhea

• Severe malnutrition

■ Conditions That Can Benefit from Boron

• Arthritis

• Cardiovascular disorders

• Female and male hormonal imbalance

• Impaired cognitive function

• Impaired immune system

• Osteopenia/osteoporosis (bone loss)

■ Recommended Dosage

1,000 micrograms daily.

■ Symptoms of Boron Toxicity

☐ Dermatitis

☐ Diarrhea

☐ Hormonal imbalance

☐ Inability to properly metabolize phosphorus

☐ Inability to properly metabolize riboflavin

☐ Lethargy

☐ Nausea

☐ Vomiting

CHROMIUM

The micronutrient chromium is essential to your health, but the body has a difficult time absorbing it when it is by itself. Combining it with another substance, such as the protein picolinate, allows it to enter the bloodstream more easily. Picolinate also increases the absorption of zinc, copper, and iron. Chromium nicotinate is also an excellent absorbable form of chromium.

Food Sources of Chromium

Chromium can be found in the following foods. However, up to 90 percent of the chromium content of food is lost in food processing. If eaten for their chromium content, the following foods should be eaten unprocessed and, most likely, along with chromium supplementation.

This list is reprinted with permission from *Clinical Nutrition: A Functional Approach* by Jeffrey Bland. Foods that contain the most chromium are listed first, followed by foods that contain progressively less chromium. The number to the left of each food describes how many milligrams of chromium are in 100 grams (3.5 ounces) of that food.

112	Brewer's yeast	11	Swiss cheese
57	Beef, round	10	Bananas
55	Calf's liver	10	Spinach
42	Whole wheat bread	10	Pork chops
38	Wheat bran	9	Carrots
30	Rye bread	8	Navy beans
26	Oysters	7	Shrimp
24	Potatoes	7	Lettuce
23	Wheat germ	5	Oranges
19	Green peppers	5	Lobster tail
16	Eggs	5	Blueberries
15	Chicken	4	Green beans
14	Apples	4	Cabbage
13	Butter	4	Mushrooms
13	Parsnips	3	Beer
12	Cornmeal	3	Strawberries
12	Lamb chops	1	Milk
11	Scallops		

◼ Functions of Chromium in Your Body

- Aids in fat loss
- Burns calories
- Decreases total cholesterol and LDL (bad) cholesterol
- Helps decrease sugar cravings
- Helps hold onto calcium and prevent osteoporosis
- Helps increase the hormone dehydroepiandrosterone (DHEA)

- Helps regulate blood sugar by making insulin work more effectively
- Increases antibodies
- Increases HDL (good) cholesterol
- Increases physical endurance
- Lowers excess cortisol
- Reduces bone loss
- Stimulates muscle development

◼ Symptoms of Chromium Deficiency

- ☐ Anxiety
- ☐ Atherosclerosis
- ☐ Decreased insulin binding, which can lead to insulin resistance and diabetes
- ☐ Elevated insulin levels
- ☐ Fatigue

- ☐ Heart disease
- ☐ Increased cholesterol and triglyceride levels
- ☐ Low blood sugar, and possibly hypoglycemia
- ☐ Neuropathy (numbness and tingling of the extremities)

◼ Causes of Chromium Deficiency

- Aging process
- Antacid use
- Excessive exercise

- Food grown in low-chromium soil
- High intake of refined sugar

- High-carbohydrate diet
- Steroid use

◼ Conditions That Can Benefit from Chromium

- Diabetes/insulin resistance
- Hypercholesterolemia (high cholesterol)
- Hypertriglyceridemia (high triglycerides)
- Hypothyroidism (low thyroid function)

- Osteoporosis/osteopenia (bone loss)
- Sarcopenia (muscle loss)
- Weight gain
- Yeast overgrowth

■ Recommended Dosage

50 to 200 micrograms daily, preferably as chromium picolinate. Higher doses have been used for specific disease processes if the individual has normal kidney function. For example:

- Insulin resistance: 600 to 1,200 micrograms.
- Sugar cravings: 300 to 600 micrograms.
- Muscle building: 1,200 micrograms.

■ Factors That Increase Chromium Absorption

- Amino acid imbalance
- Vitamin C
- Physical trauma

■ Side Effects and Contraindications

If you have compromised kidney function, be sure to speak to your healthcare provider before using a chromium supplement.

■ Symptoms of Chromium Toxicity

- ☐ Irregular heart rhythms and liver problems (These symptoms are rare.)
- ☐ Kidney damage (This has been reported from use of chromium picolinate supplements. Have your healthcare provider check your kidney function.)
- ☐ Lightheadedness
- ☐ Rashes
- ☐ Reduced control of blood sugar accompanied by stomach irritation or rash, itching, and flushing

COPPER

Copper is one of a small group of metallic elements necessary for human health. (Iron and magnesium are other examples.) The highest concentrations of copper can be found in your kidneys, liver, brain, heart, and bones. Low copper levels may inhibit iron absorption. A number of nutrition surveys have indicated that the diets of approximately 25 percent of adolescents and adults do not meet the recommended daily nutrient intake for copper.

■ Functions of Copper in Your Body

- Aids in energy production
- Aids in iron metabolism
- Assists thyroid function
- Decreases inflammation
- Helps wound healing
- Improves eye health and inhibits progression of age-related macular degeneration
- Metabolizes catecholamine (an important brain chemical)
- Metabolizes cholesterol
- Metabolizes protein
- Necessary for heart health
- Necessary for production of adrenal and ovarian hormones
- Necessary for red blood cell formation
- Necessary for skeletal mineralization
- Necessary for white blood cell formation
- Offers antioxidant protection
- Promotes healthy nerve function
- Regulates body temperature
- Regulates glucose metabolism
- Strengthens immune function
- Synthesizes connective tissue, including collagen
- Synthesizes melanin pigment
- Synthesizes myelin

■ Symptoms of Copper Deficiency

- ☐ Anemia
- ☐ Bone abnormalities
- ☐ Broken blood vessels
- ☐ Decreased hair and skin pigmentation
- ☐ Fatigue
- ☐ Hypochromic microcytic anemia
- ☐ Limb edema
- ☐ Loss of muscle tone
- ☐ Low white blood cell count

■ Causes of Copper Deficiency

- Antacid use
- Certain drugs, such as penicillamine. Speak to your healthcare provider or pharmacist to learn if any of the drugs you're taking might be causing a loss of copper.
- Diet high in phytates (found in beans, breads, matzoh, wheat germ, vanilla extract, cacao powder, oats, and nuts)
- Diet high in sugar
- Excess calcium
- Excess iron

- Excess molybdenum
- Excess vitamin C
- Excess zinc
- High-fiber foods consumed at the same time as mineral supplements

- Poor digestion
- Vegetarian diet
- Vigorous exercise

Food Sources of Copper

The following list is reprinted with permission from Jeffrey Bland's *Clinical Nutrition: A Functional Approach.* Foods that contain the most copper are listed first, followed by foods that contain progressively less copper. The number to the left of each food describes how many milligrams of copper are in 100 grams (3.5 ounces) of that food.

13.7	Oysters	0.4	Gelatin
2.3	Brazil nuts	0.3	Shrimp
2.1	Soy lecithin	0.3	Olive oil
1.4	Almonds	0.3	Clams
1.3	Hazelnuts	0.3	Carrots
1.3	Walnuts	0.3	Coconuts
1.3	Pecans	0.3	Garlic
1.2	Split peas	0.2	Millet
1.1	Beef liver	0.2	Whole wheat
0.8	Buckwheat	0.2	Chicken
0.8	Peanuts	0.2	Eggs
0.7	Cod liver oil	0.2	Corn oil
0.7	Lamb chops	0.2	Ginger root
0.5	Sunflower oil	0.2	Molasses
0.4	Butter	0.2	Turnips
0.4	Rye grain	0.1	Green peas
0.4	Pork loin	0.1	Papaya
0.4	Barley	0.1	Apple

■ Conditions That Can Benefit from Copper

- Colon cancer
- Diabetes/insulin resistance

- Hormone imbalance

- Hypercholesterolemia (high cholesterol)
- Hypothyroidism (low thyroid function)
- Malabsorption syndromes such as celiac disease and short bowel syndrome

- Osteoarthritis
- Osteoporosis/osteopenia (bone loss)
- Rheumatoid arthritis
- Wounds

■ Recommended Dosage

1.5 to 3 milligrams daily. It is very important for the body to maintain a proper ratio of zinc to copper—between 10:1 and 15:1. (See the discussion on page 119 for more information on the zinc-to-copper ratio.) The bioavailability of cupric oxide is almost zero, so it should not be taken as a supplement. Instead, use copper sulfate, copper gluconate, cupric acetate, or alkaline copper carbonate. After eating fiber-rich foods, wait two hours before taking a copper supplement.

■ Side Effects and Contraindications

Do not take copper supplements if you have Wilson's disease, a disorder that causes copper to accumulate in vital organs. Also, if you have cognitive decline, do not supplement with copper without consulting your healthcare provider.

■ Symptoms of Copper Toxicity

☐ Abdominal pain	☐ Diarrhea	☐ Kidney damage
☐ Brain damage	☐ Headaches	☐ Liver damage

■ Causes of Copper Overexposure

- Environmental exposure to copper water pipes, cookware, birth control pills, and dental materials.

IODINE

The micromineral iodine is best known for its role in making thyroid hormones, which control the body's metabolism and many other important functions. In fact, two-thirds of your body's iodine is stored in your thyroid.

This nutrient is added to many table salts—called iodized salts—to prevent iodine deficiency, the effects of which can be devastating, particularly for children. According to the World Health Organization, up to 72 percent of the world's population is affected by an iodine deficiency disorder. It is worth noting that sea salt contains very little iodine unless you purchase an iodized product.

■ Functions of Iodine in Your Body

- Fights bacteria

- Involved in energy production

- Involved in nerve function

- Maintains healthy breast tissue in women

- Needed for the development and functioning of the thyroid gland and hormones

- Promotes hair and skin growth

- Protects against toxic effects from radioactive material

- Relieves pain and soreness associated with fibrocystic breast disease

- Required for normal function of thyroid, breast, prostate, kidneys, spleen, liver, blood, salivary glands, and intestines

■ Symptoms of Iodine Deficiency

☐ Cold extremities

☐ Decreased mental capabilities

☐ Depression

☐ Dry eyes

☐ Fatigue

☐ Goiter

☐ Hypothyroidism (low thyroid function)

☐ Insomnia

☐ Neurological defects

☐ Tenderness of sternum

☐ Weight gain

■ Causes of Iodine Deficiency

- Asthma inhalers that contain fluoride or bromide

- Being born from an iodine-deficient mother

- Diets containing food grown in iodine-depleted soil

- Diets high in pasta and breads that contains bromide, which can affect iodine metabolism

- Diets low in fish or sea vegetables

- Fluoride use, which inhibits iodine binding

- Low-salt diet

- Sucralose, which contains chlorinated table sugar (Chlorinated table sugar prevents iron absorption.)

- Vegan and vegetarian diets

Food Sources of Iodine

The following list is reprinted with permission from Jeffrey Bland's *Clinical Nutrition: A Functional Approach.* Foods that contain the most iodine are listed first, followed by foods that contain progressively less iodine. The number to the left of each food describes how many milligrams of iodine are in 100 grams (3.5 ounces) of that food.

90	Clams	11	Cheddar cheese
65	Shrimp	10	Pork
62	Haddock	10	Lettuce
50	Oysters	9	Spinach
50	Salmon	9	Green peppers
46	Halibut	9	Butter
37	Sardines, canned	7	Milk
19	Beef liver	6	Cream
16	Pineapple	6	Cottage cheese
16	Tuna, canned	6	Beef
14	Eggs	3	Lamb
11	Peanuts	3	Raisins
11	Whole wheat bread		

■ Recommended Dosage

- Adults who are not pregnant: 150 micrograms daily.

- Pregnant women: 220 micrograms daily.

■ Foods That Inhibit Iodine Absorption

- Bok choy
- Broccoli
- Brussels sprouts
- Cabbage
- Cauliflower
- Horseradish
- Kale
- Mustard greens
- Radishes
- Soybeans
- Turnips

■ Side Effects and Contraindications

Before taking an iodine supplement, it is important to see your healthcare provider and have your iodine levels measured. The following are possible side effects of too much iodine:

- Acne-like skin lesions
- Increased risk of thyroid cancer
- Thyroiditis (inflammation of the thyroid gland)

IRON

The micromineral iron is a key to good health because it is involved in many vital bodily functions. It is important to note that *heme iron,* which is found in red meat, fish, and poultry, is much more readily and efficiently absorbed by the body than *non-heme* iron, which is found in vegetables and other plant foods. Despite this, the iron used to enrich iron-fortified food is non-heme iron. The absorption of this micronutrient can be improved by the consumption of the proteins found in meat, vitamin C, and several other substances. (See page 103.) Once in your body, iron is stored in hemoglobulin—the protein molecule in red blood cells that carries oxygen from your lungs to your tissues.

■ Functions of Iron in Your Body

- Essential component of hemoglobin
- Involved in immune system efficiency
- Involved in oxygen transport
- Key element in many enzymatic reactions
- Necessary for collagen synthesis
- Necessary for good cognition and behavior
- Regulates cell growth

■ Symptoms of Iron Deficiency

☐ Craving for ice

☐ Decreased cognitive functioning

☐ Decreased immune system

☐ Decreased memory

☐ Depression

☐ Fatigue

☐ Hair loss

☐ Headache

☐ Hypochromic microcytic anemia

☐ Impaired ability to maintain body temperature

☐ Impaired growth

☐ Increased blood sugar

☐ Increased body tension

☐ Increased fearfulness

☐ Inflammation of the tongue

☐ Pallor

☐ Rapid heart rate

☐ Restless leg syndrome

☐ Short attention span

☐ Shortness of breath

☐ Spoon nails (soft, concave nails)

☐ Weakness

■ Causes of Iron Deficiency

• Bleeding from any part of the body, including menstrual bleeding

• Diet high in oxalate (found in spinach, almonds and cashews, baked potatoes with skin, sweet potatoes, miso soup, beets, cocoa powder, bran cereals, and raspberries)

• Diet high in phytates (found in beans, bread, matzoh, wheat germ, vanilla extract, cacao powder, oats, and nuts)

• Excessive calcium intake

• Excessive coffee intake

• Excessive intake of black and green tea

• High levels of copper

• High levels of manganese

• High levels of zinc

• Partially digested proteins

• Polyphenolic compounds (found in certain plant foods)

• Problems in the small intestine or gastrointestinal tract

• Red wine

• Soy products

• Vegetarian diet

Foods Sources of Iron

The following list is reprinted with permission from Jeffrey Bland's *Clinical Nutrition: A Functional Approach.* Foods that contain the most iron are listed first, followed by foods that contain progressively less iron. The listed number describes how many milligrams of iron are in 100 grams (3.5 ounces) of food.

Iron in meat is more bioavailable than iron found in vegetables. Additionally, your body will absorb more iron from vegetables if they are eaten *with* meat than if they are eaten alone.

100.0	Kelp	2.3	Eggs
17.3	Brewer's yeast	2.1	Lentils
16.1	Blackstrap molasses	2.1	Peanuts
14.9	Wheat bran	1.9	Lamb
11.2	Pumpkin and squash seeds	1.9	Tofu
9.4	Wheat germ	1.8	Green peas
8.8	Beef liver	1.6	Brown rice
7.1	Sunflower seeds	1.6	Ripe olives
6.8	Millet	1.5	Chicken
6.2	Parsley	1.3	Artichokes
6.1	Clams	1.3	Mung bean sprouts
4.7	Almonds	1.2	Salmon
3.9	Prunes	1.1	Broccoli
3.8	Cashews	1.1	Currants
3.7	Lean beef	1.1	Whole wheat bread
3.5	Raisins	1.1	Cauliflower
3.4	Jerusalem artichoke	1.0	Cheddar cheese
3.4	Brazil nuts	1.0	Strawberries
3.3	Beet greens	1.0	Asparagus
3.2	Swiss chard	0.9	Blackberries
3.1	Dandelion greens	0.8	Red cabbage
3.1	English walnuts	0.8	Pumpkin
3.0	Dates	0.8	Mushrooms
2.9	Pork	0.7	Bananas
2.7	Beans	0.7	Beets
2.4	Sesame seeds, hulled	0.7	Carrots
2.4	Pecans	0.7	Eggplant

0.7	Sweet potatoes	0.5	Brown rice
0.6	Avocados	0.5	Tomatoes
0.6	Figs	0.4	Oranges
0.6	Potatoes	0.4	Cherries
0.6	Corn	0.4	Summer squash
0.5	Pineapple	0.3	Papayas
0.5	Nectarines	0.3	Celery
0.5	Watermelon	0.3	Cottage cheese
0.5	Winter squash	0.3	Apples

■ Conditions That Can Benefit from Iron

- Iron deficiency anemia
- Poor thyroid hormone function

■ Recommended Dosage

Men over the age of fifty and menopausal women should consume no supplemental iron unless instructed by their doctor. Other people can follow these guidelines:

- Males below age fifty: 10 milligrams daily.

- Pregnant women: 30 milligrams daily.

- Pre-menopausal women: 15 milligrams daily.

There are two different kinds of iron supplements: *ferrous* (such as ferrous sulfate, ferrous fumarate, and ferrous gluconate) and *ferric* (such as ferric citrate). Ferrous supplements are much more easily absorbed by the body than ferric supplements. Ferrous sulfate, the most popular iron supplement, can cause intestinal problems—such as constipation or nausea—in some users. If this occurs, change the form you are taking. Ask your healthcare provider for advice.

■ Substances That Increase Iron Absorption

- Cysteine
- Meat
- Vitamin C
- Folic acid
- Vitamin B_6
- Zinc

■ Side Effects and Contraindications

Iron supplementation decreases the absorption of some medications. Speak to your healthcare provider or pharmacist to see if it is safe to take this nutrient with your medications and if any cautions should be exercised.

■ Symptoms of Iron Toxicity

☐ Abdominal pain

☐ Decreased absorption and utilization of vitamin E (See page 32 for signs and symptoms of vitamin E deficiency.)

☐ Diabetes

☐ Gut disturbances such as nausea, vomiting, and loose stools

☐ Hair loss

☐ Hypotension (low blood pressure)

☐ Increased heart rate

☐ Irritability

☐ Lethargy

☐ Liver disease

☐ Predisposition to heart disease

☐ Headache, changes in skin color, and seizures (when iron levels are very high)

MANGANESE

Manganese is a trace mineral that is a cofactor for a large number of enzymes in the body, and therefore assists in enzyme activity and many body functions. Most Americans get the manganese they need from their diet, but because foods aren't always as nutrient-rich as you would like them to be, supplements can be important.

■ Functions of Manganese in Your Body

● Aids in protein digestion and synthesis

● Essential for a healthy nervous system

● Essential for the utilization of vitamins B and C in adrenal health

● Helps with carbohydrate metabolism

● Is a cofactor for enzymes involved in energy production

● Needed for a good immune system

● Needed for brain health

- Needed for the synthesis of cartilage, collagen, and other connective tissue
- Part of the antioxidant defense mechanism
- Required for fatty acid synthesis
- Required for the production of estrogen and progesterone
- Used for bone growth and maintenance
- Used in blood formation

■ Symptoms of Manganese Deficiency

- ☐ Decreased hair and nail growth
- ☐ Decreased HDL (good) cholesterol
- ☐ Decreased lipid metabolism (breakdown of fats)
- ☐ Impaired carbohydrate metabolism (breakdown of carbohydrates)
- ☐ Impaired coordination
- ☐ Impaired growth
- ☐ Loss of hair color
- ☐ Skeletal problems
- ☐ Skin rash

■ Causes of Manganese Deficiency

- Diet high in phytates (found in beans, bread, matzoh, wheat germ, vanilla extract, cacao powder, oats, and nuts)
- High levels of aluminum
- High levels of iron

■ Conditions That Can Benefit from Manganese

- Arrhythmias
- Arthritis
- Back pain
- Myasthenia gravis
- Osteopenia/osteoporosis (bone loss)
- Premenstrual syndrome (PMS)

■ Recommended Dosage

2.5 to 5 milligrams daily.

Food Sources of Manganese

The following list is reprinted with permission from Jeffrey Bland's *Clinical Nutrition: A Functional Approach.* Foods that contain the most manganese are listed first, followed by foods that contain progressively less manganese. The number to the left of each food describes how many milligrams of manganese are in 100 grams (3.5 ounces) of that food. Besides the foods listed below, cloves, ginger, thyme, bay leaves, and tea also contain manganese.

3.5	Pecans	0.13	Swiss cheese
2.8	Brazil nuts	0.13	Corn
2.5	Almonds	0.11	Cabbage
1.8	Barley	0.10	Peaches
1.3	Rye	0.09	Butter
1.3	Buckwheat	0.06	Tangerines
1.3	Split peas	0.06	Peas
1.1	Whole wheat	0.05	Eggs
0.8	Walnuts	0.04	Beets
0.8	Fresh spinach	0.04	Coconut
0.7	Peanuts	0.03	Apples
0.6	Oats	0.03	Oranges
0.5	Raisins	0.03	Pears
0.5	Turnip greens	0.03	Lamb chops
0.5	Rhubarb	0.03	Cantaloupe
0.4	Beet greens	0.03	Tomatoes
0.3	Brussels sprouts	0.02	Whole milk
0.3	Oatmeal	0.02	Chicken breasts
0.2	Cornmeal	0.02	Green beans
0.2	Millet	0.02	Apricots
0.19	Gorgonzola cheese	0.01	Beef liver
0.16	Carrots	0.01	Scallops
0.15	Broccoli	0.01	Halibut
0.14	Brown rice	0.01	Cucumbers
0.14	Whole wheat bread		

■ Substances That Can Lower Manganese Levels

- Diet high in phytates (found in beans, breads, matzoh, wheat germ, vanilla extract, cacao powder, oats, and nuts)
- High levels of aluminum
- High levels of iron

■ Side Effects and Contraindications

You must be cautious about consuming manganese if you have gallbladder or liver disease, which can reduce the rate at which this nutrient is removed from the body. If you have either of these disorders, consult with your doctor before starting a manganese regimen.

■ Symptoms of Manganese Toxicity

- ☐ Anxiety
- ☐ Delusions
- ☐ Disorientation
- ☐ Emotional problems
- ☐ Hallucinations
- ☐ Memory loss
- ☐ Neurological problems
- ☐ Permanent brain damage
- ☐ Slurred speech
- ☐ Tremors

MOLYBDENUM

Molybdenum is an essential micromineral. A component of three major enzymes, molybdenum is involved in several of the body's metabolism and oxidation processes. It is found in the liver, kidneys, adrenal glands, lungs, spleen, muscles, and skin.

■ Functions of Molybdenum in Your Body

- Acts as a coenzyme in alcohol detoxification
- Acts as a coenzyme in uric acid formation
- Acts as an electron transport agent in oxidation/reduction reactions
- Helps the body utilize stored iron
- Prevents copper levels from getting too high
- Used to detoxify sulfites

■ Symptoms of Molybdenum Deficiency

☐ Decreased uric acid in urine

☐ Disorientation

☐ Headache

☐ Irritability

☐ Mental disturbance

☐ Tachycardia (abnormally rapid heart rate)

☐ Visual problems

Food Sources of Molybdenum

The following list is reprinted with permission from Jeffrey Bland's *Clinical Nutrition: A Functional Approach.* Foods that contain the most molybdenum are listed first, followed by foods that contain progressively less molybdenum. The number to the left of each food describes how many milligrams of molybdenum are in 100 grams (3.5 ounces) of that food.

155	Lentils	31	Cottage cheese
135	Beef liver	30	Beef
130	Split peas	30	Potatoes
120	Cauliflower	25	Onions
110	Green peas	25	Coconut
109	Brewer's yeast	25	Pork
100	Wheat germ	24	Lamb
100	Spinach	21	Green beans
77	Beef kidney	19	Crab
75	Brown rice	19	Molasses
70	Garlic	16	Cantaloupe
60	Oats	14	Apricots
53	Eggs	10	Raisins
50	Rye bread	10	Butter
45	Corn	7	Strawberries
42	Barley	5	Carrots
40	Fish	5	Cabbage
36	Whole wheat	3	Whole milk
32	Whole wheat bread	1	Goat milk
32	Chicken		

■ Causes of Molybdenum Deficiency

Molybdenum deficiency is uncommon, and the cause is unknown except for rare inherited patterns.

■ Conditions That Can Benefit from Molybdenum

- Chronic yeast infection
- Crohn's disease

■ Recommended Dosage

45 to 200 micrograms daily.

■ Symptoms of Molybdenum Toxicity

- ☐ Copper deficiency
- ☐ Increased uric acid production
- ☐ Gout
- ☐ Kidney problems

SELENIUM

Selenium is essential to human health in trace amounts, but is harmful in excess. Each food's content of selenium depends on the soil in which it is grown. In the United States, the selenium-deficient states are Connecticut, Delaware, Illinois, Indiana, Massachusetts, New York, Ohio, Oregon, Pennsylvania, and Rhode Island. Selenium levels are also low in the District of Columbia. However, because there is such an extensive transport of food throughout the country, most people living in low-selenium areas obtain sufficient amounts of selenium. Supplements can be important for people who are unsure if they're getting the selenium they need.

■ Functions of Selenium in Your Body

- Helps prevent cancer due to its role in DNA repair
- Needed for immune system function
- Involved in thyroid function
- Reduces heavy metal toxicity
- May prevent heart disease
- Works with vitamin E as an antioxidant

■ Symptoms of Selenium Deficiency

- ☐ Cataracts
- ☐ Inflammatory disease

☐ Loss of pigment in skin and hair

☐ Low sperm count

☐ Recurrent infections

☐ Skeletal muscle problems

☐ Thyroid enlargement

☐ Weakness

■ Causes of Selenium Deficiency

- Advanced age
- Dialysis
- Gastrointestinal bypass surgery
- HIV/AIDS
- Inflammatory bowel disease

- Some medications can cause selenium deficiency. Speak to your healthcare provider or pharmacist to see if any of the drugs you're taking has the potential to lower your body's selenium level.
- Total parenteral nutrition
- Tuberculosis

■ Conditions That Can Benefit from Selenium

- Autoimmune diseases
- Cancer
- HIV/AIDS

- Infertility (in males)
- Inflammatory bowel disease
- Thyroid disease

■ Recommended Dosage

100 to 200 micrograms daily. Do not exceed 200 micrograms a day without consulting with your healthcare provider.

■ Side Effects and Contraindications

Selenium may interfere with the absorption of medications such as proton-pump inhibitors and histamine blockers. Speak to your healthcare provider or pharmacist to see if it is safe to take this nutrient with your medications and if any cautions should be exercised.

■ Symptoms of Selenium Toxicity

Selenium is a micronutrient and is needed in small quantities by the body. Large quantities can lead to toxicity, which may include the following symptoms.

☐ Bad breath

☐ Dry hair

☐ Fatigue   ☐ Irritability

☐ Hair loss   ☐ Nervous system problems

Food Sources of Selenium

The following list is reprinted with permission from Jeffrey Bland's *Clinical Nutrition: A Functional Approach.* Foods that contain the most selenium are listed first, followed by foods that contain progressively less selenium. The number to the left of each food describes how many milligrams of selenium are in 100 grams (3.5 ounces) of that food.

146	Butter	25	Garlic
141	Smoked herring	24	Barley
123	Smelt	19	Orange juice
111	Wheat germ	19	Gelatin
103	Brazil nuts	19	Beer
89	Apple cider vinegar	18	Beef liver
77	Scallops	18	Lamb chops
66	Barley	18	Egg yolk
66	Whole wheat bread	12	Mushrooms
65	Lobster	12	Chicken
63	Bran	10	Swiss cheese
59	Shrimp	5	Cottage cheese
57	Red Swiss chard	5	Wine
56	Oats	4	Radishes
55	Clams	4	Grape juice
51	King crab	3	Pecans
49	Oysters	2	Hazelnuts
48	Milk	2	Almonds
43	Cod	2	Green beans
39	Brown rice	2	Kidney beans
34	Top round steak	2	Onions
30	Lamb	2	Carrots
27	Turnips	2	Cabbages
26	Molasses	1	Oranges

SILICON

Silicon is an essential micronutrient and the third most abundant trace element in the human body. Although it is found in many forms, the only form that is useful to humans is orthosilicic acid. Most Americans get the silicon they need from their diet, but because foods aren't always nutrient-rich, supplements can be an important part of insuring good health.

◼ Functions of Silicon in Your Body

- Aids bone and cartilage development

- Responsible for elasticity of connective tissue

- Responsible for skin, hair, and nail health

- Supports and improves function of thymus gland

◼ Symptoms of Silicon Deficiency

- ☐ Brittle bones

- ☐ Insomnia

- ☐ Irritability

- ☐ Muscle cramps

- ☐ Osteopenia/osteoporosis (bone loss)

- ☐ Poor bone development in children

- ☐ Hair loss and poor hair quality

Food Sources of Silicon

The following list provides the silicon content of a number of common foods. Foods that contain the most silicon are listed first, followed by foods that contain progressively less silicon. The number to the left of each food describes how many milligrams of silicon are in 100 grams (3.5 ounces) of that food.

10.17	Bran cereal	2.25	Whole wheat bread
8.25	Raisins	2.07	Brown rice
5.44	Banana	0.33	Oranges
2.44	Green beans	0.29	Potatoes
2.42	Cornflakes	0.21	Strawberries
2.29	Carrots	0.012	Lettuce

▉ Causes of Silicon Deficiency

- Anorexia nervosa
- Chronic alcoholism
- Low dietary intake

▉ Conditions That Can Benefit from Silicon

- Acne
- Alzheimer's disease
- Boils
- Digestive disorders
- Eczema
- Hair loss and poor hair condition
- Osteopenia/Osteoporosis (bone loss)
- Psoriasis
- Slow wound healing
- Sprains and strains

▉ Recommended Dosage

1 to 2 milligrams daily. Be sure to use supplements labelled "orthosilicic acid."

▉ Side Effects and Contraindications

The silicon found in food poses no known problems. Orthosilicic acid supplements are not known to interact with any drugs and are considered safe in low doses. Silicon-containing antacids may contribute to the formation of kidney stones.

The Dangers Posed by Silicon in the Environment

Silicon is one of the most abundant elements in the universe, and it is in our environment in many forms, including silicon dioxide, or silica. This crystallized element is toxic if inhaled in abundance. Located in rock, sandstone, concrete, and paint, silica is released when these materials are crushed, drilled, or otherwise broken. The inhalation of bits of silica can cause silicosis, an irreversible and potentially fatal respiratory disease.

VANADIUM

Vanadium is needed by the body in trace amounts, and is found in most soils. Therefore, many food plants contain vanadium, and most people consume the vanadium they need in their regular daily diet. But because many of our foods are deficient in nutrients, vanadium supplements are sometimes needed to help insure good health.

■ Functions of Vanadium in Your Body

- Aids metabolism of glucose
- Improves insulin sensitivity
- Involved in metabolism of fats

■ Symptoms of Vanadium Deficiency

☐ Insulin resistance

■ Causes of Vanadium Deficiency

Deficiencies are rare and causes are unknown.

Food Sources of Vanadium

The following list is reprinted with permission from Jeffrey Bland's *Clinical Nutrition: A Functional Approach.* Foods that contain the most vanadium are listed first, followed by foods that contain progressively less vanadium. The number to the left of each food describes how many milligrams of vanadium are in 100 grams (3.5 ounces) of that food.

100	Buckwheat	10	Cabbage
80	Parsley	10	Garlic
70	Soybeans	6	Tomatoes
64	Safflower oil	5	Radishes
42	Eggs	5	Onions
41	Sunflower seed oil	5	Whole wheat
35	Oats	4	Lobster
30	Olive oil	4	Beets
15	Sunflower seeds	3	Apples
15	Corn	2	Plums
14	Green beans	2	Lettuce
11	Peanut oil	2	Millet
10	Carrots		

■ Conditions That Can Benefit from Vanadium

• Insulin resistance/diabetes

■ Recommended Dosage

10 to 50 micrograms daily. Do not take more than 50 micrograms a day without the supervision of a doctor because some of the effects of vanadium toxicity—such as bipolar disorder—are very serious.

■ Side Effects and Contraindications

Vanadium may increase the risk of bleeding when taken with prescription blood thinners, natural blood thinners, and even aspirin. Talk to your healthcare provider or pharmacist to learn if any of your medications or supplements may cause problems when taken with vanadium.

■ Symptoms of Vanadium Toxicity

☐ Bipolar disorder (exacerbation at doses above 50 micrograms)

☐ Decreased coenzyme A

☐ Depletion of chromium, lithium, and vitamin C

☐ Elevated blood pressure

☐ Increased triglyceride levels

☐ Interference with cellular energy production

☐ Low coenzyme Q_{10} levels

☐ Stomach pain, diarrhea, gas, nausea, and/or vomiting

ZINC

Although zinc is a micromineral, and therefore needed by the body only in small quantities, it is very important for overall physical and mental health. Zinc is a cofactor in over 100 enzymatic reactions in the body. A recent study revealed that zinc supplementation increases the production of insulin-like growth factor 1 (IGF-1), which is associated with growth and healthier aging.

Zinc deficiency is quite common in the developing world. In fact, about 2 billion people worldwide are believed to be zinc deficient. Even in the United States, about 12 percent of the population is thought to be at risk for this deficiency, and the percentage is higher for the elderly due to insufficient dietary intake and a decreased ability to absorb the nutrient.

■ Functions of Zinc in Your Body

- Boosts immune defenses
- Breaks down and metabolizes proteins
- Contributes to a healthy prostate
- Decreases the body's requirement for insulin
- Enhances the biochemical actions of vitamin D
- Essential component of hormones
- Essential for cell division and replication of both DNA and RNA
- Essential for fertility and reproduction
- Has anti-inflammatory effects
- Helps absorption of vitamin A
- Helps assemble proteins inside the cell
- Helps balance blood sugar levels
- Helps stabilize cell membrane and structures within the cell
- Important component of superoxide dismutase
- Improves taste and appetite
- Inhibits the enzyme that reduces levels of the male hormone dihydrotestosterone (DHT)
- Is an antioxidant
- Metabolizes carbohydrates
- Needed for the formation of bone and skin
- Needed for the proper maintenance (production and breakdown) of vitamin E
- Promotes thyroid activity
- Related to sexual maturation
- Transports vitamin A to the retina, thereby improving night vision and protecting retinal health

■ Symptoms of Zinc Deficiency

- ☐ Acne
- ☐ Anemia
- ☐ Anorexia nervosa
- ☐ Arthritis
- ☐ Behavioral disturbances (such as apathy, confusion, depression, hostility, or irritability)
- ☐ Brittle nails
- ☐ Craving for sugary foods
- ☐ Dandruff
- ☐ Decreased ability to taste
- ☐ Decreased desire for protein-rich foods
- ☐ Decreased sense of smell (anosmia)
- ☐ Decreased sexual function
- ☐ Delayed sexual maturation
- ☐ Diarrhea

☐ Eczema

☐ Enlargement of the spleen and liver

☐ Fatigue

☐ Frontal headaches

☐ Growth retardation

☐ Hair loss

☐ Immune deficiencies

☐ Impaired nerve conduction

☐ Impaired wound healing

☐ Impotence

☐ Infertility

☐ Low sperm count

☐ Memory impairment

☐ Negative nitrogen balance

☐ Nerve damage

☐ Night blindness

☐ Poor appetite

☐ Psoriasis

☐ Reduced salivation

☐ Sleep disturbances

☐ Stretch marks

☐ White spots on nails

■ Causes of Zinc Deficiency

- A large number of medications, from antibiotics to oral contraceptives, are associated with zinc deficiency. Speak to your healthcare provider or pharmacist to see if any of the drugs you're taking has the potential to lower your body's zinc levels.

- Aging (zinc absorption decreases with age)

- Alcoholism

- Anorexia nervosa

- Celiac

- Chronic renal failure

- Cirrhosis

- Cystic fibrosis

- Excess copper

- Hemolytic anemia

- HIV/AIDS

- Increased calcium ingestion

- Infection

- Inflammatory bowel disease

- Iron supplementation

- Nephrotic syndrome

- Pancreatic insufficiency

- Pancreatitis

- Rheumatoid arthritis

- Short bowel syndrome

- Smoking

- Surgery

Food Sources of Zinc

The following list is reprinted with permission from Jeffrey Bland's *Clinical Nutrition: A Functional Approach.* Foods that contain the most zinc are listed first, followed by foods that contain progressively less zinc. The number to the left of each food describes how many milligrams of zinc are in 100 grams (3.5 ounces) of that food. Black pepper, paprika, mustard, chili powder, thyme, and cinnamon are not included on the list but are also high in zinc.

148.7	Fresh oysters	1.7	Haddock
6.8	Ginger root	1.6	Green peas
5.6	Ground round steak	1.5	Shrimp
5.3	Lamb chops	1.2	Turnips
4.5	Pecans	0.9	Parsley
4.2	Split peas	0.9	Potatoes
4.2	Brazil nuts	0.6	Garlic
3.9	Beef liver	0.5	Whole wheat bread
3.5	Nonfat dry milk	0.4	Black beans
3.5	Egg yolk	0.4	Raw milk
3.2	Whole wheat	0.4	Pork chops
3.2	Rye	0.4	Corn
3.2	Oats	0.3	Grape juice
3.2	Peanuts	0.3	Olive oil
3.1	Lima beans	0.3	Cauliflower
3.1	Soy lecithin	0.2	Spinach
3.1	Almonds	0.2	Cabbage
3.0	Walnuts	0.2	Lentils
2.9	Sardines	0.2	Butter
2.6	Chicken	0.2	Lettuce
2.5	Buckwheat	0.1	Cucumbers
2.4	Hazelnuts	0.1	Yams
1.9	Clams	0.1	Tangerines
1.7	Anchovies	0.1	String beans
1.7	Tuna		

■ Conditions That Can Benefit from Zinc

- Acne
- Aging skin
- Anorexia nervosa

- Asthma
- Attention-deficit/ hyperactivity disorder (ADHD)
- Cataracts
- Colds
- Crohn's disease
- Diabetes mellitus
- Down syndrome
- Eczema
- Enlarged prostate
- Erectile dysfunction
- Furuncles (boils)
- Gastric ulcers
- Gingivitis
- Growth retardation
- Infertility
- Hansen's disease
- HIV/AIDs (in small doses)
- Hypertension
- Immune function
- Impaired sense of taste (hypogeusia)
- Infertility
- Macular degeneration
- Muscle cramps due to liver disease
- Night blindness
- Osteopenia/ osteoporosis (bone loss)
- Psoriasis
- Rheumatoid arthritis
- Sickle cell disease
- Thalassemia
- Tinnitus
- Ulcerative colitis
- Wilson's disease
- Wound healing

■ Recommended Dosage

25 to 50 milligrams. Choose one of the two forms of zinc that are best absorbed: zinc picolinate and zinc citrate. Do not use zinc sulfate, which is the least easily absorbed and may cause stomach upset. Try to take zinc at a different time of day from calcium, copper, iron, and soy, because zinc can interfere with the absorption of these substances.

It is very important for the body to maintain a proper ratio of zinc to copper—between 10:1 and 15:1. Excess zinc can lead to a copper deficiency and vice versa. So if you're taking 25 milligrams of zinc, you should be taking 1 to 2 milligrams of copper. If you're taking 50 milligrams of zinc, you should be taking 3 to 4 milligrams of copper.

■ Side Effects and Contraindications

Zinc supplements are usually safe when taken as directed above, although some people may experience nausea or upset stomach. If you experience intestinal symptoms while taking zinc, contact your healthcare provider. Symptoms may be due to elevated levels of zinc, compromised kidney function, poor gastrointestinal function, or use of a supplement that is not pharmaceutical grade. Note that while small doses of zinc help build the immune system in patients with HIV, the HIV virus also requires zinc, and a large intake of zinc may stimulate the progression of the HIV infection.

■ Substances That Decrease Zinc Absorption

- Coffee and other caffeinated beverages

- Excess copper

- Foods high in oxalate (found in spinach, almonds and cashews, baked potatoes with skin, sweet potatoes, miso soup, beets, cocoa powder, bran cereals, and raspberries)

- Foods high in phytates (found in beans, breads, matzoh, wheat germ, vanilla extract, cacao powder, oats, and nuts)

- Teas containing tannin (both green and black teas)

■ Symptoms of Zinc Toxicity

Zinc toxicity is rare, and is often due to copper deficiency. (See the discussion of copper under "Recommended Dosage.") Toxicity can lead to the symptoms that follow.

☐ Alcohol intolerance

☐ Anemia

☐ Dizziness

☐ Drowsiness

☐ Fatigue

☐ Hallucinations

☐ Increased sweating

☐ Loss of appetite

☐ Loss of muscular coordination

☐ Lowered immune function

☐ Nausea

☐ Premature heartbeats (heartbeats that occur before the regular heartbeat)

☐ Vomiting

3

Fatty Acids

Many people regard fat as an adversary to their health. It *is* true that an excessive intake of certain fats can result in serious medical problems. However, not all fats are the same. In fact, your body requires certain fatty acids—a major component of fats—to maintain health and prevent disease. Fats are also an important source of energy and help your body perform a variety of functions. Recognizing the difference between "good" and "bad" fats is crucial as you strive to achieve optimal health.

There are several different types of fats. *Saturated fats* are, for the most part, considered "bad" fats because they can raise cholesterol levels and cause unhealthy weight gain. They are primarily found in foods that come from animals, including fatty meats (such as beef and pork) and dairy products (such as whole milk and butter), and are usually solid at room temperature. However, some saturated fats are derived from plant sources. Coconut oil, for instance, is about 90 percent saturated fat—higher in sat fats than butter or lard.

Unsaturated fats come primarily from vegetable foods but also from certain fish, and they tend to be liquid at room temperature. They consist of polyunsaturated fats and monounsaturated fats, both of which are "good" fats. *Polyunsaturated fats* can positively affect your body by lowering your LDL (bad) cholesterol. However, they can also lower your HDL (good) cholesterol. (For a further discussion of cholesterol, see the inset on page 124.) *Monounsaturated fats,* on the other hand, lower LDL cholesterol but do not have an effect on HDL cholesterol.

The production of most fatty acids occurs within your body from the breakdown of fat molecules, but there are two important polyunsaturated fatty acids—omega-3 and omega-6—that cannot be manufactured in your body and must be provided through diet or taken as supplements. Hence, they are called *essential fatty acids,* or *EFAs.* Although certain low-fat diets can be healthier than diets high in fat, a major shift in food consumption to a low-fat diet may deprive your body of these essential nutrients. Starting on page 126, omega-3 and omega-6 fatty acids are described further.

Trans fatty acids are another type of unsaturated fat. In nature, they occur only in small amounts that don't have negative effects on your body. (See the inset on page 135 for an example of a naturally occurring trans fatty acid.) However, the food industry also produces this type of fat to help food stay fresh longer, to use in deep frying, and to replace more expensive shortenings such as butter and lard. As you will see later in this chapter, manufactured trans fatty acids are *very* unhealthy "bad" fats. In fact, the FDA has taken steps to remove artificial trans fats from processed foods. By January 2020, PHOs—the major source of artificial trans fats in the food supply—will no longer be allowed in foods in the United States.

As you strive to improve the fats in your diet, it is important to continue your intake of the vitamins and minerals discussed in Chapters 1 and 2. Your body requires vitamin A, the B vitamins, vitamin C, biotin, magnesium, niacin, zinc, and other nutrients to convert fatty acids into usable hormones. Protein is necessary as well. The proper intake of these nutrients as well as good fats will contribute to your good health.

Be aware that alcohol, stress, and certain medications can cause your body to use fatty acids incorrectly. At the same time, your intake of fatty acids may change the amount of medication you need. For example, increased fatty acid intake may result in your needing less Prozac or insulin. Your healthcare provider can guide you in making good decisions regarding these medications. Similarly, consult your doctor about your fatty acid consumption if you are taking a blood thinner. As you will read, some fatty acids have major effects on your blood's ability to clot. Large doses of omega-3 supplements, for instance, can act as a blood thinner.

Instead of the complete elimination of fat from your diet, you need to eat less "bad" fats while adding more "good" fats to your eating and nutrient supplementation programs. This chapter will explain which fats are good (and why), the effects they can have on your body, how much of each you can consume, and which foods contain which fats. Remember, though, that most foods contain a combination of different fats. For instance, avocados are especially high in monounsaturated fats, but also contain small amounts of polyunsaturated and saturated fats. The majority of the fats you eat should be monounsaturated or polyunsaturated.

SATURATED FATTY ACIDS

Until recently, saturated fats were all considered "bad" because they were known to have largely negative effects on overall health. Chiefly found in animal products, such as meat and dairy, these fats are the main dietary sources of high cholesterol and triglyceride levels, which increase the risk of heart disease and stroke. And like all fats, saturated fats are high in calories and can result in weight gain if eaten in excess. They are also believed to trigger inflammation.

Recent research, however, has revealed that not all saturated fats are created equal. While the saturated fat in meat and dairy is comprised of long-chain fatty acids, coconut oil's saturated fat is made of medium-chain fatty acids, which are more easily metabolized by the body. Studies have shown that unlike meat- and dairy-derived fats, coconut oil may not raise cholesterol and triglycerides, and may not cause inflammation. In fact, virgin coconut oil contains high concentrations of polyphenols—plant chemicals that have strong antioxidant and anti-inflammatory properties. Studies have further indicated that coconut oil may help prevent memory loss.

Food Sources of Saturated Fats

- Butter
- Cheese
- Coconut oil
- Combination foods containing saturated fat, such as pizza, ice cream, and cake
- Cream
- Fatty beef
- Lamb
- Lard (pig fat)
- Palm oil
- Pork
- Poultry with skin
- Processed meats such as hot dogs, salami, and sausages
- Whole milk and products made with whole or 2-percent milk

■ Disorders that Can Be Caused by a High Intake of Saturated Fats

- Atherosclerosis
- Coronary heart disease
- Decreased effectiveness of arteries
- High cholesterol levels
- Stroke
- Weight gain

Cholesterol

Cholesterol is a soft, waxy substance that is found in your bloodstream and carried through your body in lipoprotein particles. It is both made by your body and consumed in animal foods. Although necessary for life—it is required to build cell walls—the intake of too much cholesterol can clog your arteries, resulting in your heart receiving less blood and oxygen. This can cause serious cardiovascular problems.

There are two types of cholesterol: high-density lipoprotein (HDL) and low-density lipoprotein (LDL). LDL is known as the "bad" cholesterol because it can form as plaque along your arteries and increase your risk of heart disease. HDL, on the other hand, is the "good" cholesterol. Its main job is to collect, break down, and excrete the LDL that is already in your body.

Your goal for optimal health should include a low LDL count and a high HDL count. Your doctor can test your cholesterol levels from a blood sample. Ideally, your total cholesterol (LDL plus HDL) should be under 200 milligrams per deciliter (mg/dL) and your HDL should be over 40 milligrams per deciliter (mg/dL). If it is not, your doctor may need to run further tests.

If your cholesterol is high or has a sudden increase, it's generally a good idea to change your dietary habits. Although a portion of your cholesterol levels is due to heredity, limiting your intake of "bad" cholesterol while increasing exercise to elevate "good" cholesterol can lower your risk for heart disease. Throughout this book, you'll learn about vitamins and other nutrients that can further improve your cholesterol.

■ Recommended Intake

Besides getting saturated fat from food, the body can make its own from carbohydrates, so most people get more of this fat than they need. Therefore, there is no recommended intake of this fatty acid. In fact, because an excess of this saturated can be unhealthy, it is recommended that you keep your intake down to 10 percent of your daily intake of calories. To achieve this, avoid or limit most foods that are high in saturated fat, such as fatty meats and whole-milk dairy products. Instead, eat meats that are lean and high in protein, and limit your intake of dairy products. What about coconut oil? This may be healthier than other types of saturated fats, but since all fats are high in calories—fat provides nine calories per gram, while protein and carbs each contain only four per gram—it's a good idea to use coconut oil only in moderation.

MONOUNSATURATED FATTY ACIDS

Unlike animal-derived saturated fats, monounsaturated fatty acids (MUFAs) are healthy as long as they are eaten in moderation. There are several different types of MUFAs. About 90 percent are oleic acid. Others include palmitoleic acid and vaccenic acid. The best sources of monounsaturated fats include certain nuts, cooking oils made from certain plants, and avocados.

■ Functions of Monounsaturated Fatty Acids in Your Body

- Can help lower LDL (bad) cholesterol while maintaining levels of heart-healthy HDL (good) cholesterol

- Contributes the antioxidant vitamin E to the diet

- May assist in blood sugar control

- May improve blood vessel function

- Provides nutrients that help develop and maintain the cells in your body

---

Food Sources of Monounsaturated Fatty Acids

- Almonds and almond butter
- Avocados
- Brazil nuts
- Canola oil
- Cashews and cashew butter
- Hazelnuts
- Macadamia nuts
- Olive oil

- Olives, black or green
- Peanuts, peanut oil, and peanut butter
- Pecans
- Pistachio nuts
- Safflower oil
- Sesame oil
- Sunflower oil

■ Recommended Intake

Monounsaturated fats can be synthesized in the body as well as found in foods, and most people get enough of these fats. Therefore, no "recommended intake" has been set. Remember that even healthy fats should be eaten in moderation because an excessive amount can lead to weight gain. No more than 25 to 30 percent of your daily calories should come from fats, and most of these fats should be monounsaturated or polyunsaturated.

POLYUNSATURATED FATTY ACIDS

The body can produce most of the fats it needs from the foods you eat. However, the two major classes of polyunsaturated fats (PUFAs)—omega-3 and omega-6 fatty acids—cannot be synthesized by the body. Because these fats are necessary for the proper functioning of the body, they must be ingested through food or supplements. This is why both omega-3s and omega-6s are termed *essential fatty acids*.

OMEGA-3 FATTY ACIDS

Omega-3 fatty acids are used in the formation of cell membranes, assist in circulation and oxygen uptake, reduce inflammation, and do so much more. As you will realize when you see the lists of food sources of omega-3s and omega-6s, it can be difficult to get all of the omega-3s from your diet. That is why so many people don't get enough of these essential nutrients.

There are eleven different types of omega-3s. The most important of them are alpha-linolenic acid (ALA), docosahexaenoic acid (DHA), and eicosapentaenoic acid (EPA). The body is able to convert ALA into EPA and DHA, although this conversion process is not efficient and can produce only small amounts of EPA and DHA. ALA cannot be produced by the body, but fortunately, most people in the United States get adequate amounts of this fatty acid from the foods they eat.

■ Functions of Omega-3-Fatty Acids in Your Body

- Crucial for many brain functions

- Decreases inflammation

- Decreases rate of arrhythmias (irregular heartbeat)

- Diminishes build-up of plaque in arteries

- Enhances insulin function

- Helps convert nutrients from food into usable forms of energy

- Improves immune function in infants

- Involved in cell-to-cell communication

- Is an important component of brain structure and function

- Is important for mitochondrial function (which produces energy for the cells)
- Lowers triglycerides
- Makes blood less "sticky" and less likely to form dangerous clots
- May decrease homocysteine levels, decreasing the risk for heart disease
- May help treat depression
- May protect against ischemic heart disease (decreased blood flow to the heart)
- May protect the brain from stroke
- Necessary for the normal development and function of the adrenal glands, brain, eyes, inner ear, and reproductive tract
- Needed to make certain prostaglandins—hormones that affect inflammation, decrease menstrual cramps, and increase immune function
- Provides structural support for the membranes of the cell
- Raises HDL (good) cholesterol
- Reduces premenstrual syndrome (PMS) symptoms
- Used to manufacture red blood cells

■ Symptoms of Omega-3 Deficiency

☐ Allergies	☐ Excessive urination
☐ Arthritis	☐ Growth retardation
☐ Asthma	☐ Hair loss
☐ Behavioral changes	☐ Impaired immune response
☐ Brittle nails	☐ Impaired motor coordination
☐ Bumps on upper arm	☐ Inflammation
☐ Cognitive decline	☐ Learning disorders
☐ Craving fatty foods	☐ Mood swings
☐ Dandruff	☐ Thirst
☐ Depression	☐ Tingling feeling in arms or legs
☐ Dry skin	

■ Causes of Omega-3 Deficiency

- Alcoholism
- Carnitine deficiency
- Excessive consumption of omega-6 fatty acids
- High intake of saturated fats
- Inability to absorb fatty acids
- Increased intake of sugar
- Increased intake of trans fatty acids
- Insufficient intake of dietary sources of omega-3s
- Insufficient intake of nutrients needed as cofactors
- Stress
- Type 1 diabetes

Food Sources of Omega-3 Fatty Acids

Alpha-Linolenic Acid (ALA)

- Canola oil
- Dark green leafy vegetables
- Flaxseeds and flaxseed oil
- Hemp seeds and hemp oil
- Soybeans and soybean oil
- Tofu
- Walnuts and walnut oil

Docosahexaenoic Acid (DHA)

- DHA-enriched eggs
- Fatty fish, such as anchovies, herring, mackerel, salmon, sardines, and tuna
- Lamb
- Nuts

Eicosapentaenoic Acid (EPA)

- Fatty fish, such as anchovies, herring, mackerel, salmon, sardines, and tuna
- Lamb
- Nuts

■ Conditions That Can Benefit from Omega-3 Fatty Acids

- Aggressive behavior
- Alzheimer's disease
- Arthritis (rheumatoid and degenerative)
- Asthma
- Atherogenesis (fatty plaque in arteries)
- Atopic dermatitis
- Attention-deficit/hyperactivity disorder (ADHD)
- Autism

- Bipolar disorder
- Cancer of the breast, colon, lung, prostate, and skin (prevention)
- Cardiovascular disease
- Cerebral palsy
- Chronic fatigue syndrome
- Coronary heart disease
- Crohn's disease
- Cystic fibrosis
- Depression
- Down syndrome
- Eczema
- Hypercholesterolemia (high cholesterol)
- Hypertension (high blood pressure)
- Hypertriglyceridemia (high triglycerides)
- Inflammation
- Irritable bowel syndrome (IBS)
- Macular degeneration
- Malignant cardiac arrhythmias (prevention)
- Migraine headaches
- Multiple sclerosis (MS)
- Neuropathy
- Polycystic ovary syndrome (PCOS)
- Postpartum depression
- Premenstrual syndrome (PMS)
- Psoriasis
- Schizophrenia
- Stroke (prevention and recovery)
- Systemic lupus erythematosus (SLE)
- Type 2 diabetes (prevention and treatment)
- Weight loss

■ Recommended Dosage

It is important that your intake of omega-6-fatty acids and omega-3-fatty acids maintain a proper ratio—between 3:1 and 6:1—or you may become deficient in omega-3s. This is because these two essential fatty acids compete for use in the body. Unfortunately, the standard American diet is very high in omega-6-fatty acids and very low in omega-3-fatty acids, so Americans (and most people worldwide) maintain a ratio of between 10:1 and 25:1. It is paramount that you eat foods that are high in omega-3- fatty acids, and you may need to take a supplement, as well. The measurement of fatty acids is always the best way to determine the amount that you require. This test is available through several laboratories. (See Resources for contact information.) You can also ask your healthcare provider to order a fatty acids test.

- General guidelines for adults under the age of 50: 1,000 milligrams a day.
- General guidelines for adults over the age of 50: 2,000 milligrams a day.

Both fish oil and krill oil supplements supply DHA and EPA, but there are differences. Krill oil comes from small crustaceans, not fatty fish, and typically contains more EPA. And unlike the omega-3s in conventional fish oil, krill oil's omega-3s are linked to an antioxidant and other potentially beneficial substances called phospholipids. Current research suggests that fish oil is beneficial for the prevention and treatment of cardiovascular disease, and krill oil is a helpful therapy for arthritis and PMS.

When ingesting omega-3 fatty acids, take vitamin E to prevent oxidation, a process that can result in damage from free radicals. (See page 4.) To make sure that the fatty acids are converted into usable forms, also consume vitamin A, the B vitamins, vitamin C, biotin, magnesium, niacin, zinc, and protein.

Omega-3 supplements can quickly oxidize and turn rancid. To prevent this, store your omega-3s in the refrigerator. If you find yourself "burping them up," try storing them in the freezer. This will not destroy their effectiveness.

■ Side Effects and Contraindications

In large doses, omega-3-fatty acids may act as a blood thinner, particularly in doses above 3,000 milligrams a day. Speak to your healthcare provider or pharmacist to learn if blood thinners or any other medications you're taking might make it unwise to use omega-3 supplements.

The possible side effects associated with omega-3 fatty acids include the following:

- Bad breath
- Fishy taste
- Nausea
- Belching
- Loose stools
- Stomach upset

OMEGA-6 FATTY ACIDS

Like omega-3s, omega-6 fatty acids are crucial to good health and must be obtained through food and supplements because the body cannot produce them. Omega-6s play an important role in normal growth and development and in brain function. They also maintain bone health, help regulate metabolism, maintain the reproductive system, stimulate skin and hair growth, and play a role in other important body functions.

You may have read that omega-3 fatty acids help reduce inflammation, but that omega-6 fatty acids promote inflammation. It's important to understand that there are four types of omega-6 fatty acids: arachidonic acid (AA), dihomo-gamma-linolenic acid (DGLA), gamma-linolenic acid (GLA), and linoleic acid. (For more details, see the inset on page 132.) Most of our dietary omega-6s come from vegetable oil in the form of linoleic acid, and excess amounts of linoleic acid can contribute to inflammation as well as many other related health disorders. On the other hand, some omega-6s—like gamma-linolenic acid (GLA), which is absent from most diets—actually *reduce* inflammation. This is why it's usually beneficial to reduce the consumption of vegetable oils and, when necessary, to supplement your diet with gamma-linolenic acid.

■ Functions of Omega-6 Fatty Acids in Your Body

- Essential for normal development and function of the adrenal glands, brain, eyes, inner ear, and reproductive tract
- Helps convert nutrients from food into usable forms of energy
- Helps decrease nerve pain (peripheral neuropathy)
- Helps regulate inflammation
- Helps regulate metabolism
- Involved in cell-to-cell communication
- Makes blood "sticky," which allows it to clot
- Needed to make certain prostaglandins (hormones)
- Needed to nourish the skin and hair
- Provides structural support for the membranes (outer walls) of the body's cells
- Reduces premenstrual syndrome (PMS)
- Supports bone health
- Used in the manufacture of red blood cells

■ Symptoms of Omega-6 Deficiency

- ☐ Behavioral changes
- ☐ Cardiovascular abnormalities
- ☐ Dehydration
- ☐ Dry eyes
- ☐ Dry skin
- ☐ Hair loss
- ☐ Kidney problems
- ☐ Poor vision
- ☐ Reproductive problems in both men and women
- ☐ Stunted growth

■ Causes of Omega-6 Deficiency

- Chronic fat malabsorption due to a disease process, surgery, or a fat-blocking supplement

- Cystic fibrosis

Food Sources of Omega-6 Fatty Acids

Arachidonic Acid (AA)

- Beef
- Eggs

- Fish
- Poultry

Dihomo-Gamma-Linolenic Acid (DGLA)

- Human milk

Gamma-Linolenic Acid (GLA)

- Blackcurrant seed oil
- Borage seed oil

- Evening primrose oil (See page 212 to learn more about evening primrose oil.)
- Hemp oil

Linoleic Acid

- Brazil nuts
- Corn oil
- Flax oil
- Hemp oil
- Pecans
- Pine nuts

- Products made with vegetable oils, like salad dressings, mayonnaise, and other processed foods
- Safflower oil
- Sesame oil
- Soybean oil
- Sunflower oil
- Sunflower seeds

■ Conditions That Can Benefit from Omega-6 Fatty Acids

- Benign prostate hypertrophy
- Chronic fatigue syndrome
- Diabetic neuropathy

- Eczema
- Food allergies
- Hypothyroidism

- Irritable bowel syndrome (IBS)
- Leaky gut syndrome
- Lupus

- Menstrual cramps
- Multiple sclerosis (MS)
- Myasthenia gravis
- Osteoarthritis
- Osteoporosis

- Polycystic ovary syndrome (PCOS)
- Premenstrual syndrome (PMS)
- Psoriasis
- Rheumatoid arthritis

- Sjögren's syndrome
- Ulcerative colitis
- Uterine fibroids
- Yeast overgrowth

■ Recommended Dosage

As you have already read, it is important that your intake of omega-6 fatty acids and omega-3 fatty acids maintain a proper ratio—between 3:1 and 6:1—to avoid various health problems. The measurement of fatty acids is the most accurate way to determine the fatty acids that your body needs. (See page 129.)

Although the standard American diet is very high in omega-6, and excessive amounts of certain omega-6s can cause problems, the omega-6 gamma-linolenic acid (GLA) has been shown to benefit the body in many ways. This nutrient is available in supplements such as evening primrose oil and borage oil.

If you are tested for fatty acids, you will get a better idea of the amount of omega-6s that would be most appropriate for you. Part 2 recommends doses for specific conditions. A dose of 1,000 to 3,000 milligrams GLA daily is generally recommended.

■ Side Effects and Contraindications

In the form of both evening primrose oil and borage oil, gamma-linolenic acid can act as a blood thinner. If you have a bleeding disorder or are taking a medication or supplement that may thin your blood, do not take GLA supplements. If you are planning to have surgery, discontinue this therapy two weeks before the procedure. Speak to your healthcare provider or pharmacist to learn if any drugs you're taking might make it unwise to use GLA.

Do not use evening primrose oil or borage oil if you have a seizure disorder, since their use can precipitate a seizure.

These supplements can also cause some mild side effects, including the following:

- Bloating
- Diarrhea
- Headaches

- Indigestion
- Nausea
- Vomiting

TRANS FATTY ACIDS

Unsaturated fats have a tendency to oxidize and become rancid—and, therefore, inedible—rather quickly. More than a century ago, manufacturers began to *hydrogenate* these fats by adding a hydrogen molecule to them. This not only increased the shelf life of the fats by preventing oxidation but also transformed them into a solid substance that could be used as an inexpensive substitute for butter and lard. Known as trans fatty acids, or trans fats, this product has been used for decades to make cookies, crackers, bread, and frozen foods, as well as for frying.

Food Sources of Trans Fatty Acids

Foods that contain trans fatty acids will list "hydrogenated" or "partially hydrogenated" oils on their labels. Note that manufacturer's can list 0 gram of trans fat if the trans fat content is under 0.5 gram. That's why it's so important to check the ingredients list and avoid hydrogenated oils. The following foods are among the mostly likely to contain this artificial fat.

- Baked goods, including bread
- Candies, especially cream-filled
- Chocolates
- Corn chips
- Crackers
- Doughnuts
- French fries
- Fried foods
- Frozen dinners, including frozen pizza
- Margarine (particularly in stick form)
- Mayonnaise
- Microwave popcorn
- Pastries
- Potato chips
- Processed meats
- Processed oils

Unfortunately, trans fatty acids have been found to be very unhealthy. In studies, they have significantly increased bad LDL cholesterol while decreasing good HDL cholesterol. This means that these artificial products greatly increase the risk of heart disease. Trans fatty acids are so unhealthy that for many years, they have been completely banned in some European countries. In the United States, current FDA regulations state that PHOs, the major source of artificial trans fats in our foods, will be banned in 2020. In the meantime, it's important to avoid foods that contain even small amounts of these fats. Check the label, looking for partially or fully hydrogenated oils. When you see either of these terms in the ingredients list, you know that the food contains trans fats.

It's important to understand that some trans fatty acids occur naturally, although usually in very small quantities. In fact, natural trans fats have been part of the human diet since we began eating meat and dairy from cattle, sheep, and goats. Fortunately, studies have determined that a moderate amount of these fats is not harmful. Conjugated linoleic acid (CLA), one type of natural trans fat, has actually been found to be beneficial, as described in the inset below. The rest of this section will look at the more common trans fats: the ones that are manufactured by companies in order to preserve foods for longer shelf life and to serve as a substitute for more expensive solid fats.

Conjugated Linoleic Acid

Conjugated linoleic acid (CLA) is a naturally occurring trans fatty acid. Unlike manufactured fatty acids, CLA can have positive effects on your overall health. It is currently marketed as a dietary supplement because it has been shown to aid in weight loss. When used for this purpose, CLA should be consumed in quantities of 3,000 to 4,000 milligrams a day.

CLA is beneficial in many other ways, as well. It is an antioxidant, lowers cholesterol, fortifies the immune system, and improves insulin sensitivity. It is also believed to fight breast and colon cancer. For these preventative measures, 100 to 500 milligrams of CLA should be consumed daily.

CLA is found in low quantities in beef, kangaroo meat, and lamb. However, in order to ingest the suggested dosages, it is best to take CLA supplements.

■ Disorders that Can Be Caused by High Intake of Trans Fatty Acids

- Clogged arteries
- Decreased HDL (good) cholesterol
- Heart disease

- Increased LDL (bad) cholesterol

- Increased triglycerides

- Interference with your body's ability to make its own DHA (an omega-3 essential fatty acid)

- Leaking cell membranes, which can disrupt cellular metabolism and allow toxins to enter your cells

- "Stickier" blood, which can increase blood clots

- Type 2 diabetes

■ Recommended Intake of Trans Fatty Acids

You are surrounded by foods that contain artificial trans fatty acids. Regardless of your current health status, it is important for your future well-being to avoid these compounds, which have only negative effects on health.

4

Amino Acids

There are 40,000 *proteins* in your body, and they are necessary for a wide range of functions. Protein is a component of every one of your cells. It is used to build and repair tissue; to make hormones, enzymes, and other chemicals in the body; and to form bones, muscles, cartilage, blood, and skin. Although carbohydrates are the body's preferred source of energy, when needed, protein can also be turned into energy.

The building blocks of proteins are *amino acids,* which are linked together in chains. Most of the 40,000 proteins in your body are made from only twenty amino acids. These *standard amino acids* are included in the genetic code of every living being. After the proteins are constructed by your body, however, some of these amino acids become attached to other functional groups (such as phosphates or lipids), at which point they are structurally changed into different amino acids. These, too, are vital for health.

Amino acids are divided into three categories. Some are called *essential amino acids* because your system cannot manufacture them on its own, so they must be consumed in foods or supplements. Others are termed *nonessential amino acids* because, although they are important for your health, they are made in sufficient quantities by your body, so it is not essential to ingest them. The last group is called *conditionally essential amino acids.* These can be made by your body under normal conditions but may have to be ingested through diet or supplements when factors such as illness, fever, diet, or chemotherapy prevent the body from manufacturing them. Moreover, a process such as detoxification—which uses amino acids to neutralize toxic compounds—may use up the amino acids the body has made. Table 4.1 shows which amino acids fall into which of these three groups.

TABLE 4.1. AMINO ACIDS		
Essential Amino Acids	**Conditionally Essential Amino Acids**	**Nonessential Amino Acids**
Histidine	Arginine	Alanine
Isoleucine	Cysteine	Asparagine
Leucine	Cystine	Aspartic acid
Lysine	Glutamine	5-HTP
Methionine	Glycine	Glutamate
Phenylalanine	Proline	Serine
Threonine	Taurine	
Tryptophan	Tyrosine	
Valine		

If your body is not getting the amino acids it needs, you may have an amino acid deficiency. The list below identifies a number of symptoms that may characterize such a deficiency, and within each entry presented in this chapter, you will find deficiency symptoms specific to that amino acid. Your doctor can perform an amino acid analysis test to determine the dosages of amino acids you should take. If you are deficient in one or two amino acids, you can buy supplements from a pharmaceutical grade company. (See page 485.) If you are deficient in several amino acids, your doctor can contact a *compounding pharmacist,* who can formulate amino acids into a prescription that meets your needs. The Professional Compounding Centers of America can help you find a compounding pharmacist near you. (See page 485.)

■ Symptoms of an Amino Acid Deficiency

☐ Aggressive behavior

☐ Alcoholism

☐ Anxiety

☐ Arthritis

☐ Attention-deficit/hyperactivity disorder (ADHD)

☐ Blood sugar disorders

☐ Chronic fatigue

☐ Craving for carbohydrates and sugar

☐ Depression

☐ Fibromyalgia

☐ Food or chemical allergies

☐ Frequent colds

- ☐ Frequent headaches
- ☐ Hyperactivity
- ☐ Immune dysfunction
- ☐ Insomnia
- ☐ Mental or emotional problems
- ☐ Mood swings

- ☐ Neurological disorders
- ☐ Obsessive compulsive disorder (OCD)
- ☐ Panic attacks
- ☐ Premenstrual syndrome (PMS)
- ☐ Recurrent ear infections

When you are buying amino acids, be sure to buy only those of pharmaceutical grade. You should also attempt to buy *free amino acids*, which are amino acids that are in their purest form and do not need to be digested before being utilized. These nutrients are absorbed directly into the bloodstream and immediately put to use by your body.

You will see that most amino acids come in two forms: D- and L- (such as D-carnitine and L-carnitine). The D-amino acid is a mirror image of the L-amino acid. They are very similar, and both can be taken as supplements. However, the L- form is preferable because it is the form that can be incorporated into proteins. (Note that the amino acids glycine and taurine are each available in only one form. Although you may see supplements labeled "L-taurine," there is no D-taurine.)

This chapter focuses on some of the most important amino acids found in your body. Be aware that your body needs vitamin B$_6$ (pyridoxine) to metabolize most amino acid supplements. (See page 48 for more information on this vitamin.) Also be aware that if you have diabetes, hypertension, kidney disease, or liver disease, you should consult a physician before taking any amino acid supplements.

ALANINE

Alanine is one of the most simply structured amino acids and also one of the most widely used in the body. Like most of the amino acids discussed in this chapter, it is required for the biosynthesis of proteins, including receptor, transport, and structural proteins. But alanine plays roles in many other vital processes as well. For instance, it is required for the synthesis of all enzymes and also for the process of gluconeogenesis, which results in the generation of glucose from certain non-carbohydrate substances.

Alanine is nonessential and requires vitamin B_6 for metabolism. It can be manufactured in the body from pyruvate and branched-chain amino acids such as valine, leucine, and isoleucine.

■ Functions of Alanine in Your Body

- Aids in the production of the amino acid carnosine
- Is converted to glucose when energy is needed or blood sugar levels decrease
- Forms part of DNA
- Helps form neurotransmitters (chemical "messengers" in the brain)
- Helps generate glucose, which provides the body with energy
- Is an inhibitory neurotransmitter in the brain
- Is involved in the production of antibodies
- Is needed for protein production
- Is required for the metabolism of the amino acid tryptophan
- Plays a role in muscle endurance during aggressive exercise

■ Symptoms of Alanine Deficiency

☐ Fatigue   ☐ Poor exercise endurance

☐ Hypoglycemia (low blood sugar)

Food Sources of Alanine

- Beans
- Brown rice
- Corn
- Dairy products
- Duck
- Eggs
- Fish
- Legumes
- Nuts
- Sausage
- Seeds
- Soy
- Turkey
- White meat chicken

■ Causes of Alanine Deficiency

- Poor dietary intake of foods high in alanine.

■ Conditions That Can Benefit from Alanine

- Hypoglycemia (low blood sugar)   • Poor exercise endurance

■ Recommended Dosage

200 to 600 milligrams daily. Since alanine can be made in the body, most people do not need to take supplements of this amino acid. However, individuals with hypoglycemia tend to have low levels of alanine and may benefit from increased intake.

■ Side Effects and Contraindications

Check with your doctor before starting an amino acid regimen if you have diabetes, hypertension, kidney disease, or liver disease. Also, alanine may interact with some heart medications and with drugs for erectile dysfunction. The safety of supplementation has not been established for children or patients that are pregnant or breastfeeding. Some people have reported tingling of the skin after taking large doses of alanine. These symptoms usually subside within ninety minutes.

ARGININE

Arginine is a conditionally essential amino acid, which means that usually—but not always—it can be made by your body in sufficient amounts. When the body is under stress, though, this nutrient may have to be consumed through diet or supplements.

Like most amino acids, arginine is used in the synthesis of protein, but it also performs other important functions throughout the body. For instance, it is vital for muscle metabolism and liver function; it is involved in cell regulation and neurotransmission; and it aids in ammonia clearance as part of the urea cycle.

■ Functions of Arginine in Your Body

- Aids in ammonia clearance as part of the urea cycle
- Aids in the healing of wounds
- Builds muscle while decreasing body fat
- Decreases platelet stickiness
- Enhances fat metabolism
- Enhances immune function by increasing natural killer cell activity
- Expands blood vessels, reducing blood pressure
- Increases circulation
- Increases human growth hormone (HGH) production
- Increases insulin sensitivity

- Increases sperm count
- Inhibits plaque accumulation in the arteries
- Is an anti-inflammatory
- Is important for gut health
- Is needed for protein production
- Reduces pain from claudication (pain in extremities due to poor circulation)

- Used in cell regulation
- Used in neurotransmission
- Used to produce nitric oxide, which allows for better blood flow
- Used to treat liver disorders
- Vital for secretion of glucagon and insulin

◼ Symptoms of Arginine Deficiency

- ☐ Angina (chest pain)
- ☐ Chronic inflammatory disorders
- ☐ Cirrhosis of the liver
- ☐ Constipation

- ☐ Coronary artery disease
- ☐ Fatty liver disease
- ☐ Hair loss and breakage
- ☐ High ammonia levels

- ☐ Hypertension (high blood pressure)
- ☐ Insulin resistance/ diabetes
- ☐ Poor wound healing
- ☐ Skin rash
- ☐ Weight gain

Food Sources of Arginine

- Asparagus
- Avocados
- Beans
- Broccoli
- Chocolate
- Corn
- Dairy products
- Eggs

- Fish
- Green peas
- Legumes
- Meat
- Nuts
- Oatmeal
- Onions
- Potatoes

- Raisins
- Sesame seeds
- Spinach
- Sunflower seeds
- Swiss chard
- Whey
- Whole grains

◼ Causes of Arginine Deficiency

- Calorie-restricted diets
- Poor digestion of protein

- Poor intake of foods and nutrients that make ornithine, which is needed by the body to make arginine
- Poor intake of foods high in arginine

■ Conditions That Can Benefit from Arginine

- Anal fissures
- Anemia associated with kidney disease
- Cerebral vascular disease
- Chronic cyclosporine nephrotoxicity
- Chronic yeast infection
- Congestive heart failure
- Coronary heart disease
- Diabetic foot ulcers
- Erectile dysfunction
- Extreme weight loss due to HIV (prevention)
- Fatty liver disease
- Hyperhomocysteinemia (high homocysteine level)
- Hypertension (high blood pressure)
- Hypertriglyceridemia (high triglyceride levels)
- Insulin resistance/diabetes
- Intermittent claudication (cramping pain in the legs)
- Interstitial cystitis
- Low sperm count and motility
- Malaria
- Migraine headaches (arginine can be taken with ibuprofen)
- Polycystic ovary disease
- Poor wound healing
- Pressure ulcers in hip-fracture patients (prevention)
- Raynaud's disease
- Senile dementia
- Sickle cell disease
- Stress and anxiety
- Systemic sclerosis

■ Recommended Dosage

1,000 to 3,000 milligrams daily. You may want to have your healthcare provider measure your amino acid levels to determine the exact amount of arginine that your body needs.

■ Side Effects and Contraindications

Check with your doctor before starting an amino acid regimen if you have diabetes, hypertension, kidney disease, or liver disease. Also note that arginine can cause an increase in outbreaks of herpes simplex infections: cold sores and genital herpes. The addition of the amino acid lysine to the supplementation program can limit this effect. (See page 165 to learn about lysine.)

Arginine can interact badly with certain drugs, ranging from cholesterol-lowering agents to medications used to treat erectile dysfunction. Speak to your healthcare provider or pharmacist to learn if any of the drugs you're taking might make it unwise to take arginine.

Since arginine can affect your blood pressure, discontinue this supplement two weeks before surgery. The following are other side effects that can result from arginine supplementation:

- Abdominal pain
- Bitter taste in the mouth
- Bloating
- Diarrhea
- Gout

- Hypotension (low blood pressure)
- Nausea
- Tightness in chest
- Worsening of allergies
- Worsening of asthma

ASPARAGINE

A nonessential amino acid, asparagine can be made in the body from aspartic acid and adenosine triphosphate. When necessary, the body can convert asparagine back into aspartic acid, which plays a major role in metabolism.

■ Functions of Asparagine in Your Body

- Forms part of the DNA
- Helps protect the liver
- Involved in the metabolism of ammonia
- Metabolizes carbohydrates via the Krebs cycle

- Needed for protein production
- Needed for the development and function of the brain
- Promotes mineral absorption in the intestinal tract
- Transports nitrogen in the body

■ Symptoms of Asparagine Deficiency

- ☐ Allergies
- ☐ Fatigue

■ Causes of Asparagine Deficiency

- Poor dietary intake of foods high in asparagine.

Food Sources of Asparagine

- Asparagus
- Beef
- Cheese
- Chicken
- Dairy products
- Eggs
- Fish
- Legumes
- Nuts
- Pork
- Potatoes
- Sausage
- Seeds
- Soy
- Turkey

■ Conditions That Can Benefit from Asparagine

- Fatigue

■ Recommended Dosage

Since asparagine can be made in the body, most people do not need to take supplements. A deficiency of this amino acid is very rare. Have your doctor order an amino acid test to determine if your level is optimal.

■ Side Effects and Contraindications

Check with your doctor before starting an amino acid regimen if you have diabetes, hypertension, kidney disease, or liver disease. The safety of supplementation has not been established for children or for individuals that are pregnant or breastfeeding.

ASPARTIC ACID

Aspartic acid is an amino acid as well as an *excitatory neurotransmitter*, which is a chemical that stimulates brain activity. A nonessential amino acid, it is made in the body from glutamic acid. In addition, the body can convert the amino acid asparagine into aspartic acid.

Aspartic acid is required for the biosynthesis of all body proteins, amino acid metabolism, and the detoxification of ammonia in the urea cycle. It is also used as an energy source, increases stamina and resistance to fatigue, and more.

Recently, some men have used D-aspartic acid in an effort to increase testosterone levels. Although one study showed that this supplement can significantly increase testosterone levels, aspartic acid may cause serious side effects, including an increase in the amino acid homocysteine, which can lead to heart disease, memory loss, prostate or breast cancer, depression, and bone loss. Therefore, this is not a recommended use of aspartic acid.

■ Functions of Aspartic Acid in Your Body

- Forms part of the DNA and RNA
- Involved in the metabolism of ammonia
- Involved in the urea cycle
- Is an excitatory neurotransmitter
- May enhance endurance
- May play a role in the immune system
- Metabolizes carbohydrates via the Krebs cycle
- Necessary for the production of glucose
- Needed for protein production
- Needed for the development and function of the brain

■ Symptoms of Aspartic Acid Deficiency

☐ Depression

☐ Fatigue

■ Causes of Aspartic Acid Deficiency

- Poor dietary intake of foods high in aspartic acid

Food Sources of Aspartic Acid

- Beef
- Chicken
- Cottage cheese
- Fish
- Pork
- Ricotta cheese
- Sausage
- Turkey

■ Conditions That Can Benefit from Aspartic Acid

- Depression
- Fatigue
- Low sperm count and motility

■ Recommended Dosage

Since aspartic acid can be made in the body, most people do not need to take supplements. A deficiency of this amino acid is very rare. Have your doctor order an amino acid test to determine if your level is optimal.

■ Side Effects and Contraindications

Check with your doctor before starting an amino acid regimen if you have diabetes, hypertension, kidney disease, or liver disease. The following are possible side effects of aspartic acid use:

- Acne
- Depression
- Diarrhea
- Elevated levels of homocysteine
- Elevated levels of testosterone
- Headache
- Mood swings

■ Symptoms of Aspartic Acid Toxicity

☐ Depression   ☐ Epilepsy   ☐ Stroke

BRANCHED-CHAIN AMINO ACIDS (BCAAs)

Isoleucine, leucine, and valine are all *branched-chain amino acids (BCAAs)*. The term "branched-chain" refers to the chemical structure of these nutrients.

All three BCAAs are essential, which means that the body must obtain them from foods or supplements. Although the BCAAs have many functions, they are best known for their role in building the protein in muscle and reducing muscle breakdown. They are found in abundance in muscle tissue.

■ Functions of BCAAs in Your Body

- Contributes to the synthesis of the amino acids glutamate and gamma-aminobutyric acid (GABA)
- Helps regulate energy during strenuous muscle activity
- Involved in the control mechanisms for neurotransmitters (chemical "messengers" in the brain)
- Needed for the regulation of glucose
- Prevents the decrease of muscle protein synthesis that can occur with stress
- Promotes wound healing
- Required for the synthesis of all enzymes and proteins
- Stimulates the growth and repair of muscle tissue
- Stimulates the increase of lean body mass in response to exercise
- Used in the production of blood cells

■ **Symptoms of BCAA Deficiency**

☐ Alopecia (hair loss)

☐ Confusion

☐ Depression

☐ Dizziness

☐ Fatigue

☐ Headaches

☐ Hypoglycemia (low blood sugar)

☐ Inability to build muscle

☐ Irritability

☐ Loss of muscle mass

Food Sources of Isoleucine

- Avocados
- Beans (especially soy)
- Cereals (especially millet)
- Cheese
- Corn
- Eggs
- Grains
- Green peas
- Lentils
- Meats
- Milk
- Nuts
- Potatoes
- Seeds
- Spinach
- Swiss chard

Food Sources of Leucine

- Asparagus
- Avocados
- Broccoli
- Cereals (especially millet)
- Cheese
- Corn
- Eggs
- Fish
- Gelatin
- Grains
- Green peas
- Lentils
- Meats
- Milk
- Mushrooms
- Nuts
- Potatoes
- Seeds
- Spinach
- Sweet potatoes
- Swiss chard
- Tomatoes
- Wheat germ

Food Sources of Valine

- Avocados
- Beets
- Broccoli
- Cereals (especially buckwheat, millet, and oatmeal)
- Cheese
- Chocolate
- Corn
- Green peas
- Milk
- Peanuts
- Potatoes
- Spinach
- Sweet potatoes
- Swiss chard

■ Causes of BCAA Deficiency

- Increased loss of BCAAs by the kidneys in times of stress
- Increased usage of BCAAs
- Low protein intake
- Poor digestion

■ Conditions That Can Benefit from BCAAs

- Amyotrophic lateral sclerosis (ALS)
- Burns
- Insulin resistance/diabetes
- Major physical trauma
- Mania
- Muscle tissue damage
- Poor wound healing
- Post-surgery recovery
- Sepsis
- Sleep apnea
- Spinocerebral degeneration
- Stress-induced decrease of muscle protein synthesis (prevention)
- Traumatic brain injury (TBI)

■ Recommended Dosage

1 to 5 grams daily of each BCAA, depending on the reason they are being taken. The three BCAAs should be taken together rather than individually, because supplementation of a single BCAA can cause a deficiency in the other two.

■ Side Effects and Contraindications

Check with your doctor before starting an amino acid regimen if you have diabetes, hypertension, kidney disease, or liver disease.

Note that BCAA supplementation can reduce the effectiveness of certain drugs, such as the Parkinson's disease medication levodopa. Speak to your healthcare provider or pharmacist to learn if any drugs you're taking might make it unwise to take BCAAs.

BCAAs compete for transport across the blood-brain barrier (BBB) with the amino acids tryptophan, tyrosine, and phenylalanine, and can therefore decrease the uptake of these substances. The decrease in these amino acids directly affects the synthesis and release of serotonin and catecholamines, which affect mood and the management of stress. If you have depression, anxiety, or manic attacks, work with your healthcare provider before taking BCAAs.

■ Symptoms of High BCAAs

☐ Confusion

☐ Depression

☐ Diabetic microangiopathy (disease of the small blood vessels)

☐ Dizziness

☐ Fatigue

☐ Headaches

☐ Hypoglycemia (low blood sugar)

☐ Increased urination

☐ Irritability

■ Causes of High BCAAs

Taking excessively high amounts of BCAAs can cause levels to be too high, as can insulin resistance, diabetes, and a deficiency of vitamin B_6. If your BCAA levels are elevated, discontinue the BCAAs you are taking. If insulin resistance or diabetes may be the cause, see your healthcare provider for treatment and make sure you are not deficient in B_6.

CARNOSINE

Carnosine is an amino acid that is formed when a beta-alanine molecule and a histidine molecule join together.

Carnosine is a powerful antioxidant. Stored in the brain, heart, and muscles, it protects the body from *glycation,* a process that can lead to the formation of *advanced glycation end products (AGEs),* which accelerate aging and have been linked to many chronic disorders. One study showed that carnosine was the only antioxidant to significantly protect cellular chromosomes from the oxidative damage associated with glycation. Carnosine has also been shown to inhibit glycation in eye lens protein, thereby helping to prevent and treat cataracts.

Do not confuse this nutrient with the similar-sounding supplement *carnitine,* which is discussed on page 270.

■ Functions of Carnosine in Your Body

- Binds metal ions that cause tissue damage

- Blocks the aging effects of glycation

- Helps maintain memory

- Is an antioxidant

- Protects muscle tissue from lactic acid

- Regulates levels of copper and zinc

■ Symptoms of Carnosine Deficiency

☐ Cataract formation

☐ Cognitive decline

☐ Dry eyes

☐ Hypertension (high blood pressure)

■ Causes of Carnosine Deficiency

● Poor dietary intake of foods containing carnosine.

● Poor dietary intake of foods containing beta-alanine and histidine.

Food Sources of Carnosine

● Beef   ● Chicken   ● Pork   ● Turkey

■ Conditions That Can Benefit from Carnosine

● Aging

● Alzheimer's disease

● Atherosclerosis

● Autism

● Brain injury

● Cataracts

● Diabetes mellitus

● Dry eyes

● Hypertension

● Skin aging

● Stroke

● Wound healing

■ Recommended Dosage

1,000 to 2,000 milligrams daily. If you have dry eyes, you can use eye drops that contain carnosine.

■ Side Effects and Contraindications

Check with your doctor before starting an amino acid regimen if you have diabetes, hypertension, kidney disease, or liver disease. Also be aware that if you take too much carnosine, it can result in hyperactivity.

CYSTEINE

Cysteine is a conditionally essential amino acid that is made from the amino acids serine and methionine. Usually, the body is able to produce as much cysteine as it needs. This compound's many important functions include helping synthesize protein and serving as one of the building blocks of glutathione, which has been referred to as "the mother of all antioxidants."

The amino acid *cystine* is formed when two cysteine molecules join together. The conversion of cysteine into cystine occurs as required by the body. Unlike the amino acid from which it is derived, cystine is rarely used as a dietary supplement.

■ Functions of Cysteine in Your Body

- Aids in cancer protection by stimulating natural killer cells
- Aids in healing after surgery
- Boosts your immune system
- Breaks down homocysteine, an amino acid that can contribute to heart disease
- Breaks up mucus, making it easier to relieve congestion
- Builds muscle
- Decreases the toxicity of some chemotherapy drugs, such as ifosfamide and doxorubicin
- Detoxifies the body of mercury, lead, and cadmium
- Enhances immune function
- Helps destroy acetaldehyde and free radicals produced by smoking and drinking
- Helps synthesize proteins
- Involved in communication between cells
- Is an antioxidant
- Prevents hair loss
- Promotes hair growth
- Promotes metabolism of fats and production of muscle
- Promotes wound healing
- Reduces inflammation
- Vital to the production of glutathione, a strong antioxidant

■ Symptoms of Cysteine Deficiency

- ☐ Apathy
- ☐ Decreased focus and memory
- ☐ Depression
- ☐ Dizziness
- ☐ Dry skin
- ☐ Edema
- ☐ Fatigue
- ☐ Frequent colds
- ☐ Headaches
- ☐ Joint pain
- ☐ Lethargy
- ☐ Liver damage
- ☐ Loss of pigmentation of hair
- ☐ Rashes
- ☐ Sleep disorders
- ☐ Slow growth in children
- ☐ Weakness

■ Causes of Cysteine Deficiency

• Poor dietary intake of foods that contain cysteine

Food Sources of Cysteine

• Beans	• Fish	• Onions
• Broccoli	• Garlic	• Red peppers
• Brussels sprouts	• Legumes	• Seafood
• Dairy products	• Meat	• Seeds
• Eggs	• Nuts	• Soy

■ Conditions That Can Benefit from Cysteine

• Alzheimer's disease

• Amyotrophic lateral sclerosis (ALS)

• Angina

• Chronic fatigue syndrome

• COPD/bronchitis

• Cough (cysteine breaks up and liquefies mucus)

• *H. pylori* infection

• Hair loss

• Hangover

• High levels of lipoprotein (a), a risk factor for coronary disease

• HIV

• Hyperhomocysteinemia (high levels of homocysteine)

• Infertility due to clomiphene-resistant PCOS

• Keratoconjunctivitis

• Poor wound healing

• Pulmonary fibrosis

• Recurrent miscarriage (use cysteine with folic acid)

• Sjogren's syndrome

■ Recommended Dosage

Cysteine is used as a therapy for several disorders. Doses of 250 to 2,000 milligrams a day of n-acetyl cysteine (NAC)—the form most frequently used by the body—have been taken safely. Do not take D-cysteine, D-cystine, or 5-methyl cysteine, because they can be toxic.

Cysteine supplements should be taken with vitamin C (500 to 1,000 milligrams). This will help prevent an increase in kidney stone production from cysteine precipitation. Long-term use of n-acetyl cysteine may lead to depletion of zinc and copper. Therefore, it's important to take a multivitamin when taking cysteine.

■ Side Effects and Contraindications

Check with your doctor before starting an amino acid regimen if you have diabetes, hypertension, kidney disease, or liver disease. Do not use cysteine if you have an active peptic ulcer.

N-acetyl-cysteine strongly potentiates the effect of nitroglycerin and related medications, and caution should be used in people receiving these medications since it may cause hypotension (low blood pressure). Speak to your healthcare provider or pharmacist to learn if cysteine might cause problems if taken with any of your medications.

Cysteine can cause the following side effects:

- Abdominal pain
- Abnormal taste
- Anorexia
- Asthma
- Blurred vision
- Constipation

- Diarrhea
- Dizziness
- Dry mouth
- Facial flushing
- Headache
- Indigestion

- Nausea
- Shortness of breath
- Skin rash
- Sweating
- Vomiting

GLUTAMATE

Glutamate is found in both plant and animal protein, and is the most abundant free amino acid in the body. It can be made by the body from aspartic acid, ornithine, arginine, proline, and alpha-ketoglutarate, and can be converted into both gluatmine and GABA. Aside from being an important amino acid, glutamate is also the chief excitatory neurotransmitter, which means it increases the activity of the nerve cells. Under normal conditions, this substance plays an important role in learning and memory. If too much glutamate is present, however, it can actually be damaging to nerve cells and the brain as a whole. In fact, excessively high levels of glutamate are more common than glutamate deficiency.

When you read about glutamate, you may come across related terms. Glutamate is glutamic acid to which a mineral ion has been attached. Sometimes these two terms are used interchangeably. Monosodium glutamate (MSG) is a sodium salt of glutamic acid.

■ Functions of Glutamate in Your Body

- As an excitatory neurotransmitter, it sends signals to the brain that helps cognitive function, memory, learning, and other brain processes
- Balances blood sugar levels
- Decreases sugar cravings
- Enhances immune function
- Enhances pain control
- Improves mental alertness
- Increases energy
- Involved in sensory perception and motor skills
- Maintains digestive health
- Maintains muscle health
- Necessary to protein synthesis
- Neutralizes toxins
- Plays a role in the body's ability to adapt to environmental and genetic influences
- Promotes healing
- Promotes healthy acid-alkaline balance
- Promotes weight loss
- Supports motor skills

■ Symptoms of Glutamate Deficiency

Glutamate deficiency is rare, but when it does occur, you may experience the following symptoms.

- ☐ Anxiety
- ☐ Decreased ability to concentrate
- ☐ Depression
- ☐ Insomnia
- ☐ Low energy
- ☐ Mental exhaustion
- ☐ Sugar cravings

Food Sources of Glutamate

- Bacon
- Beans
- Brown rice
- Chicken
- Cottage cheese
- Duck
- Eggs
- Fish
- Granola
- Ham
- Nuts
- Parsley
- Sausage
- Spinach
- Turkey
- Yogurt

■ Causes of Glutamate Deficiency

- Poor dietary intake of foods high in glutamate

■ Conditions That Can Benefit from Glutamate

- Cognitive decline
- Depression

■ Recommended Dosage

Since glutamate can be made in the body, this amino acid doesn't usually have to be supplemented. Have your doctor order an amino acid test to determine if your level is optimal.

■ Side Effects and Contraindications

Do not take glutamate without consulting a healthcare professional. If you are sensitive to monosodium glutamate (MSG), avoid glutamate, because it may exacerbate your symptoms.

■ Conditions Associated With Elevated Glutamate Levels

- Alzheimer's disease
- Amyotrophic lateral sclerosis (ALS)
- Anxiety disorder
- Attention-deficit/hyperactivity disorder (ADHD)
- Autism
- Bipolar disorder
- Epilepsy
- Fibromyalgia/chronic fatigue syndrome
- Gout
- Increase in chronic pain
- Insomnia
- Mania
- Migraine headaches
- Mood lability (exaggerated changes in mood)
- Panic disorder
- Parkinson's disease
- Post traumatic stress disorder (PTSD)
- Restless leg syndrome
- Schizophrenia
- Seizures
- Treatment-resistant depression

■ Ways to Lower Glutamate

- Decrease intake of foods high in glutamate
- Lower mercury levels with chelation therapy (see your healthcare provider)
- Lower stress levels

- Take the following supplements: n-acetyl cysteine (NAC), magnesium, melatonin, and vitamin D. (Have your doctor measure your vitamin D and melatonin levels to prescribe the proper amounts.)

GLUTAMINE

Glutamine is used to synthesize protein and is also involved in many metabolic processes. A conditionally essential amino acid, glutamine can be produced by the body but can become depleted when used in overabundance, such as during intense physical activity or stress. Fortunately, this nutrient can be found in dairy, eggs, meat, and several other common foods.

■ Functions of Glutamine in Your Body

- Balances blood sugar levels
- Controls *intestinal permeability*—the passing of material from the GI tract through the gut wall to the rest of the body
- Fights cold and flu
- Helps prevent leaky gut syndrome
- Helps synthesize protein
- Helps the brain dispose of ammonia
- Improves mental alertness
- Increases energy
- Increases growth hormone
- Is a fuel source for the immune system
- Is a precursor for GABA, a neurotransmitter (see page 294)
- Is an inhibitory neurotransmitter
- Is needed for DNA synthesis
- Is needed for gut health
- Is needed for the metabolism and maintenance of muscle
- Neutralizes toxins
- Promotes a healthy acid-alkaline balance
- Promotes growth
- Promotes weight loss
- Promotes wound healing and tissue repair
- Protects the body from stress
- Stops food cravings
- Supports glutathione

■ Symptoms of Glutamine Deficiency

- ☐ Anxiety
- ☐ Decreased immune system
- ☐ Depression
- ☐ Insomnia
- ☐ Lack of concentration

■ Causes of Glutamine Deficiency

- Intense exercise
- Nutritional deficiencies

Food Sources of Glutamine

- Asparagus
- Beans
- Bone broth
- Brown rice
- Dairy products
- Eggs
- Fish
- Legumes
- Meat
- Nuts
- Seafood
- Seeds
- Soy
- Spinach
- Spirulina
- Whole grains

■ Conditions That Can Benefit from Glutamine

- Acute pancreatitis/chronic pancreatitis
- Alcoholism
- Attention-deficit/hyperactivity disorder (ADHD)
- Bone marrow transplant (to improve recovery)
- Burns
- Chronic yeast infections
- Crohn's disease
- Cystinuria
- Dysbiosis/leaky gut syndrome
- HIV (to prevent weight loss)
- Irritable bowel syndrome (IBS)
- Mucositis secondary to chemotherapy
- Muscle and joint pain secondary to chemotherapy
- Neuropathy
- Radiation colitis (prevention)
- Short bowel syndrome
- Sickle cell anemia
- Stomach ulcers
- Stress
- Ulcerative colitis
- Weight gain

■ Recommended Dosage

500 to 3,000 milligrams daily.

■ Side Effects and Contraindications

If you have a sensitivity to monosodium glutamate (MSG), use glutamine with caution because the body metabolizes glutamine into glutamate. Also use with caution if you take medications for seizures. Speak to your healthcare provider or pharmacist to learn if any drugs you're taking might make it unwise to take glutamine supplements.

Until more is known about glutamine supplementation, it is recommended that people who have nerve-damaging chronic neurological diseases, such as ALS and multiple sclerosis, and those who have had recent neurological surgeries limit their intake of supplemental glutamine and/or have glutamine and glutamate levels measured, and supplement according to lab levels. Do not use glutamine if you have cirrhosis or hepatic encephalopathy, since it may worsen these conditions. Do not take glutamine if you have manic episodes.

GLUTATHIONE

Glutathione is a tripeptide composed of three amino acids: cysteine, glutamic acid, and glycine. Because the body can manufacture glutathione, it is considered nonessential. You can get this important nutrient from supplements and your diet, but it is relatively rare in foodstuffs.

Although glutathione benefits the body in many ways, it is perhaps best known as the strongest antioxidant produced by the body—and one that is found in every cell in the body. In its capacity as an antioxidant, it protects cells from damage by oxidation and free radicals. Around the age of forty, glutathione levels commonly begin to diminish.

■ Functions of Glutathione

- Acts as a neuromodulator (a substance released by neurons to alter the activity of other neurons)

- Acts as a neurotransmitter

- Decreases sugar cravings

- Displaces glutamate from its binding site

- Enhances liver and brain detoxification of toxic chemicals and heavy metals

- Helps facilitate cellular magnesium and glucose uptake

- Helps to recycle other antioxidants, such as vitamins C and E

- Is a powerful antioxidant

- Is part of amino acid transport

- Plays a role in protein and prostaglandin synthesis

- Stimulates the production of interleukin 1 and 2, which help regulate the immune system

- Used in DNA synthesis and repair

■ Symptoms of Glutathione Deficiency

☐ Asthma

☐ Compromised immune system

☐ Depression

☐ Dizziness

☐ Faster progression of HIV

☐ Fatigue

☐ Headaches

☐ Hemolytic anemia (destruction of red blood cells)

☐ Joint pain

☐ Reduced focus and memory

☐ Sleep disorders

■ Causes of Glutathione Deficiency

- Acetaminophen use

- Aging process

- Cadmium, arsenic, lead, mercury, iron, copper, and cobalt toxicity

- Cigarette smoking

- Excessive intake of alcohol

- Overly processed chemical-laden foods (such as luncheon meats that contain nitrites or nitrates)

- Poor dietary intake of foods that increase glutathione levels

---

Food Sources of Glutathione

These foods may increase glutathione levels:

- Apples
- Asparagus
- Avocados
- Bananas
- Broccoli
- Cantaloupe
- Carrots
- Cauliflower
- Cucumbers
- Garlic

- Grapefruit
- Green bell peppers
- Lemons
- Mangoes
- Melons
- Onions
- Okra
- Oranges
- Papaya

- Peaches
- Potatoes
- Red bell peppers
- Spinach
- Squash
- Strawberries
- Tomatoes
- Walnuts
- Watermelon
- Zucchini

■ Conditions That Can Benefit from Glutathione

- Aging process

- Allergic rhinitis

- Amyotrophic lateral sclerosis (ALS)

- Anxiety
- Autism
- Cardiovascular disease
- Chronic fatigue syndrome
- Chronic otitis media
- Chronic stress
- Cirrhosis of the liver
- COPD/asthma/acute respiratory distress syndrome (ARDS)
- Diabetes/insulin resistance

- Hepatitis C
- HIV
- Hypertension
- Meniere's disease
- Multiple sclerosis
- Parkinson's disease
- Toxic metals and chemicals
- Ulcerative colitis

■ Recommended Dosage

There are several ways to take glutathione or increase its production:

- Take 500 to 3,000 milligrams of n-acetyl cysteine (NAC) daily to increase glutathione levels. The cysteine in NAC can precipitate and cause kidney stones to form if you are predisposed to cysteine stone formation. To avoid this complication, take 500 to 1,000 milligrams of vitamin C a day. Long-term use of n-acetyl cysteine may lead to depletion of zinc and copper. Therefore, it's important to take a multivitamin when taking cysteine.

- Take 250 to 500 milligrams of liposomal glutathione in the morning in the form of a liquid or lozenge.

- To increase the production of the enzyme necessary to synthesize glutathione, take curcumin and/or quercetin.

■ Side Effects and Contraindications

Check with your doctor before starting an amino acid regimen if you have diabetes, hypertension, kidney disease, or liver disease. Glutathione is contraindicated in people with sulfite sensitivity since it is converted in part to sulfite.

GLYCINE

Glycine is a conditionally essential amino acid that is produced by the body but can be depleted through increased needs for detoxification. It is, however, available in both foods and supplements. This substance has many functions in the body, ranging from its role in the metabolism of proteins to its anti-inflammatory activity.

◼ Functions of Glycine in Your Body

- Acts as an anti-inflammatory
- Aids the absorption of calcium
- Calms aggression
- Decreases muscle wasting
- Decreases sugar cravings
- Enhances the neurotransmitters (messengers) in the brain
- Helps create muscle tissues
- Helps form collagen
- Is a precursor to components of the cell membrane
- Is an inhibitory neurotransmitter (reduces the activity of nerve cells)
- Is important to the manufacture of glucose from glycogen in your liver
- Needed for prostate gland function
- Needed to maintain the nervous system
- Stimulates detoxification in the liver
- Used for the formation of glutathione
- Used in the metabolism of proteins
- Used in the synthesis of DNA, hemoglobin, and RNA

◼ Symptoms of Glycine Deficiency

☐ Anxiety

Food Sources of Glycine

The following are common foods that contain glycine. Meat, fish, poultry, and dairy are the best sources, but some plant foods do contain small amounts of this amino acid.

- Beans
- Cabbage
- Cauliflower
- Chicken
- Dairy products
- Fish
- Kale
- Meat
- Pumpkin
- Soybeans
- Spinach
- Turkey
- Wheat germ

■ Causes of Glycine Deficiency

- Food additives and pharmaceuticals that require glycine for detoxification
- Impaired pathways in the body of detoxification, tissue repair, and the generation of glucose
- Poor dietary intake of foods high in glycine

■ Conditions That Can Benefit from Glycine

- Bipolar disorder
- Cancer (prevention)
- Chronic fatigue syndrome
- Diabetic leg ulcers (use topically)
- Epilepsy
- Gastrointestinal side effects of aspirin use (prevention)
- Insomnia
- Kidney disease (prevention)
- Poor memory
- Prostate enlargement (prevention)
- Schizophrenia
- Spasticity
- Stroke

■ Recommended Dosage

500 to 3,000 milligrams daily. Dosage is best determined by your healthcare provider, who can perform amino acid testing.

■ Side Effects and Contraindications

Check with your doctor before starting an amino acid regimen if you have diabetes, hypertension, kidney disease, or liver disease. Some drugs, such as clozapine, may be less effective when taken with glycine. Speak to your healthcare provider or pharmacist to learn if glycine will cause a problem when used with the drugs you are taking. Pregnant and breastfeeding women should avoid taking glycine.

Most people do not experience side effects when taking glycine. However, there have been a few reports of the following side effects:

- Drowsiness
- Nausea
- Soft stools
- Upset stomach
- Vomiting

HISTIDINE

The amino acid histidine is unique because although most adults can manufacture it in the liver, children cannot produce it and must consume it through their diets. For that reason, it is considered an essential amino acid, although some people term it semi-essential. An adequate intake of histidine is especially important during periods of accelerated growth, such as infancy.

Histidine can be converted into histamine, which is a substance that plays a major role in allergic reactions and the dilation of blood vessels. Histamine is part of the body's natural allergic response to substances such as pollen.

◼ Functions of Histidine in Your Body

- Able to turn minerals into forms that can be used by the body

- Can be converted to histamine

- Dilates blood vessels

- Helps absorb and transport zinc

- Important for proper immune function

- Is a mild anti-inflammatory

- May be an antioxidant

- Needed for the body's response to allergens

- Needed for the growth and repair of tissues

- Needed for the maintenance of the myelin sheath, which protects nerve cells from damage

- Needed for the production of red and white blood cells

- Needed for the synthesis of enzymes and proteins

- Plays a crucial role in sexual function

- Used to make gastric juices

◼ Symptoms of Histidine Deficiency

- ☐ Cataracts
- ☐ Eczema
- ☐ Indigestion
- ☐ Joint pain
- ☐ Poor allergic response

◼ Causes of Histidine Deficiency

- Excessive supplementation of lysine or arginine, which compete with histidine for absorption

- Folic acid deficiency, which leads to increased breakdown of histidine

- Malabsorption of histidine

- Poor dietary intake of histidine-rich foods
- Salicylates and steroids, which decrease histidine levels

Food Sources of Histidine

- Bananas
- Beans
- Beef
- Cheese
- Chicken

- Eggs
- Fish
- Milk and other dairy products
- Nuts

- Pork
- Potatoes
- Seeds
- Soy
- Turkey

■ Conditions That Can Benefit from Histidine

- Allergic reactions
- Nerve damage
- Osteoarthritis
- Rheumatoid arthritis
- Sexual dysfunction

■ Recommended Dosage

Dosage is best determined by your healthcare provider, who can perform amino acid testing.

■ Side Effects and Contraindications

Check with your doctor before starting an amino acid regimen if you have diabetes, hypertension, kidney disease, or liver disease. Do not take histidine if you have active ulcers or if you have high hydrochloric acid (HCL) levels, since histidine increases the production of HCL in the stomach. Pregnant and breastfeeding women should avoid taking histidine supplements. The symptoms of histidine toxicity include copper deficiency and elevated levels of LDL (bad) cholesterol.

LYSINE

Lysine is an essential amino acid that must be consumed daily in the form of food or supplements. Your body needs lysine for growth and maintenance and many other important functions. Fortunately, it is found in meat, dairy products, vegetables, legumes, and more.

■ Function of Lysine in Your Body

- Aids in the production of antibodies
- Functions as an antiviral to help fight herpes outbreaks (cold sores or genital herpes)
- Helps maintain bone health by enhancing calcium absorption and decreasing calcium excretion
- Helps protect the lens of the eye
- Helps support immune defense
- Lowers triglyceride levels, the main constituent of body fat
- Maintains nitrogen balance
- Needed for making enzymes
- Needed for the synthesis of collagen and elastin
- Plays an important role in the production of carnitine
- Promotes the release of growth hormone
- Regulates the mammary glands, ovaries, and pineal gland
- Required for growth and tissue repair

■ Symptoms of Lysine Deficiency

☐ Anemia	☐ Fever blisters	☐ Irritability
☐ Apathy	☐ Hair loss	☐ Loss of energy
☐ Bloodshot eyes	☐ High triglyceride levels	☐ Muscle loss
☐ Carnitine deficiency		☐ Stomach ulcers
☐ Depression	☐ Inability to concentrate	☐ Stunted growth
☐ Edema		☐ Weakness
☐ Fatigue	☐ Infertility	

■ Causes of Lysine Deficiency

- Carnitine deficiency
- Excessive arginine or histidine supplementation, which competes for absorption
- Poor dietary intake of foods containing lysine
- Prolonged stress

Food Sources of Lysine

- Asparagus
- Avocados
- Beans
- Beef
- Cheese
- Chicken
- Chocolate
- Corn
- Dairy products

- Eggs
- Fenugreek seed
- Fish
- Green peas
- Legumes
- Lentils
- Lima beans
- Mushrooms
- Nuts

- Pork
- Potatoes
- Seafood
- Soy
- Spinach
- Spirulina
- Turkey
- Whole grains

■ Conditions That Can Benefit from Lysine

- Anxiety
- Diabetes
- Herpes infection
- Hypertriglyceridemia (high triglycerides)

- Muscle weakness
- Osteoporosis/osteopenia (bone loss)
- Schizophrenia

■ Recommended Dosage

500 to 1,500 milligrams daily. Have your doctor measure your amino acid levels to determine if you are deficient in this important amino acid. For people with the herpes virus, lysine can be used to limit the occurrence and severity of the outbreaks. During an outbreak, increase your lysine intake to 3,000 milligrams a day until it has resolved.

■ Side Effects and Contraindications

Check with your doctor before starting an amino acid regimen if you have diabetes, hypertension, kidney disease, or liver disease. Do not take lysine for more than six months, because it can cause an imbalance of arginine unless arginine is also supplemented. If you are allergic to eggs, milk, or wheat, use lysine supplementation with caution or not at all.

Lysine supplementation can cause gastrointestinal problems such as abdominal pain and diarrhea.

METHIONINE

Methionine is a sulfur-containing essential amino acid that cannot be synthesized by the body and must be obtained from the diet on a daily basis. Most people do not need to take methionine supplementation, because this nutrient is available in so many common foods.

Like many amino acids, methionine is vital for normal metabolism and growth and has many other important functions in the body. It is required for the biosynthesis of all enzymes, all proteins, and many other vital compounds. It is also necessary for genetic expression, muscle movement, normal brain and nerve function, and much more.

■ Functions of Methionine in Your Body

- Acts as an antioxidant, as the sulfur removes harmful free radicals

- Detoxifies the body of lead and other heavy metals

- Facilitates the breakdown of fats, helping to prevent fat accumulation in the liver and arteries

- Is a component of SAMe (S-adenosylmethionine)

- Is essential to genetic expression

- Is needed for normal brain and nerve function

- Is needed for normal metabolism and growth

- Is needed for the absorption, transportation, and availability of selenium and zinc

- Is needed for the formation of acetylcholine, carnitine, choline, collagen, cysteine, epinephrine, glutathione, lecithin, melatonin, nucleic acids, serine, and taurine

- Is needed for the normalization of urinary pH, helping to keep the urinary environment unfavorable to bacterial growth

- Provides sulfur and other compounds required for normal metabolism and growth

- Vital for the formation of proteins, body tissues, and enzymes

- Works with other amino acids to form creatine, an important constituent of muscles

■ Symptoms of Methionine Deficiency

☐ Apathy

☐ Edema (tissue swelling)

☐ Lethargy

☐ Liver damage

☐ Loss of pigmentation in hair

☐ Muscle weakness and loss

☐ Skin lesions

☐ Slow growth in children

☐ Weakness

■ Causes of Methionine Deficiency

- High dietary intake of foods containing tannin (barley, beans, beer, berries, chocolate, cider, grapes, nuts, pomegranates, red wine, rhubarb, sorghum, and tea)

- Poor dietary intake of foods containing methionine.

Food Sources of Methionine

- Avocados
- Cheese
- Cottage cheese
- Duck
- Eggs
- Fish

- Lentils
- Meat
- Milk
- Peanuts
- Pork
- Pumpkin

- Sausage
- Seafood
- Sunflower seeds
- Wild game

■ Conditions That Can Benefit from Methionine

- Alcoholism
- Alkaline urine (urine should be acidic)
- Allergies
- Asthma
- Copper poisoning

- Depression
- Drug withdrawal
- Liver damage due to acetaminophen use (prevention)
- Parkinson's disease
- Poor wound healing

■ Recommended Dosage

100 mg to 2,000 milligrams daily. A common dose for the average person is 100 milligrams. If you do begin a methionine regimen, be sure to get enough folate, vitamin B_6, and vitamin B_{12} to prevent a build-up of homocysteine, a

substance that increases the risk of heart disease, depression, memory loss, bone loss, and some forms of cancer.

■ Side Effects and Contraindications

Check with your doctor before starting an amino acid regimen if you have diabetes, hypertension, kidney disease, or liver disease. Use methionine only under the direction of a healthcare provider if you have one of the genetic markers for MTHFR.

A high intake of methionine can counter the effects of certain drugs, such as levodopa which is used for Parkinson's disease. Speak to your healthcare provider or pharmacist to learn if methionine supplements can cause problems when used with any of the drugs you're taking.

Do not use large doses of methionine if you have schizophrenia, since it can cause symptoms to worsen. High doses of methionine can also cause brain damage and death and promote the growth of some tumors. Speak to your healthcare provider about the right dose for you.

PHENYLALANINE

Phenylalanine is an essential amino acid. It is converted to the amino acid tyrosine in the liver. Although tyrosine is not essential, if adequate amounts are not made in the body, they must be provided by the diet. Tyrosine is converted into the neurotransmitters dopamine, norepinephrine, and epinephrine. If tyrosine levels are low, the symptoms mimic low levels of phenylalanine.

Although phenylalanine is necessary for optimal health, too much of this amino acid can be toxic and extremely dangerous. Likewise, low levels of phenylalanine can be hazardous to your health.

■ Functions of Phenylalanine in Your Body

- Decreases depression
- Enables the overall nervous system to operate efficiently
- Helps to regulate a number of hormones that are produced by the thyroid, adrenal gland, and pituitary gland
- Improves alertness and memory
- Regulates the release of cholecystokinin (CCK), the hormone that signals the brain to feel satisfied after eating
- Stimulates pain relief

■ Symptoms of Phenylalanine Deficiency

- ☐ Apathy
- ☐ Cataracts
- ☐ Confusion
- ☐ Decreased alertness
- ☐ Decreased sexual interest

- ☐ Depression
- ☐ Edema
- ☐ Fat loss
- ☐ Lack of appetite
- ☐ Liver damage

- ☐ Loss of pigmentation in hair
- ☐ Low levels of proteins
- ☐ Muscle loss
- ☐ Skin lesions
- ☐ Weakness

■ Causes of Phenylalanine Deficiency

- Excessive intake of caffeine
- Lack of phenylalanine-rich foods in the diet

Food Sources of Phenylalanine

- Almonds
- Avocados
- Bananas
- Beans
- Cheese
- Chocolate
- Corn

- Dairy products
- Eggs
- Fish
- Green peas
- Legumes
- Lentils
- Lima beans

- Meat
- Nuts
- Potatoes
- Soy
- Spinach
- Sweet potatoes
- Whole grains

■ Conditions That Can Benefit from Phenylalanine

- Alcohol withdrawal
- Attention-deficit/hyperactivity disorder (ADHD)
- Chronic pain
- Depression

- Osteoarthritis
- Parkinson's disease (do not use with levodopa)
- Rheumatoid arthritis
- Tyrosinemia (genetic disorder)

■ Recommended Dosage

500 to 3,000 milligrams daily. Your healthcare provider can order neurotransmitter testing and amino acid testing for more precise dosing. Phenylalanine is best taken with food.

■ Side Effects and Contraindications

Check with your doctor before starting an amino acid regimen if you have diabetes, hypertension, kidney disease, or liver disease. Phenylalanine should not be taken if you have phenylketonuria (PKU), if you are pregnant, or if you have schizophrenia.

Phenylalanine can interact with certain medications, ranging from MAO inhibitors to levodopa. Speak to your healthcare provider or pharmacist to learn if any of the drugs you're taking might make it unwise to use phenylalanine supplements.

The symptoms of phenylalanine toxicity can include:

- Agitation
- Hypertension
- Nerve damage
- Headache
- Insomnia

PROLINE

Proline is a conditionally essential amino acid that can be synthesized by the body from the amino acid glutamate in the presence of vitamin C. This substance can become depleted when large amounts are used, but you can get more of the proline your body needs from animal foods and dairy products.

This amino acid's best-known function is to synthesize collagen, which is used in the construction of arteries, ligaments, and tendons. Proline also helps regenerate cartilage, repair skin damage and wounds, and repair joints.

■ Functions of Proline in Your Body

- Combats arteriosclerosis (hardening of the arteries) by enabling the walls of the blood vessels to release fat
- Improves skin texture and promotes new cell formation
- Is needed to make collagen, the main structural protein found throughout the body
- Promotes tissue repair after soft tissue trauma
- Strengthens cartilage, connective tissue, joints, and tendons

■ Symptoms of Proline Deficiency

- ☐ Early signs of aging/skin wrinkling
- ☐ Sagging skin
- ☐ Stiff joints

■ Causes of Proline Deficiency

- Poor dietary intake of foods containing proline

Food Sources of Proline

- Bone broth
- Chicken
- Cottage cheese
- Dairy products
- Duck
- Eggs
- Pork
- Ricotta cheese
- Turkey

■ Conditions That Can Benefit from Proline

- Alzheimer's disease and other neurological diseases
- Arteriosclerosis (prevention)
- Arthritis
- Wrinkled skin (prevention)

■ Recommended Dosage

This amino acid doesn't usually have to be supplemented, so ask your doctor to test your amino acid levels before taking supplemental proline.

■ Side Effects and Contraindications

Check with your doctor before starting an amino acid regimen if you have diabetes, hypertension, kidney disease, or liver disease.

SERINE

The amino acid serine is nonessential; it is made by the body from the amino acid glycine, with folic acid, vitamin B_6, and vitamin B_3. Serine is used in many body functions, including the metabolism of fats and fatty acids, the growth of muscle and tissue, and the maintenance of the immune system.

■ Functions of Serine in Your Body

- Aids in muscle formation
- As a precursor to cysteine, is needed for the synthesis of glutathione
- Helps maintain a healthy immune system
- Helps manufacture the nerve cell sheath

- Is essential to good memory
- Needed for DNA synthesis
- Needed for the metabolism of fats and fatty acids
- Plays a part in the production of immunoglobulins and antibodies
- Required for the proper metabolism of methionine
- Stabilizes cell membranes
- Used in the formation of neurotransmitters (chemical "messengers" in the brain)

■ Symptoms of Serine Deficiency

☐ Cognitive decline

☐ Elevated levels of homocysteine, which can lead to heart disease, memory loss, prostate or breast cancer, depression, and bone loss

☐ Neurological problems such as cerebral palsy, congenital microcephaly, epilepsy, and seizures

☐ Problems with methionine metabolism

■ Causes of Serine Deficiency

Serine deficiency is a rare inherited disorder that prevents the body from manufacturing serine. Although this disease can be extremely serious, it is also very rare, and often goes undetected. Once diagnosed, however, serine deficiency is treatable. Other causes of serine deficiency include the following:

- Impaired ability to detoxify
- Increased demand for glutathione
- Kidney transplant resulting in mild elevation of creatinine

---

Food Sources of Serine

- Dairy products
- Eggs
- Pork
- Soy
- Tuna fish
- Turkey

■ Conditions That Can Benefit from Serine

- Possibly Alzheimer's disease
- Possibly amyotrophic lateral sclerosis (ALS)
- Serine deficiency

■ Recommended Dosage

Have your doctor order an amino acid test to determine the daily dosage. A common form of supplementation is phosphatidylserine.

■ Side Effects and Contraindications

Check with your doctor before starting an amino acid regimen if you have diabetes, hypertension, kidney disease, or liver disease.

TAURINE

Taurine is a conditionally essential amino acid, meaning that although it can usually be manufactured by the body, under certain conditions—such as illness and stress—the body may not be able to produce as much as is needed. In those cases, taurine supplementation can be helpful. Taurine is also found in animal foods, such as meat and dairy, as well as in some energy drinks.

Unlike most other amino acids, taurine is not used to build proteins. However, this sulfur-containing nutrient is one of the most abundant amino acids in the brain, retina, muscle tissue, and organs, and is used in numerous biological and physiological processes. Adequate levels of taurine decrease the risk of developing heart disease, hypertension, congestive heart failure, and epilepsy.

■ Functions of Taurine in Your Body

- Aids in glucose metabolism by increasing the activity of insulin receptors
- Aids in wound healing
- Decreases triglycerides
- Has antioxidant effects
- Helps regulate calcium levels
- Helps the liver detoxify damaging substances
- Improves fat metabolism in the liver
- Improves lung health
- Improves sensitivity to insulin
- Is a natural diuretic
- Is an inhibitory neurotransmitter (reduces activity of nerve cells)
- Lowers blood pressure
- Lowers LDL (bad) cholesterol
- Needed for kidney function
- Needed for the formation of bile acids
- Prevents blood clots
- Protects cell membranes from damage

- Stabilizes heart rhythms
- Stabilizes membranes
- Strengthens the heart muscle
- Supports the immune system

◼ Symptoms of Taurine Deficiency

- ☐ Allergies
- ☐ Angina
- ☐ Anxiety
- ☐ Chemical sensitivities
- ☐ Congestive heart failure
- ☐ Hyperactivity
- ☐ Hypercholesterolemia (high cholesterol)
- ☐ Hypertension (high blood pressure)
- ☐ Impaired brain function
- ☐ Insulin resistance/diabetes
- ☐ Irregular heart rhythm
- ☐ Night blindness
- ☐ Seizures
- ☐ Weight gain

◼ Causes of Taurine Deficiency

- Impaired detoxification
- Maldigestion of fat
- Stress
- Some medications can cause a taurine deficiency. Speak to your healthcare provider or pharmacist to learn if any of the drugs you're taking might be causing taurine loss.
- The following conditions and treatments can cause a taurine deficiency: aging process, cancer, congestive heart failure, diabetes, kidney disease, liver disease, obesity, and radiation.
- Vegetarian or vegan diet

◼ Conditions That Can Benefit from Taurine

- Allergies
- Attention-deficit/hyperactivity disorder (ADHD)
- Cardiac arrhythmia (irregular heart rhythm)
- Chemical sensitivities
- Chronic hepatitis
- Congestive heart failure (CHF)
- Cystic fibrosis
- Diabetic nephropathy (kidney disease related to diabetes)

- Diabetic neuropathy (numbness and tingling of the extremities due to diabetes)

- Diabetic retinopathy (eye disease related to diabetes)

- Hearing loss

- Heart disease, including arterial thickening and stiffness

- Hypercholesterolemia (high cholesterol)

- Hypertension (high blood pressure)

- Insulin resistance/diabetes

- Nonalcoholic fatty liver disease

- Psoriasis

- Seizure disorder

- Tinnitus (ringing in the ears)

- Weight gain

Food Sources of Taurine

- Beef
- Brewer's yeast
- Chicken (especially dark meat)
- Dairy products
- Eggs
- Fish
- Lamb
- Organ meats, such as liver
- Shellfish
- Turkey

▣ Recommended Dosage

Have your doctor order an amino acid test to determine the daily dosage. 1 to 4 grams a day is a common dose with normal kidney function.

▣ Side Effects and Contraindications

Taurine should not be taken with aspirin or salicylates. Speak to your healthcare provider or pharmacist to see if taurine might interact with any of your other medications. People with bipolar disorder should not take taurine, as it may exacerbate the condition.

Taurine is generally safe and causes no negative side effects when taken in prescribed amounts. Possible mild side effects can include the following:

- Dizziness

- Headache

- Itching

- Nausea

THREONINE

Threonine, an essential amino acid, is used as a building block to construct many of the body's proteins, as well as the important amino acids glycine and serine. It is also vital for proper functioning of the central nervous system, and it supports the immune system by aiding in the production of antibodies.

■ Functions of Threonine in Your Body

- Decreases spasms in leg muscles
- Helps metabolize fat
- Helps produce antibodies that boost the immune system
- Is a precursor of the amino acid glycine, which is a neurotransmitter (a chemical "messenger" in the brain)
- Needed for proper digestion
- Needed for the formation of tooth enamel, collagen, and elastin
- Prevents the build-up of fat in the liver
- Stabilizes blood sugar levels
- Stimulates the growth of the thymus gland

■ Symptoms of Threonine Deficiency

- ☐ Confusion
- ☐ Depression
- ☐ Hypoglycemia (low blood sugar)
- ☐ Immunosuppression
- ☐ Increased liver fat
- ☐ Indigestion
- ☐ Irritability
- ☐ Mental health deterioration
- ☐ Reduced growth

■ Causes of Threonine Deficiency

- High cortisol levels
- Increased need for glutathione
- Poor dietary intake of foods containing threonine

■ Conditions That Can Benefit from Threonine

- Amyotrophic lateral sclerosis (ALS)
- Familial spastic paraparesis
- Multiple sclerosis (MS)
- Spinal spasticity

Food Sources of Threonine

- Beans
- Chicken
- Corn
- Cottage cheese
- Dairy products
- Eggs
- Fish
- Green peas
- Legumes
- Meat
- Nuts
- Potatoes
- Seafood
- Spinach
- Turkey
- Watercress
- Whole grains

■ Recommended Daily Dosage

Have your doctor order an amino acid test to determine the daily dosage.

■ Side Effects and Contraindications

Check with your doctor before starting an amino acid regimen if you have diabetes, hypertension, kidney disease, or liver disease. Threonine is generally safe when taken in prescribed amounts. Possible mild side effects include:

- Headache
- Nausea
- Skin rash
- Stomach upset

TRYPTOPHAN

Tryptophan is an essential amino acid that must be consumed in the diet or as a supplement because the body cannot manufacture it. The primary function of this amino acid is to help synthesize protein, but it is needed for other functions as well. Perhaps the best known of these is serving as a precursor to serotonin—a neurotransmitter that is vital for the regulation of appetite, sleep, and mood.

■ Functions of Tryptophan in Your Body

- Acts as a mood stabilizer
- Is a precursor for the compound tryptamine
- Is a precursor for the neurotransmitter serotonin
- Decreases intestinal inflammation
- Helps with insomnia
- Is an inhibitory neurotransmitter (reduces activity of nerve cells)
- Necessary for protein synthesis
- Necessary for the growth of infants

- Necessary for the production of vitamin B$_3$ (niacin)

- Necessary for the release of growth hormone

- Suppresses appetite

■ Symptoms of Tryptophan Deficiency

- ☐ Aggression
- ☐ Anxiety
- ☐ Cognitive decline
- ☐ Decreased zinc levels
- ☐ Depression

- ☐ Impaired growth
- ☐ Increased pain sensitivity
- ☐ Insomnia
- ☐ Pellagra
- ☐ Weight gain

■ Causes of Tryptophan Deficiency

- Aging process
- Elevated serotonin synthesis
- Poor intake of foods high in tryptophan
- Poor intake of foods high in vitamin B$_3$ (tryptophan may be used to make B$_3$, depleting the body's tryptophan)
- Pro-inflammatory cytokines, which can cause tryptophan to degrade in the blood

---

Food Sources of Tryptophan

- Beans
- Brown rice
- Chicken
- Dairy products
- Eggs

- Fish
- Grains
- Lentils
- Meats
- Milk

- Nuts
- Pork
- Seeds
- Turkey

■ Conditions That Can Benefit from Tryptophan

- Anxiety disorder
- Attention-deficit/hyperactivity disorder (ADHD)
- Bruxism (grinding of teeth)

- Depression
- Facial pain
- Inflammatory bowel disease (IBD)
- Insomnia

- Obsessive compulsive disorder (OCD)
- Parkinson's disease
- Premenstrual dysphoric disorder (PMDD)
- Schizophrenia

- Serotonin deficiency
- Sleep apnea
- Tourette syndrome
- Weight gain

■ Recommended Dosage

5 to 50 milligrams daily. Tryptophan works best when taken with vitamin B_6.

■ Side Effects and Contraindications

Check with your doctor before starting an amino acid regimen if you have diabetes, hypertension, kidney disease, or liver disease. Do not take tryptophan if you are pregnant or breastfeeding.

Some medications, such as MAO inhibitors, can interact poorly with tryptophan. Speak to your healthcare provider or pharmacist to learn if any drugs you're taking might make it unwise to take tryptophan.

TYROSINE

Tyrosine is a conditionally essential amino acid, which means that although it can be manufactured by the body, under certain conditions, the body may not be able to produce what is required. The body synthesizes tyrosine from phenylalanine. People with a condition known as phenylketonuria cannot convert phenylalanine into tyrosine and must obtain tyrosine from their diet or from supplements.

Tyrosine is a building block for proteins. It is also the precursor of several neurotransmitters, including dopamine, epinephrine, and norepinephrine; of the thyroid hormones T3 and T4; and of melanin, the pigment in the skin, hair, and eyes.

■ Functions of Tyrosine in Your Body

- Has antioxidant activity
- Helps form the pigment melanin

- Helps regulate growth metabolism
- Improves mental performance in stressful situations

- Improves mood in stressful environmental situations such as cold or high altitudes
- Is the precursor of the neurotransmitters dopamine, epinephrine, and norepinephrine
- Is the precursor of the thyroid hormones
- Lowers blood pressure
- Suppresses chronic fatigue
- Suppresses appetite
- Used to maintain mitochondrial function (energy production)

■ Symptoms of Tyrosine Deficiency

- ☐ Aggression
- ☐ Anxiety
- ☐ Apathy
- ☐ Blood sugar imbalance
- ☐ Depression
- ☐ Edema
- ☐ Fat loss
- ☐ Fatigue
- ☐ Flu-like symptoms
- ☐ Lethargy
- ☐ Liver damage
- ☐ Loss of pigmentation in hair
- ☐ Low blood pressure
- ☐ Low serum levels of essential proteins
- ☐ Mood disorders
- ☐ Muscle loss
- ☐ Poor temperature regulation
- ☐ Restless leg syndrome
- ☐ Skin lesions
- ☐ Stress
- ☐ Unexplained weight gain
- ☐ Weakness

■ Causes of Tyrosine Deficiency

- Medications such as estrogen and antiandrogen therapies can cause tyrosine deficiency. Speak to your healthcare provider or pharmacist to learn if any drugs you're taking might be causing tyrosine loss.

- Nutritional deficiencies, including inadequate amounts of folate; vitamins B_3, B_6, B_{12}, C, and D; iron; and copper

- Phenylketonuria (condition that prevents the body from turning phenylalanine into tyrosine)

- Poor dietary intake of foods high in phenylalanine

- Poor dietary intake of foods high in tyrosine

■ Conditions That Can Benefit from Tyrosine

- Alcohol and cocaine withdrawal
- Alzheimer's disease

- Attention-deficit/hyperactivity disorder (ADHD)
- Caffeine and nicotine withdrawal
- Chronic fatigue syndrome
- Depression
- Erectile dysfunction
- Hepatocellular carcinoma
- Hypothyroidism
- Narcolepsy
- Obesity
- Parkinson's disease
- Poor adaptation to stress
- Premenstrual syndrome (PMS)
- Reward deficiency syndrome
- Schizophrenia
- Wrinkles (apply to the skin)

Food Sources of Tyrosine

- Almonds
- Avocados
- Bananas
- Beans
- Cheese
- Corn
- Cottage cheese
- Dairy products
- Eggs
- Fish
- Legumes
- Lima beans
- Meat
- Milk
- Nuts
- Potatoes
- Pumpkin seeds
- Seafood
- Soy
- Spinach
- Whey
- Whole grains

■ Recommended Dosage

500 to 2,000 milligrams daily. Start at 100 milligrams a day and increase the dose gradually.

■ Side Effects and Contraindications

Check with your doctor before starting an amino acid regimen if you have diabetes, hypertension, kidney disease, or liver disease. Do not take tyrosine if you have malignant melanoma. Furthermore, use only under the direction of a healthcare provider if you have Grave's disease.

Some drugs, from thyroid hormone replacement to antidepressants, should not be taken with tyrosine. Speak to your healthcare provider or pharmacist to learn if tyrosine can be used in combination with the medications you are taking.

Some people experience hypertension (high blood pressure), hypotension (low blood pressure), or migraine headaches when taking tyrosine supplementation. If any of these manifestations occur, discontinue use. Other possible side effects of tyrosine include:

- Arthralgia (a form of joint pain)
- Fatigue
- GI upset
- Heartburn
- Insomnia
- Nausea
- Nervousness

5

Herbs

An herb is a plant whose leaves, seeds, roots, berries, bark, or flowers are used for culinary or medicinal purposes. There is no strict division between herbs that are used in the kitchen and those that are employed for healing. Most culinary herbs have medicinal uses, as well. The healing properties of herbs are thought to be largely due to their *phytonutrients*—chemical compounds found only in plants that develop to protect the plant, but also offer benefits to human beings. In fact, more than 40 percent of the medications used today have been based on phytonutrients, and it is estimated that nearly 80 percent of the world's population uses herbs for some aspect of primary health care.

In this chapter, we will explore the healing powers of a number of herbs, each of which can help you achieve optimal health in a different way. Some have properties that reduce inflammation, some improve memory and brain function, some boost your immune system, some improve the health of your heart, and some have other beneficial effects on your body and mind.

Because plants have long been known to have medicinal properties, in recent years, pharmaceutical companies have begun to isolate the most active ingredients in various herbs and sell them individually. Most people now agree, however, that important substances are left behind when these targeted ingredients are extracted. The other ingredients may have any of a number of purposes, such as curbing or enhancing the main ingredient's full effect. Some herbalists even believe that medicinal plants should be used only as they are found in nature.

Regardless of whether you choose pharmaceutical grade herbal supplements or whole herbs, you must utilize them correctly and appropriately. Because herbs are natural, they are often considered safer than prescription drugs. But herbs contain potent substances that can potentially have harmful effects—especially when taken without consideration for proper guidelines and precautions, or when taken with certain medications. (See "Mixing Supplements, Drugs, and Food" on page 9.) Always read all directions before taking an herbal supplement. You should also consult your doctor before starting any supplement regimen—particularly if you have kidney or liver disease or are pregnant or nursing. Your pharmacist is another good source of information about herb and drug interactions.

Be aware that unlike prescription drugs, the contents of dietary supplements such as herbs are not regulated by the U.S. government. Always read the full ingredient list before ingesting any herb, looking specifically for the elements discussed in the section "Buying Herbal Supplements," below.

BUYING HERBAL SUPPLEMENTS

Dietary supplements are not regulated by the Food and Drug Administration (FDA), so it is up to you—and your healthcare provider—to be fully aware of what you are putting in your body. Familiarize yourself with the following tests, which will help you determine a product's quality and potential effectiveness. Every herbal supplement you take should pass each test. First check the side of the product's packaging for the applicable information. If the facts are not there or are unclear, you can call the company or visit its website. If the answers to your questions remain unavailable after checking these sources, it's best to avoid the products of that company. After all, most companies that properly examine their products will make the results readily available to their customers. (For more information on buying high-quality supplements, see the inset on page 18 of Chapter 1.)

Authenticity

Buy only those herbal supplements that have clearly labeled lists of ingredients and amounts. Unfortunately, these lists are not always reliable. Some companies identify the herbs they use based on the plant's appearance, which can lead to mistakes, because many herbs look alike. Less reputable companies may even knowingly turn a blind eye to this problem due to the high cost of certain medicinal herbs. More reliable companies use tests, such as a technique called thin layer chromatography (TLC), to scientifically identify the product's compounds and verify that the correct herb is being packaged.

Potency

A supplement's potency refers to its concentration of active ingredients. This detail is very important. After all, low potency usually means that the product will provide you with little or no results—and some herbal supplements are very expensive. There are tests the company can perform to determine a product's potency. One such test is the high-performance liquid chromatography (HPLC), which separates and identifies the product's molecules.

In order for a supplement to be potent, it must be absorbed by your body. To test how well it can be absorbed, drop an herbal supplement into a glass of water and watch what happens. The herbs should dissolve. An herb that doesn't dissolve will probably not have consistent potency since it will not be well absorbed.

Purity

An herbal supplement is not pure if it contains any extraneous material or if its composition has been altered in any way. You can request that a company provide you with laboratory certificates ensuring that its product's purity has been tested.

Examining and tasting the product may allow you to determine if the product may have been adulterated. The following are some examples of qualities that would suggest your supplement is impure.

- If it has a gritty texture when chewed, it probably contains improper ingredients.

- If it is darker in color than usual or tastes particularly bitter, the herbs may have been burnt—which destroys the herb's active components and their effectiveness.

- If it tastes sweet or is sticky to the touch, a high percentage of the supplement may be made of sugar rather than the proper ingredients.

Safety

It is very important that the safety of a product be thoroughly tested. Some companies do not perform these tests. Other companies perform the tests on a random sampling of their products. The companies from which you buy herbal supplements should test every batch of herbs they put on the market. When a product passes this inspection, the company is usually given a Certificate of Analysis (COA). You can request proof of this certificate before purchasing a company's products.

USING HERBS

There are a variety of different ways to utilize medicinal herbs, and we explore several possibilities below. I suggest experimenting with each of the following options before determining which you will use regularly.

Compresses

You can make a *compress* by soaking a clean cloth in an herbal solution. (For instructions on making herbal solutions, see "Decoctions and Infusions," below.) Wring out the cloth to remove excess liquid. Then apply the compress to your body. If you have a specific pain, apply the cloth to that area, such as your head or back. The herbs will be absorbed into your skin, and your blood vessels will transport the active ingredients throughout your body.

Decoctions and Infusions

While most people are acquainted with herbal teas, there are two other water-based preparations that can help you benefit from the healing qualities of herbs. Both decoctions and infusions are stronger than herbal teas.

A *decoction* is an herbal solution made by cooking hard and woody parts of a plant that would not yield the plant's active compounds through steeping. To make a decoction, first break up pieces of the bark, roots, or seeds of the plant. Do not cut or crush the plant pieces, since vital constituents can be lost. Place from one teaspoon to one tablespoon of the plant pieces per cup of cold water in a pot made from a nonreactive material, such as stainless steel or enamel. (Do not use aluminum.) Turn the heat to medium and simmer the decoction with the lid off until the volume of the liquid is reduced by one quarter. (For instance, if you start with a pint of water, or sixteen ounces, simmer the mixture until you have twelve ounces left.) Allow the decoction to cool, and strain out the plant pieces before using the solution to make a compress or a drink. Store in the refrigerator for no more than seventy-two hours.

Unlike decoctions, water-based *infusions* are not simmered and do not use the tough woody parts of the plant. However, they are allowed to steep for a longer period of time than teas—sometimes, overnight.

To make an infusion, place one tablespoon of dried flowers, leaves, or stems or three tablespoons of fresh herbs in a ceramic teapot or mug for each cup you wish to brew. Pour one cup of boiling water over the herbs, cover the teapot or mug, and allow the herbs to steep for ten to fifteen minutes or overnight. Strain out the plant pieces before drinking or using to make a compress. If you want to avoid the straining process, place the herbs in a muslin tea bag or stainless steel tea infuser before adding the water. Store for up to forty-eight hours in the refrigerator.

Teas

An herbal tea is made specifically for drinking, and therefore is steeped for a shorter period than an infusion to avoid a bitter-tasting brew. To prepare the tea, place one teaspoon of dried flowers, leaves, or stems or two teaspoons of fresh herbs in a ceramic pot or mug for each cup you wish to brew. Pour one cup of boiling water over the herbs, and allow the herbs to steep uncovered for five minutes. Strain out the plant pieces before drinking, adding honey for flavor and sweetness if desired, but adding no milk. If you want to avoid the straining process, place the herbs in a muslin tea bag or stainless steel tea infuser before adding the water. Drink hot or cold, storing in the refrigerator for up to twenty-four hours.

Most people find it beneficial to drink one cup of herbal tea three times a day. To change the taste and intensity, experiment using more or less of the herb.

Poultices

A *poultice* is a paste made of ground herbs and oil or warm water that is applied directly to the skin or wrapped in a piece of thin cloth and applied to the skin. Usually, the poultice is kept in contact with the skin for several hours with the goal of relieving inflammation and soreness. You may want to reheat the poultice when it cools off. Poultices are usually effective for twenty-four hours.

Tablets and Capsules

Herbs can be bought in tablet or capsule form. You can either take them with a glass of water or dissolve them in hot water before drinking. Tablets and capsules are undoubtedly the most convenient way to take herbs.

ALOE VERA

The cactus-like aloe vera plant (*Aloe barbadensis*), which is native to southern Africa, is easy to recognize by its spear-shaped leaves, which grow from the base of the plant. The clear gel-like center of the plant's leaves is extracted and used for skin burns, infections, and wounds, and is applied as a topical ointment, gel, or spray. It can also be taken orally, although this has been less studied than the topical treatment. The yellowish liquid found between the gel and outer leaf is latex. This can be dried and ingested.

Aloe vera contains seventy-five active constituents, including vitamins, minerals, enzymes, sugars, lignin, salicylic acids, and amino acids.

■ Functions of Aloe Vera in Your Body

- Encourages healing by increasing the collagen content of the wound
- Has antibiotic and antiseptic properties
- Protects against radiation damage to the skin
- Reduces inflammation
- Relieves pain from certain skin conditions
- Slows aging of the skin by binding moisture to it
- Strengthens the immune system
- Works as a laxative by increasing intestinal water content and stimulating mucus secretion and intestinal peristalsis (wavelike movements)

■ Conditions That Can Benefit from Aloe Vera

Topical Aloe Vera

- Burns
- Canker sores
- Dandruff
- Eczema
- Frostbite
- Genital herpes (male)
- Herpes simplex
- Lichen planus
- Pressure ulcers
- Psoriasis
- Radiation dermatitis
- Seborrheic dermatitis
- Skin infections
- Various wounds

Oral Aloe Vera (Juice or Capsules)

- Acne
- AIDS
- Asthma
- Cancer prevention
- Constipation
- Diabetes
- Frostbite
- Immune weakness
- Inflammation
- Inflammatory bowel disease (IBD)
- Peptic ulcer disease

■ Recommended Dosage

Aloe vera can be applied topically in the form of a cream or gel, consumed as a juice, or taken as an oral supplement.

- Creams and gels with aloe vera (topical aloe vera) vary in dosage. Some creams for minor burns have only 0.5 percent aloe vera, while others used for skin conditions such as psoriasis may contain as much as 70 percent aloe vera.

- Aloe vera juice: 25 milliliters (about 1 ounce) up to four times daily.

- Oral supplement: 500 to 800 milligrams daily of standardized acemannan (aloe vera's active ingredient).

■ Side Effects and Contraindications

High oral doses of aloe or aloe latex are dangerous. Do not exceed the manufacturer's recommendations.

Topical Aloe Vera

Test any aloe vera topical product—including gel taken directly from the plant—on a small area first to test for a possible allergic reaction. Do not use it on deep surgical wounds. Do not use if you are allergic to latex. Possible side effects can include:

- Burning
- General dermatitis (rare)

- Redness
- Stinging

Oral Aloe Vera (Juice or Capsules)

Oral aloe vera lowers potassium levels, which can be especially dangerous if you're taking certain medications, such as digoxin or furosemide. Speak to your healthcare provider or pharmacist to learn if any drugs you're taking might make it unwise to use oral aloe vera. Do not take aloe vera if you have low potassium levels.

Do not use oral aloe vera if you are allergic to plants in the Liliaceae (lily) family or to latex.

Oral aloe vera may cause the following side effects:

- Abdominal cramps
- Diarrhea
- Hepatitis

- Nausea
- Red-colored urine
- Worsening of constipation

ASHWAGANDHA

Grown in India, Pakistan, and Sri Lanka, ashwagandha (*Withania somnifera*) is part of the nightshade family. The roots of ashwagandha are known to improve resistance to emotional and physical stress and to benefit the body in other ways, as well.

Herbs to Treat Inflammation

Herbs can help the body heal a variety of ailments. The herbs on the following list, for example, have anti-inflammatory properties. They can help decrease both inflammation and the pain that's associated with it. For suggestions on buying herbal supplements as well as various ways to utilize them, see pages 186 to 189.

One of the ways in which herbs combat inflammation is to act as COX-2 inhibitors—substances that directly target COX-2, an enzyme responsible for inflammation and pain. There are COX-2 inhibitor medications that work very well but may have side effects, such as increased blood pressure. When botanicals block the action of COX-2, there is less of a tendency to have undesirable consequences. In the list below, some of the herbs are marked as being natural COX-2 inhibitors. The other herbs help relieve inflammation in other ways. To learn more about the herbs listed below, read the full entries presented in this chapter.

- Aloe vera (*Aloe barbadensis*).
- American skullcap (*Scutellaria lateriflora*). Natural COX-2 inhibitor.
- Boswellia (*Boswellia serrata*).
- Cayenne pepper (*Capsicum annuum*). Natural COX-2 inhibitor.
- Chinese skullcap (*Scutellaria baicalensis*). Natural COX-2 inhibitor.
- Curcumin/Turmeric (*Curcuma longa*). Natural COX-2 inhibitor.
- Feverfew (*Tanacetum parthenium*). Natural COX-2 inhibitor.
- Ginger (*Zingiber officinale*). Natural COX-2 inhibitor.
- Ginkgo biloba (*Ginkgo biloba*).
- Green tea (*Camellia sinensis*). Natural COX-2 inhibitor.
- Licorice root (*Glycyrrhiza glabra*).
- Rosemary (*Rosmarinus officinalis*). Natural COX-2 inhibitor.
- Thyme (*Thymus vulgaris*). Natural COX-2 inhibitor.
- White willow (*Salix alba*). Natural COX-2 inhibitor.

■ Functions of Ashwagandha in Your Body

- Activates the immune system
- Enhances endurance and strength
- Has antibacterial properties
- Has anti-inflammatory properties
- Has cytotoxic (cell-killing) and tumor-sensitizing actions
- Helps preserve adrenal function
- Helps with stress reduction
- Increases libido and sexual performance
- Increases muscle mass
- Is an antioxidant
- Lowers cholesterol
- Protects the liver

■ Conditions That Can Benefit from Ashwagandha

- Anxiety
- Asthma
- Back pain
- Constipation
- Coronary heart disease
- Depression
- Fever
- Fibromyalgia
- Hiccups
- Hypercholesterolemia (high cholesterol)
- Hypothyroidism (underactive thyroid)
- Infection (antibacterial and antifungal)
- Inflammation
- Insomnia
- Insulin resistance
- Memory loss
- Mood swings
- Osteoarthritis
- Stress
- Tardive dyskinesia (involuntary muscle movements)
- Weakness

■ Recommended Dosage

Ashwagandha is available in capsule form or can be made into a tea.

- Capsule: 500 to 2,000 milligrams daily.
- Dried root prepared in tea: 3 to 4 grams daily.

■ Side Effects and Contraindications

The following side effects may occur when using ashwagandha:

- Diarrhea
- Nausea
- Vomiting

ASTRAGALUS

Astragalus (*Astragalus membranaceus*) belongs to the pea family. The astragalus root contains an isoflavone that can enhance metabolism and digestion, as well as treat related problems. Astragalus also contains triterpenoid saponins, substances that are believed to lower cholesterol levels and have antioxidant effects. Furthermore, this herb contains polysaccharides that strengthen the immune system.

■ Functions of Astragalus in Your Body

- Enhances digestion by strengthening the intestine's movement and muscle tone
- Helps regulate the immune system
- Improves sperm motility
- Increases blood flow
- Is an antioxidant
- Lowers blood pressure
- Lowers blood sugar
- Lowers cholesterol
- Protects the liver
- Protects the nerves

■ Conditions That Can Benefit from Astragalus

- Allergies
- Angina
- Asthma
- Cancer (as adjunct to chemotherapy and to decrease side effects)
- Cerebral ischemia (insufficient blood flow to the brain)
- Chronic fatigue syndrome
- Chronic kidney disease
- Cognitive decline
- Congestive heart failure
- Cough, colds, and upper respiratory tract infections
- Diabetes
- Exposure to toxins
- Fibromyalgia
- HIV/AIDS
- Hypercholesterolemia (high cholesterol)
- Hypertension (high blood pressure)
- Kidney dysfunction caused by lithotripsy treatments
- Male infertility
- Stress
- Stroke (post-stroke treatment)
- Viral infection (prevention and treatment)

■ Recommended Dosage

Dose depends on health status, age, renal function, and weight. The following are common doses:

- 250 to 500 milligrams of standardized extract three to four times daily.

- 2 to 4 milliliters 1:1 fluid extract three times daily.

■ Side Effects and Contraindications

Do not take astragalus after an organ transplant or if you have an allergy to gum tragacanth.

Astragalus may interact with medications that affect the immune system, such as drugs taken by organ transplant recipients and some cancer patients. It can also interact with steroids and lithium. Speak to your healthcare provider or pharmacist to learn if astragalus might interact with any of the drugs you're taking.

Although astragalus is considered safe for most adults, commonly reported side effects include gastrointestinal issues such as diarrhea.

BILBERRY

The bilberry (*Vaccinium myrtillus*) is a relative of the blueberry, and its berries and leaves have been used for medicinal purposes for centuries. The berries of the plant have a high concentration of antioxidants called anthocyanins, which are known to provide many health benefits. One of the bilberry's most important functions is safeguarding eye function, but it is believed to enhance well-being in a number of other ways, as well.

■ Functions of Bilberry in Your Body

- As an antioxidant, protects the eye against free radical damage

- Decreases inflammation

- Has antibacterial properties

- Has antiviral properties

- Helps your eyes adapt to the dark

- Improves circulation

- Improves failing eyesight

- Reduces the effects of diabetic retinopathy

- Reduces the risk of cardiovascular disease by decreasing LDL (bad) cholesterol and increasing HDL (good) cholesterol

- Slows the progression of cataracts

- Stabilizes DNA

■ Conditions That Can Benefit from Bilberry

- Atherosclerosis
- Cataracts
- Chronic fatigue syndrome
- Constipation
- Diabetes
- Diabetic retinopathy (eye disease due to diabetes, both prevention and treatment)
- Diarrhea
- Doxorubicin-induced cardiotoxicity (prevention)
- Dry eye
- Eye fatigue and strain
- Glaucoma

- Gout
- Hemorrhoids
- Hypercholesterolemia (high cholesterol)
- Kidney disease
- Liver damage (prevention)
- Macular degeneration
- Osteoarthritis
- Poor circulation
- Problems with night vision
- Retinitis pigmentosa
- Ulcerative colitis
- Urinary tract infection
- Varicose veins

■ Recommended Dosage

60 to 120 milligrams twice a day.

■ Side Effects and Contraindications

Bilberry may interfere with iron absorption. If you are anemic, discuss bilberry supplementation with your healthcare provider before starting a regimen. High doses should be used with caution in people with bleeding disorders.

BITTER MELON

Bitter melon (*Momordica charantia*), also called bitter gourd, is a tropical fruit widely used in Asia, Africa, and South America. This fruit is best known for its ability to lower blood sugar, and it has been used for this purpose for centuries. A study of one of bitter melon's active components, polypeptide-p (an insulin-like protein), found it to be a more potent hypoglycemic agent than the medication tolbutamide. Bitter melon is also known to offer a range of other health benefits.

▪ Functions of Bitter Melon in Your Body

- Has anticancer actions
- Has antibacterial properties
- Has anti-inflammatory properties
- Is antiviral
- Is antiprotozoal and anti-parasitic
- Lowers blood sugar
- Lowers lipids
- Promotes wound healing
- Reduces pain

▪ Conditions That Can Benefit from Bitter Melon

- Cancer
- HIV/AIDS
- Infection
- Insulin resistance/diabetes
- Wounds

▪ Recommended Dosage

Bitter melon can be taken as a capsule or consumed as a juice.

- Capsule: 500 to 1,000 milligrams daily.
- Juice: 50 to 100 milliliters daily.

▪ Side Effects and Contraindications

Do not use bitter melon if you are pregnant or breastfeeding. Do not use if you are male and are trying to initiate a pregnancy, since it may decrease sperm activity, or if you are female and trying to get pregnant. If you have blood sugar problems, monitor your blood sugar on a regular basis while using this supplement, since it lowers blood sugar.

Generally, bitter melon causes few side effects. When they do occur, they can include:

- Abdominal pain
- Diarrhea
- Headache
- Low blood sugar

BLACK COHOSH

Black cohosh (*Actaea racemosa*) is native to North America and has a long history of use. It is known as a pain reliever and is particularly helpful for muscle soreness. Moreover, black cohosh is often recommended to women going through menopause. It is believed that this plant may lessen the duration and severity of certain menopausal symptoms, including hot flashes, night sweats, anxiety, and vaginal dryness.

■ Functions of Black Cohosh in Your Body

- Lowers blood pressure
- Lowers LDL (bad) cholesterol
- May relieve mild depression
- Relieves muscle soreness
- Helps to decrease some menopausal symptoms, such as hot flashes and vaginal dryness

■ Conditions That Can Benefit from Black Cohosh

- Cardiovascular problems
- Fibrocystic breast disease
- Menopausal symptoms
- Menstrual migraines (with soy and dong quai)
- Muscle pain
- Osteoarthritis
- Osteoporosis
- Premenstrual syndrome (PMS)
- Prostate cancer
- Rheumatoid arthritis
- Uterine fibroids

■ Recommended Dosage

40 to 160 milligrams daily for no longer than six months.

■ Side Effects and Contraindications

Do not use black cohosh if you have liver damage or drink alcohol excessively. Do not use during pregnancy, since it may stimulate uterine contractions; and avoid if you have hormonally related breast, ovarian, or endometrial cancer. Use with caution if you have fibroids or endometriosis.

A number of side effects are possible with black cohosh, including:

- Abdominal pain
- Decreased heart rate
- Diarrhea
- Dizziness
- Headache
- Impaired circulation
- Joint pain
- Nausea
- Shortness of breath
- Tremors
- Vertigo
- Vision changes
- Vomiting
- Weight gain

BOSWELLIA

The boswellia tree (*Boswellia serrata*) grows in mountainous regions of India, North Africa, and the Middle East, and for thousands of years, its resin has been used both as incense and in medicine. The extract of the tree is a powerful anti-inflammatory that has been found effective in treating a number of inflammatory conditions—such as osteoarthritis, rheumatoid arthritis, and asthma—and in relieving the pain often associated with these conditions. Boswellia also appears to suppress tumor growth and to have other beneficial properties.

■ Functions of Boswellia in Your Body

- Has strong anti-inflammatory properties
- Is toxic to cancer cells
- Lowers blood sugar levels
- Lowers cholesterol levels
- Raises levels of HDL (good) cholesterol
- Reduces pain
- Regulates the immune system

■ Conditions That Can Benefit from Boswellia

- Acute respiratory distress syndrome (ARDS)
- Asthma
- Cancer
- Chronic bronchitis
- Cystic fibrosis
- Hypercholesterolemia (high cholesterol)
- Insulin resistance/diabetes
- Irritable bowel disease
- Osteoarthritis
- Peptic ulcer disease
- Psoriasis
- Rheumatoid arthritis

■ Recommended Dosage

300 to 500 milligrams of an extract standardized to contain 30 to 40 percent boswellic acids, taken two to three times daily. The complete effect may take several weeks.

■ Side Effects and Contraindications

Do not use boswellia if you are pregnant. It may stimulate blood flow in the uterus and pelvis and therefore may increase menstrual flow and induce miscarriage. Boswellia may also interact with NSAIDs, including aspirin. Speak to your healthcare provider or pharmacist to learn if the actions of any of the drugs you're taking might be affected by boswellia.

Common side effects of boswellia include the following:

- Acid reflux
- Diarrhea
- Nausea
- Skin rashes

BUTCHER'S BROOM

Butcher's broom (*Ruscus aculeatus*) is a shrub that grows in the Mediterranean regions of Europe. The young stems and roots have for many years been used medicinally and are now especially valued as a treatment for inflammatory conditions and poor circulation.

■ Functions of Butcher's Broom in Your Body

- Improves venous blood flow
- Is a natural anticoagulant
- Is a vasoconstrictor
- Is an anti-inflammatory

■ Conditions That Can Benefit from Butcher's Broom

- Hemorrhoids
- Orthostatic hypotension (decrease in blood pressure when changing position)
- Varicose veins (enlarged, twisted veins)
- Venous insufficiency (failure of veins to circulate blood)

■ Recommended Dosage

Butcher's broom can be taken orally as a supplement or used as a topical cream to treat hemorrhoids.

- Oral supplement: 7 to 11 milligrams daily of standardized ruscogenin (butcher's broom extract).
- Topical cream for hemorrhoids: Apply twice a day.

■ Side Effects and Contraindications

Butcher's broom is a natural anticoagulant. If you have a bleeding disorder or are taking a medication or supplement that may thin your blood, do not take or apply this herb. If you are planning to have surgery, discontinue this herbal therapy two weeks before the procedure.

This supplement can interact with MAO inhibitors and alpha blockers. Speak to your healthcare provider or pharmacist to learn if any drugs you're taking may make it unwise to use butcher's broom. Do not use butcher's broom during pregnancy or if you are breastfeeding.

Possible side effects of butcher's broom include the following:

- Loose and frequent bowel movements
- Nausea
- Stomach upset
- Uterine contractions

CAT'S CLAW

Cat's claw (*Uncaria tomentosa*) is a vine that grows in the tropical areas of Central and South America. Its name is derived from its claw-like thorns.

There are two different species of cat's claw: *Uncaria guianensis* and *Uncaria tomentosa*. This discussion deals with the latter, which has been found to have numerous medicinal uses due to its powerful anti-inflammatory and antioxidant effects.

■ Functions of Cat's Claw in Your Body

- Boosts immune system function
- Can cleanse and treat the gastrointestinal tract
- Improves mental abilities
- Improves white blood cell function
- Is a diuretic
- Is an anti-inflammatory
- Is an antioxidant
- Lowers blood pressure
- May inhibit the growth of cancer cells since it has anti-proliferative effects and supports apoptosis (programmed cell death)

■ Conditions That Can Benefit from Cat's Claw

- AIDS
- Alzheimer's disease
- Asthma
- Cancer (treatment of glioblastoma and neutropenia after chemotherapy)
- Chronic fatigue syndrome
- Crohn's disease
- Diarrhea
- Diverticulitis
- Gastric ulcers

- Gastritis
- Hay fever
- Hemorrhoids
- Inflammation
- Leaky gut syndrome

- Rheumatoid arthritis
- Shingles
- Ulcers
- Wound healing

■ Recommended Dosage

- 200 milligrams daily.

■ Side Effects and Contraindications

Do not take cat's claw if you have leukemia or if you are pregnant or nursing. Cat's claw can lower blood pressure, so use with caution if you are taking a drug that lowers blood pressure.

Cat's claw has mild blood-thinning effects. If you have a bleeding disorder or are taking a medication or supplement that may thin your blood, do not take this herb. If you are planning to have surgery, discontinue this herbal therapy two weeks before the procedure. Speak to your healthcare provider or pharmacist to learn if any drugs you're taking might make it unwise to use cat's claw.

Use this herb with caution if you have had an autoimmune disease, skin grafts, tuberculosis, or have had an organ transplant. Also use with caution if you have kidney or liver disease.

The following are possible side effects of cat's claw supplementation:

- Allergies that can cause kidney inflammation and rashes
- Altered heart rhythm
- Ataxia (lack of muscle coordination)

- Diarrhea
- Hormonal changes
- Nausea
- Stomach discomfort

CAYENNE/CAPSAICIN

Cayenne (*Capsicum annuum*) is popular as a cooking spice. However, cayenne also has a number of healing abilities, including the potential to improve the function of the circulatory and digestive systems and to significantly reduce pain.

Many of cayenne's health benefits are thought to be the result of the fruit's active component, capsaicin, although it also contains a range of nutrients, from vitamins A and C to carotenoids. Capsaicin is thought to ease pain in a unique way. The compound stimulates nerve endings so they release substance P, which transmits pain signals to the brain. When a nerve ending has released all of its substance P reserves, pain signals are no longer sent to the brain until substance P has been replenished. The sensation of pain then decreases or resolves.

In the discussion below, I recommend using oral cayenne supplements or a topical cream. If you also want to include cayenne peppers in your diet, keep in mind that these peppers are very potent. After handling them, wash your hands thoroughly. If you have a difficult time getting cayenne off your skin, wash it with vinegar. Avoid contact between cayenne and your eyes, any open wounds, or your mucous membranes.

■ Functions of Cayenne/Capsaicin in Your Body

- Aids digestive health by increasing digestive fluid production and delivering enzymes to the stomach

- Diminishes the awareness of pain

- Has anti-inflammatory actions

- Improves blood flow and circulation

- Is an antioxidant

- Lowers blood sugar levels

- Lowers LDL (bad) cholesterol

■ Conditions That Can Benefit from Cayenne/Capsaicin

- Cluster headaches

- Heart disease

- Indigestion

- Inflammation

- Insulin resistance/diabetes

- Irregular heartbeat (arrhythmia)

- Muscle cramps

- Nerve pain

- Obesity

- Osteoarthritis

- Peripheral neuropathy (numbness and tingling of the extremities) due to diabetes

- Poor appetite

- Psoriasis

- Rheumatoid arthritis

- Shingles

- Sore throat

■ Recommended Dosage

Cayenne/capsaicin can be taken orally or used topically.

- Capsule: 20 to 100 milligrams, three times a day.

- Topical cream: Apply a thin coat three times a day for three weeks.

■ Side Effects and Contraindications

Oral Cayenne/Capsaicin

Individuals who are allergic to latex, bananas, kiwis, chestnuts, and avocados may also be allergic to cayenne and should avoid this pepper. Pregnant and nursing mothers should avoid cayenne and its active ingredient, capsaicin.

Capsaicin can interact with a large number of medications, from ACE inhibitors to antacids and pain relievers. Speak to your healthcare provider or pharmacist to learn if any drugs you're taking might make it unwise to use supplemental capsaicin.

Supplements may cause the following side effects:

- Heartburn
- Stomach irritation
- Vomiting

- Nausea
- Ulcers

If any of these symptoms occur, stop taking capsaicin. Symptoms of cayenne toxicity can include:

- Gastroenteritis
- Kidney damage
- Liver damage

Topical Cayenne/Capsaicin

Topical capsaicin can cause burning or itching in some individuals. This usually subsides after several uses. If it does not, discontinue use. Test the capsaicin cream on a small area of your skin before applying it to larger areas.

Do not use capsaicin with a heating pad, and do not apply capsaicin cream immediately before or after a hot shower, as this can increase the burning sensation.

CHAMOMILE

Chamomile (*Matricaria recutita*) is one of the oldest and best-known medicinal herbs. Its flowers have been used for their calming and anti-inflammatory effects, as a pain reliever, and as a sleep aid for ages. Yet chamomile has many other healthful functions, such as treating stomach disorders and fighting cancer.

■ Functions of Chamomile in Your Body

- Acts as a sleep aid/sedative
- Aids digestion
- Decreases inflammation
- Has anti-cancer properties
- Has anti-spasmodic effects

- Has calming effects
- Is a muscle relaxant
- Relieves pain
- Relieves stress

■ Conditions That Can Benefit from Chamomile

- Anxiety
- Arthritis
- Cancer (breast, ovarian, prostate, and skin)
- Carpal tunnel syndrome
- Common cold
- Constipation
- Diabetes
- Eczema
- Gastric acidity
- Hay fever
- Headache
- Hemorrhoids

- Indigestion
- Insomnia
- Irritable bowel syndrome (IBS)
- Menstrual cramps
- Mucositis as complication of chemotherapy
- Muscle spasm
- Postpartum depression
- Sinusitis
- Stomachache
- Stress
- Ulcers
- Wounds

■ Recommended Dosage

Chamomile is commonly made into a tea and consumed three to four times daily. The tea can also be cooled and applied to inflamed skin or wounds three to four times a day.

If you prefer to take a chamomile supplement, take from 400 to 1,000 milligrams daily in capsule form.

■ Side Effects and Contraindications

Chamomile is a natural blood thinner. If you have a bleeding disorder or are taking a medication or supplement that may thin your blood, do not take this herb. If you are planning to have surgery, discontinue this herbal therapy two weeks before the procedure. Also avoid taking chamomile if you are taking cyclosporine. Speak to your healthcare provider or pharmacist to learn if any drugs you're taking might make it unwise to use chamomile.

Do not use chamomile if you are pregnant. Also avoid it if you are allergic to plants such as ragweed, chrysanthemums, marigolds, or daisies. Do not take if you have a hormonally related cancer, such as breast, prostate, uterine, or ovarian.

A sleep aid, chamomile may make you quite drowsy. Do not drink alcohol or other sedatives after ingesting chamomile.

CURCUMIN/TURMERIC

Turmeric (*Curcuma longa*) has been used in India for over four thousand years as both a spice and a medicinal. Recently, science has revealed that the source of turmeric's ability to protect health is its main active ingredient, curcumin. Because of curcumin, turmeric has a wide range of beneficial properties.

■ Functions of Curcumin in the Body

- Has anti-cancer activity
- Improves and helps maintain brain function
- Improves digestion
- Increases the body's antioxidant capacity
- Is a powerful anti-inflammatory
- Lowers blood sugar levels
- Lowers LDL (bad) cholesterol, total cholesterol, and triglyceride levels

■ Conditions That Can Benefit from Curcumin

- Cancer
- Cognitive decline/Alzheimer's disease
- Gas and bloating
- Hypercholesterolemia (high cholesterol)
- Hypertriglyceridemia (high triglycerides)
- Insulin resistance/diabetes
- Irritable bowel syndrome (IBS)
- Multiple sclerosis (MS)
- Osteoarthritis
- Parkinson's disease
- Ulcerative colitis
- Uveitis (inflammation in the middle layer of the eye)

■ Recommended Dosage

400 to 600 milligrams daily. Choose a formula that includes piperine, a compound found in black pepper, or bioperine, which works like piperine. Curcumin is poorly absorbed when taken on its own, and these additions boost absorption.

■ Side Effects and Contraindications

If you are pregnant or breastfeeding, do not take curcumin supplements. Also avoid this supplement if you have gallstones, since it stimulates the gallbladder to produce bile.

Curcumin can have blood-thinning effects. If you have a bleeding disorder or are taking a medication or supplement that may thin your blood, do not take this herb. If you are planning to have surgery, discontinue this herbal therapy two weeks before the procedure.

Curcumin can also interact with blood sugar-lowering and immunosuppressant medications, as well medications that decrease stomach acid. Speak to your healthcare provider or pharmacist to learn if any drugs you're taking might make it wise to avoid curcumin.

Although curcumin does not cause significant side effects, the following can occur:

- Diarrhea
- Dizziness
- Nausea
- Stomach upset

DANDELION

The dandelion (*Taraxacum officinale*) is a rich source of vitamins, fiber, calcium, potassium, iron, manganese, phosphorus, zinc, and many other nutrients, as well as beneficial phytonutrients such as sterols, tannins, and asparagin. Perhaps this is why the plant has long been used as not only a food but also a powerful medicine.

■ Functions of Dandelion in Your Body

- Acts as a laxative
- Builds the immune system
- Has anti-inflammatory action
- Helps regulate blood sugar
- Functions as a mild diuretic
- Is a prebiotic (fuel for probiotic bacteria)
- Is an antioxidant

- Lowers cholesterol and triglycerides

- Optimizes liver function and protects the liver from toxins

- Prevents gallbladder issues by increasing bile excretion

- Promotes healthy digestion

- Reduces the risk of cancer

■ Conditions That Can Benefit from Dandelion

- Acne

- Arthritis

- Cancer

- Constipation

- Eczema

- Heartburn

- HIV/AIDS

- Hypercholesterolemia (high cholesterol)

- Hypertriglyceridemia (high triglycerides)

- Indigestion

- Insulin resistance/diabetes

- Liver problems

- Psoriasis

■ Recommended Dosage

100 milligrams standardized powdered leaf extract, one to two times daily.

■ Side Effects and Contraindications

If you are pregnant or breastfeeding, do not use dandelion. Also avoid this supplement if you have gallbladder obstruction or another serious disease of the gallbladder, or if you have peptic ulcer. Do not use if you have severe liver disease or liver failure.

Dandelion can have blood-thinning effects. If you have a bleeding disorder or are taking a medication or supplement that may thin your blood, do not take this herb. If you are planning to have surgery, discontinue this herbal therapy two weeks before the procedure.

Dandelion can also interact with quinolones and proton pump inhibitors. Speak to your healthcare provider or pharmacist to learn if any drugs you are taking might make it unwise to use dandelion.

Avoid dandelion if you are allergic to plants such as ragweed, chrysanthemums, marigolds, or daisies.

ECHINACEA

The North American plant echinacea was long used as traditional medicine by Native Americans of the Great Plains. Now, scientific research shows that this herb is notable in its ability to enhance the immune system and help ward off colds and resist infections. Echinacea is also used in topical preparations that are applied to the skin.

▪ Functions of Echinacea in Your Body

- Boosts immune system function
- Fights colds and flu
- Helps heal damaged skin
- Is an anti-inflammatory
- Protects skin from sun damage

▪ Conditions That Can Benefit from Echinacea

- Acne
- Allergies
- Bronchial asthma
- Burns
- Cancer
- Candidiasis
- Common colds (prevention and treatment)
- Compromised immune system
- Eczema
- Flu
- Halitosis (bad breath)
- Herpes
- Radiation-induced leukopenia (low white blood cell count)
- Sore throat
- Urinary tract infections
- Wounds

▪ Recommended Dosage

- For general well-being: 250 to 500 milligrams orally every day for no longer than eight weeks in a row.

- To fight a cold whose symptoms have already begun: 1 to 2 grams orally every day. Start as soon as possible after noticing the symptoms, and continue treatment for three weeks.

- To heal a burn or wound: Apply echinacea cream to injured area daily. If improvement is not seen after one week, discontinue therapy. If symptoms worsen, see your healthcare provider immediately.

■ Side Effects and Contraindications

Do not use echinacea if you have an autoimmune disease or tuberculosis. Also avoid if you are allergic to plants such as ragweed, chrysanthemums, marigolds, daisies, or dandelions.

For most people, short-term use of echinacea is safe. The most common possible side effects are digestive tract symptoms such as nausea and stomach pain. Anaphylaxis, asthma exacerbation, and angioedema (swelling that affects the deeper layers of the skin) have been reported in rare cases.

ELEUTHERO

Eleuthero (*Eleutherococcus senticosus*)—a species of shrub found in China, Korea, Japan, and Russia—has long been used by natural healers to increase energy, enhance endurance, and boost immunity. For many years, it was called Siberian ginseng because its effects are similar to those of ginseng. That name is now rarely used in the United States because it implies that the herb is part of the Panax genus (like American and Asian ginseng), while it actually belongs to the genus Eleutherococcus. Regardless of the controversy over its name, this herb is used to treat a variety of ailments.

■ Functions of Eleuthero in Your Body

- Acts as a stimulant
- Acts as an adaptogen to help your body manage stress
- Aids the immune system by increasing T-cell and natural killer cell activity
- Improves endurance
- Improves learning ability
- Increases mental awareness
- Increases physical performance and stamina
- Increases tolerance to excessive heat, noise, and workload
- Is an anti-inflammatory
- Is an antioxidant
- Promotes healing

■ Conditions That Can Benefit from Eleuthero

- Anxiety
- Chronic fatigue
- Common cold and flu
- Crohn's Disease
- Diabetes
- Fibromyalgia
- Herpes simplex type 2 infection

- Hypercholesterolemia (high cholesterol)
- Inflammation
- Insomnia

- Joint pain
- Kidney disease
- Liver disease
- Memory loss

Ephedra: A Potentially Dangerous Herb

Many of the herbs in this chapter can have side effects, but most can be avoided if you prudently adhere to the medical advice offered by your doctor and pharmacist. Unfortunately, there are other herbs that can have more serious consequences. Some are even banned in the United States by the Food and Drug Administration (FDA). One such herb is ephedra. At the height of its popularity, ephedra—and one of its main active ingredients, ephedrine—was responsible for over half the herb-related deaths in the country.

Although originally used for a variety of purposes, ephedra was mainly being sold as a stimulant and appetite suppressant in the mid-1990s. Many bodybuilders and dieters utilized the herbal supplement, which boosts the metabolism; burns stored fat; and creates a speedy, energetic feeling in the user. It was advertised as a natural supplement, which led many people to conclude that the pills were safe.

A short time later, a growing number of ephedra-related deaths began to surface in the news. The fatalities were largely linked to the dangerous effects ephedra can have on the heart, which include heart attack, stroke, and cardiac arrest. Some ephedra-taking athletes, provided with extra energy that allowed them to practice far beyond what was healthy, died of heat stroke. Many other users experienced a number of less serious side effects, including increased anxiety, insomnia, irritability, and nausea.

Interestingly, studies have shown that ephedra, when properly used, is actually fairly safe. The Chinese have been using the herb for thousands of years. However, the supplement has very high potential for addiction and over-use. It was also found to be ineffective at promoting long-term weight loss!

The FDA first became concerned with ephedra in 1997, but it was the high-profile death of Baltimore Orioles pitcher Steve Bechler in 2003 that set the wheels in motion to ban the product. Since April 2004, the sale of ephedra in the United States has been illegal. There have also been lawsuits filed against certain companies that sold ephedra, claiming that unsubstantiated statements were made in the marketing of these diet pills. Several of these lawsuits have been settled—in favor of the plaintiffs.

- Osteoarthritis
- Premenstrual syndrome (PMS)
- Rheumatoid arthritis
- Stress

◼ Recommended Dosage

500 to 1,000 milligrams daily. Eleuthero can be taken for three months, followed by three to four weeks off.

◼ Side Effects and Contraindications

Do not use eleuthero if you have a history of heart disease, hypertension, sleep apnea, narcolepsy, mania, or schizophrenia, or if you are pregnant or breast-feeding. Women who have a history of estrogen-sensitive cancers or uterine fibroids should probably avoid eleuthero since it has mild estrogenic effects. Consult your healthcare provider if you have an autoimmune disease before using this herb.

Eleuthero can have a blood-thinning effect. If you have a bleeding disorder or are taking a medication or supplement that may thin your blood, do not take this herb. If you are planning to have surgery, discontinue this herbal therapy two weeks before the procedure.

Eleuthero can also interact with drugs taken to treat an autoimmune disease, drugs taken after organ transplant, steroids, digoxin, lithium, and sedatives (especially barbiturates). Speak to your healthcare provider or pharmacist to learn if any drugs you're taking might make it unwise to use eleuthero.

Eleuthero can lower blood sugar levels. If you are being treated for insulin resistance or diabetes, monitor your blood sugar levels often to make sure that they don't get too low.

EVENING PRIMROSE OIL

The evening primrose (*Oenthera biennis*) is an interesting plant. Throughout the summer, the flowers of this North American native live for only one day, blooming in the morning and dying at night. Evening primrose oil is made from the seeds of the flowers and is rich in the omega-6 fatty acid known as gamma-linolenic acid (GLA). (To learn more about omega-6 fatty acids, see page 130.) Taken as a supplement in capsule form, this oil provides many health benefits.

■ Functions of Evening Primrose Oil in Your Body

- Acts as an anti-inflammatory
- Can help with weight loss

- Can prevent thrombosis (blood clots within a blood vessel) from forming
- Lowers blood pressure

■ Conditions That Can Benefit from Evening Primrose Oil

- Acne
- Allergies
- Alzheimer's disease
- Arthritis
- Asthma
- Attention-deficit/hyperactivity disorder (ADHD)
- Cancer
- Chronic fatigue syndrome
- Chronic headaches
- Diabetes
- Dry eyes
- Eczema
- Endometriosis
- Fibrocystic breast disease
- Heart disease
- Hypercholesterolemia (high cholesterol)
- Hypertension (high blood pressure)

- Intermittent claudication (cramping pain in the legs)
- Irritable bowel syndrome (IBS)
- Mastalgia (breast pain)
- Menopausal symptoms
- Multiple sclerosis (MS)
- Neurodermatitis
- Neuropathy secondary to diabetes
- Obesity
- Osteoporosis
- Peptic ulcer
- Premenstrual syndrome (PMS)
- Psoriasis
- Raynaud's syndrome
- Rheumatoid arthritis
- Schizophrenia
- Tardive dyskinesia (involuntary body movements)
- Ulcerative colitis

■ Recommended Dosage

1,000 to 3,000 milligrams daily. For a more precise dose, ask your healthcare provider to test your fatty acid levels.

■ Side Effects and Contraindications

Evening primrose oil can act as a blood thinner. If you have a bleeding disorder or are taking a medication or supplement that may thin your blood, do not take this herb. If you are planning to have surgery, discontinue this herbal therapy two weeks before the procedure. Speak to your healthcare provider or pharmacist to learn if any drugs you're taking might make it unwise to use evening primrose oil.

Do not use evening primrose oil if you have a seizure disorder, since its use can precipitate a seizure.

This supplement can also cause some mild side effects, including the following:

- Bloating
- Headaches
- Nausea
- Diarrhea
- Indigestion
- Vomiting

EYEBRIGHT

Since the Middle Ages, eyebright (*Euphrasia offcinalis*) has been used, both internally and externally, to treat eyes that are burning, itchy, or irritated due to colds and allergies. Research has shown that the positive effects of this herb are associated with the plant's ethanol and ethyl acetate compounds.

■ Functions of Eyebright in Your Body

- Decreases the allergic response by blocking the release of histamine
- Has antibacterial properties
- Has anti-inflammatory properties
- Stimulates the production of proteins used by the body in healing

■ Conditions That Can Benefit from Eyebright

- Allergies
- Blepharitis (inflammation of the eyelids)
- Conjunctivitis
- Hay fever
- Sinusitis
- Stye

■ Recommended Dosage

Eyebright can be found in commercial eye drops or eyewash, either alone or in combination with other eye-healthy substances. Make sure to purchase a sterile product at a reputable store or compounding pharmacy, and use according to package directions. Usually, these products are used three times a day for one week or longer, or as instructed by your healthcare provider.

Eyebright is also available in capsules. Use them according to the manufacturer's directions.

■ Side Effects and Contraindications

Eyebright can cause allergic reactions in some individuals. Get emergency medical help if you experience any of the following allergic symptoms:

- Difficulty breathing
- Hives
- Swelling of the face, lips, tongue, or throat

Also stop using eyebright and call your healthcare provider at once if you experience:

- Eye redness or swelling
- Increased sensitivity to light
- Vision disturbances
- Watery or itchy eyes

Other side effects of eyebright supplements can include the following:

- Confusion
- Constipation
- Headache
- Insomnia
- Nausea
- Sneezing and coughing
- Sweating
- Tooth pain

FENUGREEK

Fenugreek (*Trigonella foenum-graecum*) is an annual herb with green leaves, small white flowers, and pungent, aromatic seeds. While both the leaves and seeds are used in cooking, only the seeds are used for medicinal purposes. Valued by traditional healers for many years, fenugreek is now recommended to lower blood sugar levels, improve digestion, and perform a variety of other functions.

■ Functions of Fenugreek in Your Body

- Improves digestion
- Is an anti-inflammatory

- Is an antioxidant
- Is chemoprotective (protects healthy tissue from anticancer drugs)
- Lowers blood pressure
- Lowers blood sugar levels
- Lowers cholesterol levels
- Lowers triglyceride levels
- Promotes milk flow in breastfeeding
- Protects the kidneys
- Protects the liver
- Stimulates the immune system

■ Conditions That Can Benefit from Fenugreek

- Boils
- Bronchitis and chronic cough
- Cancer
- Canker sores
- Constipation
- Depression
- Dysmenorrhea (painful menstrual cycles)
- Erectile dysfunction
- Gastritis
- *H. pylori* infection
- Hair loss
- Hypercholesterolemia (high cholesterol)
- Hypertriglyceridemia (high triglycerides)
- Insulin resistance/diabetes
- Loss of appetite
- Male infertility
- Obesity
- Parkinson's disease
- Peripheral neuropathy (numbness and tingling of the extremities)
- Polycystic ovary syndrome (PCOS)
- Upset stomach

■ Recommended Dosage

2.5 grams twice a day. Fenugreek is also sometimes used as a poultice.

■ Side Effects and Contraindications

Fenugreek has mild blood-thinning effects. If you have a bleeding disorder or are taking a medication or supplement that may thin your blood, do not take this herb. If you are planning to have surgery, discontinue this herbal therapy two weeks before the procedure.

Fenugreek can inhibit iron absorption, so if you are taking iron, separate the use of these two supplements by two hours. Speak to your healthcare provider or pharmacist to learn if any drugs you're taking might make it unwise to use fenugreek.

If you are taking thyroid medication or your thyroid function is not optimal, consult your doctor before using this herb. Fenugreek can decrease the conversion of thyroid hormone T4 to active T3 and impact thyroid function.

Fenugreek can cause a severe and potentially life-threatening reaction in people who are allergic to chickpeas, peanuts, green peas, or soybeans. Avoid this herb if you have an allergy to any of these substances, and seek treatment immediately if you experience the following symptoms:

- Difficulty swallowing
- Dizziness
- Facial swelling and/or flushing
- Hives
- Shortness of breath
- Vomiting
- Weakness
- Wheezing

Mild to moderate side effects of fenugreek may include the following:

☐ Bloating   ☐ Diarrhea   ☐ Gas

FEVERFEW

Feverfew (*Tanacetum parthenium*), a plant that grows throughout Europe and North and South America, was used in traditional medicine chiefly to treat fevers and headaches. The name, in fact, comes from the Latin word *febrifugia*, which means "fever reducer." But this herb is now believed to have wide-ranging medicinal benefits.

■ Functions of Feverfew in Your Body

- Acts as a sedative
- Has anti-cancer effects
- Inhibits histamine release
- Inhibits muscle spasms
- Inhibits serotonin release
- Is an anti-inflammatory
- Is an anti-spasmodic
- Is heart protective
- Reduces fever
- Regulates the immune system to better fight bacteria and fungi
- Stimulates menstrual flow

■ Conditions That Can Benefit from Feverfew

- Allergies
- Anemia
- Arthritis
- Asthma
- Cancer
- Common cold
- Diarrhea
- Dizziness
- Earache

- Fever
- Infertility
- Insect bites
- Irregular menstrual cycles
- Migraine headache
- Muscle tension
- Nausea and vomiting

- Osteoporosis
- Psoriasis
- Rheumatoid arthritis
- Stomachache
- Tinnitus (ringing in the ears)
- Toothache
- Upset stomach

■ Recommended Dosage

100 to 300 milligrams up to four times daily, standardized to contain 0.2 to 0.4 percent parthenolide, feverfew's active compound.

■ Side Effects and Contraindications

Do not use feverfew if you are allergic to plants such as ragweed, chrysanthemums, marigolds, or daisies. Also avoid feverfew if you are pregnant or breastfeeding.

Feverfew can have blood-thinning effects. If you have a bleeding disorder or are taking a medication or supplement that may thin your blood, do not take this herb. If you are planning to have surgery, discontinue this herbal therapy two weeks before the procedure. Speak to your healthcare provider or pharmacist to learn if any drugs you're taking might make it unwise to use feverfew.

One study showed that patients who had switched to a placebo after taking feverfew for several years experienced the following symptoms: headache, insomnia, joint pain and stiffness, muscle stiffness, nervousness, poor sleep patterns, tension, and fatigue. This phenomenon is called "post-feverfew" syndrome. Do not abruptly stop taking this herb if you have used it for more than one week. Wean off feverfew slowly.

This plant can cause contact dermatitis if the leaves are chewed, leading to symptoms such as inflammation of the oral mucosa and tongue, lip swelling, and loss of taste. Avoid chewing the leaves, and if these symptoms occur, immediately contact a healthcare provider.

Feverfew is generally safe, but symptoms can include:

- Abdominal pain
- Diarrhea
- Gas
- Indigestion
- Mouth ulcers
- Nausea
- Nervousness
- Vomiting

GARLIC

For thousands of years, garlic (*Allium sativum*) has been known to offer a variety of medicinal benefits. This pungent bulb is packed with nutrients, including amino acids, vitamins, trace minerals, flavonoids, enzymes, and two hundred additional compounds. Most of garlic's health benefits, though, are the result of its sulfur compounds, the most famous of which is allicin, an antibacterial that is produced when the garlic is crushed or chopped. Because allicin is most effective immediately after its formation, garlic should be eaten soon after it is prepared. Garlic supplements containing allicin are also available.

■ Functions of Garlic in Your Body

- Balances blood sugar levels
- Boosts your immune system by increasing natural killer cell activity
- Decreases LDL (bad) cholesterol and increases HDL (good) cholesterol
- Decreases plasma viscosity
- Increases cellular glutathione synthesis
- Increases nitric oxide, which increases blood flow
- Is a natural blood thinner
- Is a powerful anti-inflammatory
- Is an antioxidant
- Lowers blood pressure
- Lowers homocysteine, decreasing the risk of heart disease, osteoporosis, depression, and memory loss
- Lowers triglyceride levels
- May decrease the risk of prostate cancer

■ Conditions That Can Benefit from Garlic

- Atherosclerosis
- Cancer (colon, esophageal, and stomach)
- Common cold (prevention)
- Heart disease

- Hypercholesterolemia (high cholesterol)
- Hyperhomocysteinemia (high homocysteine)
- Hypertension (high blood pressure)
- Infection

▪ Recommended Dosage

10 milligrams allicin or a total allicin potential of 4,000 micrograms (equal to one clove of garlic).

▪ Side Effects and Contraindications

Garlic is a blood thinner. If you are taking a blood-thinning medication or a supplement that is a blood thinner, do not take garlic supplements and do not eat large amounts of garlic. Garlic can also interact with blood pressure medication. Speak to your healthcare provider or pharmacist to learn if any drugs you're taking might make it unwise to take garlic supplements.

Pregnant women should not take large doses of garlic—fresh or in supplement form—since sizeable amounts of garlic can cause uterine contractions.

Possible side effects of garlic ingestion include the following:

- Abdominal pain
- Allergic conjunctivitis, rhinitis, or bronchospasms
- Bad breath
- Bloating
- Diarrhea
- Dizziness
- Gas
- Headache
- Heartburn
- Nausea/vomiting
- Profuse sweating

GINGER

Ginger (*Zingiber officinale*) has been used for culinary and medicinal purposes for thousands of years. The root (or rhizomes) of the ginger plant can be consumed fresh or cooked; powdered and used as a flavoring or to make tea; infused into an oil; or juiced. Medicinal forms of ginger include teas, tinctures, capsules, and lozenges.

Ginger has been extensively studied and found to contain many beneficial substances. Of these, the best known are gingerols and shogaols, both of which exhibit a host of biological activities.

◼ Functions of Ginger in Your Body

- Accelerates gastric emptying and stimulates stomach contractions
- Balances the immune system
- Decreases dizziness
- Decreases nausea and vomiting
- Enhances wound healing
- Has anti-ulcer activity
- Improves heart function
- Improves insulin sensitivity
- Is an antihistamine
- Is an antioxidant
- Is antifungal
- Is anti-inflammatory
- Is antimicrobial
- Is antiviral
- Lowers blood pressure
- Prevents platelets from sticking together and forming blood clots
- Protects healthy tissues from anti-cancer drugs
- Protects the kidneys
- Protects the liver
- Reduces anxiety
- Relaxes smooth muscle cells
- Stimulates the flow of saliva, bile, and gastric secretions

◼ Conditions That Can Benefit from Ginger

- Allergies
- Asthma
- Indigestion
- Insulin resistance/diabetes
- Mastitis (inflammation of breast tissue)
- Menstrual cramps
- Migraine headache (prevention and treatment)
- Motion sickness
- Nausea
- Osteoarthritis
- Post-exercise induced muscle pain
- Rheumatoid arthritis
- Stomach cramps
- Ulcerative colitis
- Weight gain
- Wounds

◼ Recommended Dosage

500 milligrams twice a day. Do not take more than 4 grams of ginger a day, including food sources.

■ Side Effects and Contraindications

Ginger can act as a blood thinner. If you have a bleeding disorder or are taking a medication or supplement that may thin your blood, do not take this supplement. If you are planning to have surgery, discontinue this herbal therapy two weeks before the procedure. Speak to your healthcare provider or pharmacist to learn if any drugs you're taking might make it unwise to take ginger supplements.

It is rare to have side effects from ginger, but some may occur. Taking ginger in capsule form or with meals may help you avoid the following side effects:

- Diarrhea
- Heartburn
- Stomach upset

Used topically, ginger may cause contact dermatitis. If this occurs, discontinue use.

GINKGO BILOBA

For thousands of years, leaves from the *Ginkgo biloba* tree—also called the maidenhair tree—have been used in Chinese medicine to improve health. Now, westerners take ginkgo supplements to boost circulation, enhance mood and memory, and improve other functions of the mind and body.

■ Functions of Ginkgo in Your Body

- Acts as an anti-inflammatory
- Acts as an antioxidant to prevent membrane damage
- Helps control blood sugar levels
- Helps prevent memory loss and improve brain function
- Improves circulation through blood-thinning and vessel-dilating actions
- Improves mood by increasing serotonin receptors
- Increases oxygen to the brain by improving circulation
- Lowers cholesterol
- May increase acetylcholine synthesis, which improves memory

■ Conditions That Can Benefit from Ginkgo

- Allergies
- Altitude sickness (prevention)

- Alzheimer's disease
- Asthma
- Anxiety disorder
- Cancer (prevention)
- Chronic fatigue syndrome
- Depression
- Diabetic nephropathy (diabetic kidney disease)
- Diabetic retinopathy (diabetic eye disease)
- Glaucoma
- Heart disease
- Hypercholesterolemia (high cholesterol)
- Impotence/erectile dysfunction
- Lyme disease
- Macular degeneration
- Memory loss
- Migraine headaches (when used with magnesium, coenzyme Q_{10}, and B_2)
- Multiple sclerosis (MS)
- Peripheral vascular disease, claudication, or decreased circulation, all of which can result in leg pain
- Premenstrual syndrome (PMS)
- Raynaud's disease
- Schizophrenia
- Tardive dyskinesia (involuntary body movements)
- Tinnitus (ringing in the ears)
- Vertigo

■ Recommended Dosage

60 to 120 milligrams daily.

■ Side Effects and Contraindications

Ginkgo biloba may interact with a wide range of drugs, including blood thinners, MAO inhibitors, blood pressure medications, and more. Speak to your healthcare provider or pharmacist to learn if any drugs you're taking might make it unwise to use ginkgo supplements. Do not take ginkgo if you are pregnant.

Rarely, Stevens-Johnson syndrome, a severe skin reaction, is associated with ginkgo supplementation. More commonly, side effects of this supplement include the following:

- Diarrhea
- Dizziness
- Headache
- Nausea
- Racing heart
- Restlessness
- Stomachache
- Vomiting

Stop taking ginkgo biloba if you experience any of these symptoms.

GINSENG

Ginseng is a family of herbs well known for its strong medicinal benefits. There are two popular types of this plant: American ginseng and Asian ginseng, which is often called Korean or Chinese ginseng. The two varieties have many similar medicinal effects, and both contain ginsenosides, the active ingredients in ginseng. Both varieties are also adaptogens, which means that they help you adapt to stress by exerting a normalizing effect on your body's processes. This is why the herb can, for instance, correct both low and high levels of cortisol. Yet the two ginseng varieties are sufficiently different in their effects to warrant separate discussions.

Note that Siberian ginseng, or eleuthero (*Eleutherococcus senticosus*), is a different plant and does not have the same active ingredients. (See page 210 for a discussion of eleuthero.)

AMERICAN GINSENG

American ginseng (*Panax quinquefolium*), which grows chiefly in North America, is valued for several biological activities, including the management of stress, boosting the immune system, and increasing energy.

■ Functions of American Ginseng in Your Body

- Helps control menopausal symptoms
- Increases energy
- Is an adaptogen that helps the body manage stress
- Is an antioxidant
- Lowers blood sugar levels
- Lowers insulin levels
- May improve memory
- Strengthens the immune system

■ Conditions That Can Benefit from American Ginseng

- Attention-deficit/hyperactivity disorder (ADHD)
- Cancer-related fatigue
- Cognition problems
- Common cold (prevention)
- Diabetic neuropathy (numbness and tingling of the extremities due to diabetes)
- Heart disease
- Hypercortisolism (high cortisol)
- Hypocortisolism (low cortisol)

- Hypertension (high blood pressure)
- Insulin resistance/diabetes

■ Recommended Dosage

125 to 500 milligrams. Take ginseng with food so that it doesn't lower your blood sugar levels too dramatically. Do not take this supplement consistently for more than one year.

■ Side Effects and Contraindications

Do not take ginseng if you are taking warfarin or another blood-thinning medication, as ginseng can decrease the effectiveness of the medication. Also avoid ginseng if you are pregnant or breastfeeding, or if you have a history of breast cancer or other hormone-sensitive conditions.

American ginseng can interact with a wide range of drugs, including blood thinners, MAO inhibitors, diabetes medication, drugs used to treat ADHD, and more. Speak to your healthcare provider or pharmacist to learn if any of the medications you're taking might make it unwise to use American ginseng supplements.

Ginseng can make the effects of caffeine stronger, possibly causing nervousness, sweating, insomnia, or irregular heartbeat. Avoid caffeine or stop taking ginseng if you experience these symptoms.

Common side effects of ginseng include the following:

- Anxiety
- Breast pain
- Diarrhea
- Euphoria
- Headache
- Hypertension (high blood pressure)
- Insomnia
- Nosebleed
- Restlessness
- Vaginal bleeding
- Vomiting

ASIAN GINSENG

Asian ginseng (*Panax ginseng*), also called Chinese ginseng and Korean ginseng, is available in two forms: red and white. These forms are derived from the same species but are different because of the way the plant is processed. Both are dried, but red ginseng is steamed after drying. Although both forms are common, red ginseng is preferred for medicinal purposes because the processing actually raises the level of certain ginsenosides in the plant.

■ Functions of Asian Ginseng in Your Body

- Aids in lowering cholesterol and triglycerides
- Decreases bloating and fullness
- Decreases depression
- Enhances heart function
- Enhances liver function
- Helps increase physical endurance
- Helps relieve anxiety
- Helps relieve insomnia and restlessness
- Improves glucose control
- Improves mood
- Increases energy
- Increases mental abilities
- Is an adaptogen that helps the body manage stress
- Is an antioxidant
- May improve memory
- Strengthens the immune system
- Supports adrenal function

■ Conditions That Can Benefit from Asian Ginseng

- Acne
- AIDS
- Cancer (prevention and decrease of chemotherapy side effects)
- Chronic fatigue syndrome
- Chronic obstructive pulmonary disease (COPD)
- Depression
- Erectile dysfunction
- Hair loss
- Hearing loss due to medications such as cisplatin and aminoglycosides (prevention)
- Hypercholesterolemia (high cholesterol)
- Hypercortisolism (high cortisol level)
- Hypertriglyceridemia (high triglycerides)
- Hypocortisolism (low cortisol level)
- Insulin resistance/diabetes
- Memory loss (prevention)
- Stomach ulcers (prevention)
- Wounds

■ Recommended Dosage

125 to 500 milligrams. Take ginseng with food so that it doesn't lower your blood sugar levels too dramatically. Do not take this supplement consistently for more than one year.

■ Side Effects and Contraindications

Do not take Asian ginseng if you have bipolar disorder, because this supplement can increase the risk of mania. Also avoid ginseng if you are pregnant or breastfeeding, or if you have a history of breast cancer or other hormone-sensitive conditions.

Asian ginseng can interact with a wide range of drugs, including blood thinners, MAO inhibitors, ACE inhibitors, drugs used after organ transplants, drugs used to treat ADHD, and more. Speak to your healthcare provider or pharmacist to learn if any medications you're taking might make it unwise to use ginseng supplements.

Asian ginseng may make the effects of caffeine stronger, possibly causing nervousness, sweating, insomnia, or irregular heartbeat. Avoid caffeine or stop taking ginseng if you experience these symptoms.

Common side effects of ginseng include the following:

- Breast pain
- Diarrhea
- Euphoria
- Headache
- Hypertension (high blood pressure)
- Nosebleed
- Vaginal bleeding
- Vomiting

GOLDENSEAL

One of the top-selling herbs in the United States, goldenseal (*Hydrastis canadensis*) is native to North America, and its roots have a range of medicinal uses. The benefits of goldenseal are derived from the plant's many constituents, which include amino acids; alkaloids such as berberine, hydrastine, and canalidine; and more. Generally, the alkaloid content is used as a marker for standardization and quality control.

■ Functions of Goldenseal in Your Body

- Boosts immune function
- Cleans and treats sore or inflamed gums and canker sores
- Has potent cancer cell-killing activity
- Helps to detoxify the body
- Improves digestive issues through antimicrobial activity
- Is an anti-inflammatory
- Kills pathogens in the body, including bacterium, fungus, and virus
- Lowers blood glucose levels
- Relieves congestion
- Stimulates antibodies

■ Conditions That Can Benefit from Goldenseal

- Alcohol-related liver disease
- Allergies
- Alzheimer's disease (decreases beta-amyloid peptides)
- Arthritis
- Atherosclerosis
- Bladder infection
- Canker sores, recurrent
- Colds
- Congestive heart failure
- Constipation
- Depression
- Diarrhea
- Eczema
- Hypercholesterolemia (high cholesterol)
- Indigestion
- Inflammation
- Insulin resistance/diabetes
- Irregular heartbeat (arrhythmia)
- Polycystic ovary syndrome (PCOS)
- Psoriasis
- Radiation-induced intestinal symptoms (prevention)
- Radiation-induced lung injury (prevention)
- Sore throat
- Stomach problems
- Vaginitis/yeast infections
- Wounds

■ Recommended Dosage

Goldenseal can be taken orally—as a capsule, tea, or liquid extract—or used as a topical cream. Orally, take 250 to 500 milligrams two to three times a day. Be sure to take B-complex vitamin supplements during treatment, and do not take goldenseal for longer than two weeks. Then, allow a break of at least two weeks before using goldenseal again.

If using a topical cream, follow the manufacturer's directions.

■ Side Effects and Contraindications

Do not take goldenseal if you are pregnant or nursing, if you have kidney or liver disease, or if you have high blood pressure.

Goldenseal can interact with a wide range of drugs, including blood thinners, tetracycline antibiotics, medication used after organ transplants, digoxin, and more. Speak to your healthcare provider or pharmacist to learn if any medications you're taking might make it unwise to use goldenseal.

Although allergic reactions to goldenseal are rare, they have been occasionally reported. Stop taking this supplement and seek medical attention if you experience any of the following symptoms:

- Breathing difficulty
- Closing of the throat
- Hives
- Swelling of the lips, tongue, or face

Large doses of goldenseal can be toxic and can cause cardiac damage, paralysis, respiratory failure, seizures, and even death. If you experience any of the following side effects, stop taking goldenseal and see your doctor.

- Anxiety
- Diarrhea
- Hypotension (low blood pressure)
- Nausea/vomiting
- Seizures
- Shortness of breath

GOTU KOLA

Gotu kola (*Centella asiatica*) has been used since ancient times in traditional Indian and Chinese medicine. The leaves are the most valuable part of the plant as they contain vitamins B and C, proteins, minerals, and powerful phytonutrients such as carotenoids, flavonoids, saponins, volatile oils, tannins, and polyphenols. This gives gotu kola significant medicinal powers whether consumed as a green leafy vegetable, a juice, or a nutritional supplement.

Functions of Gotu Kola in Your Body

- Aids in wound healing
- Enhances and strengthens connective tissue
- Has a sedative effect
- Has antimicrobial activity
- Helps tone the skin
- Improves memory, mental alertness, and concentration
- Is a diuretic
- Is an antioxidant
- Strengthens blood vessels

Conditions That Can Benefit from Gotu Kola

- Alzheimer's disease
- Anal fissure
- Anxiety
- Asthma
- Burns
- Cellulite

- Insomnia
- Hemorrhoids
- Keloids
- Leprosy (used outside of North America)
- Lupus
- Memory loss
- Psoriasis
- Radiation dermatitis
- Scleroderma
- Stomach ulcers
- Stretch marks
- Varicose veins/ venous insufficiency
- Wounds

■ Recommended Dosage

Gotu kola is available in several forms:

- Capsules or tablets: 60 to 180 milligrams, two to three times a day. Standardized extracts should contain about 40 percent asiaticoside, 29 to 30 percent asiatic acid, 29 to 30 percent madecassic acid, and 1 to 2 percent madecassoside—three of the active components in gotu kola.

- Ointments: Apply two to three times a day until the lesion heals (not to be used long-term).

- Tinctures: 10 to 20 milliliters a day.

■ Side Effects and Contraindications

Do not take gotu kola if you have liver disease, as there is some concern that this supplement might worsen liver damage. Speak to your healthcare provider or pharmacist to learn if any drugs you're taking might make it unwise to use this herb.

Gotu kola can cause allergic reactions. Get medical help immediately if you experience any of these symptoms:

- Burning sensation of the skin
- Difficulty breathing
- Rash
- Swelling of the face, lips, tongue, or throat

Other side effects, not from allergic reaction, can include the following:

- Dizziness
- Drowsiness
- Headache
- Nausea
- Stomach upset

GREEN COFFEE BEAN EXTRACT

Extracted from "green coffee"—coffee that has not been roasted—this supplement contains the plant chemical chlorogenic acid, which is present in higher levels in green coffee than in roasted beans. Chlorogenic acid has been shown to effectively lower blood sugar. In one study, standardized green coffee bean extract reduced after-meal blood sugar by 32 percent. The extract has been found to potentially benefit the body in other ways, as well.

■ Functions of Coffee Bean Extract in Your Body

- Has antimicrobial activity
- Lowers after-meal glucose surges (blood sugar levels)
- Promotes weight loss

■ Conditions That Can Benefit from Coffee Bean Extract

- Hypertension (high blood pressure)
- Insulin resistance/diabetes
- Periodontal disease
- Weight gain

■ Recommended Dosage

400 milligrams daily.

■ Side Effects and Contraindications

Green coffee bean extract contains caffeine. If you are sensitive to caffeine, this may not be the right supplement for you. Possible side effects include:

- Increased heart rate
- Insomnia
- Nausea
- Nervousness
- Restlessness
- Upset stomach
- Vomiting

GREEN TEA AND EGCG

Green tea has been popular in eastern countries such as China, India, and Japan for much of recorded history, and more recently, it has become popular in the western world, as well. It is recognized for a wide range of medicinal benefits, which can be attributed to the many organic compounds it contains. The most significant of green tea's components is believed to be *epigallocatechin gallate*, or EGCG. One of a group of plant phenols described as tannins, EGCG is a powerful antioxidant that minimizes oxidative damage in the cells, helps protect against cancer, enhances cognition, and benefits the cardiovascular system.

Green tea and black tea both come from the plant *Camellia sinensis*, but are different because of the processing used after harvest. While black tea goes through a lengthy process that includes oxidation of the leaves to form complex flavor compounds, green tea is simply steamed and dried. Therefore, more of the active compounds found in the tea plant are preserved in green tea. Benefits can be gained both by drinking brewed green tea and by taking EGCG supplements.

■ Functions of Green Tea in Your Body

- Aids communication between cells
- Has a high content of antioxidants
- Has antibacterial effects
- Has antiviral effects
- Improves alertness
- Improves heart health
- Inhibits growth of cancerous cells

- Is an anti-inflammatory
- Lowers blood pressure
- Lowers LDL (bad) cholesterol
- Lowers triglyceride levels
- May encourage weight loss
- Regulates blood sugar levels
- Restricts the development of dangerous blood clots

■ Conditions That Can Benefit from Green Tea

- Allergies
- Amyloidosis (when heart involvement is present)
- Arthritis
- Asthma
- Cancer (prevention and treatment)
- Cardiovascular disease
- Depression

- Diabetes
- Diarrhea
- Excess weight
- Genital warts
- Hypercholesterolemia (high cholesterol)
- Hypertriglyceridemia (high triglycerides)
- Infection

- Irritable bowel syndrome (IBS)
- Kidney stone formation (prevention)

- Obesity
- Tooth decay and gingivitis
- Ulcerative colitis

■ Recommended Dosage

To benefit from green tea, you can either drink brewed tea or take supplements of EGCG:

- Consume three to five cups of green tea a day. Choose your favorite from among the many great-tasting green teas now available. Do not take green tea directly with iron supplements since the tannins in the tea may bind to iron and decrease its absorption.

- Take 200 to 400 milligrams daily of EGCG. 200 milligrams of EGCG that is 98 percent polyphenols is equal to two to three cups of green tea.

■ Side Effects and Contraindications

Do not drink green tea or use EGCG if you are taking a MAO inhibitor. Green tea can interact with a number of drugs, from lithium to acetaminophen to many antibiotics. Speak to your healthcare provider or pharmacist to learn if any drugs you're taking might make it unwise to drink large amounts of this tea or take a green tea supplement. Be aware, too, that green tea may reduce the body's ability to absorb folic acid and iron. If you have liver disease, do not drink green tea or take EGCG without contacting your healthcare provider.

Unless the product is marked "decaffeinated," green tea and EGCG contain caffeine. Although the amount of this substance is small compared with that found in coffee, it can cause insomnia and restlessness in some people. Decrease the amount of tea consumed if the caffeine seems to be causing a problem. Because of the caffeine, use with caution if you have high blood pressure, cardiac arrhythmia (irregular heartbeat), anxiety, psychiatric disorders, insomnia, or liver disease.

Some people have allergic reactions to green tea. If you experience any signs of allergy, seek medical help immediately. The most common symptoms are the following:

- Anxiety
- Closing of the throat
- Constipation or diarrhea

- Difficulty breathing
- Headache
- Hives

- Loss of appetite
- Nausea
- Swelling of the lips, tongue, or face

GUGULIPID

Gugulipid comes from the mukul myrrh tree (*Commiphora mukul*), which is native to Arabia and India. The tree exudes a resin, volatile oils, and gum that contain active compounds known as guggulsterones. Used in Ayurevedic medicine for hundreds of years, gugulipid is valued chiefly for its ability to lower both cholesterol and triglyceride levels, although it has other uses, as well.

■ Functions of Gugulipid in Your Body

- Has anti-acne effects comparable to those of tetracycline
- Has anti-cancer effects, such as inhibiting proliferation and inducing apoptosis (cell death)

- Is an anti-inflammatory
- Lowers cholesterol
- Lowers triglycerides
- Promotes weight loss

■ Conditions That Can Benefit from Gugulipid

- Acne
- Cancer
- Cognitive decline
- Heart disease
- Hypercholesterolemia (high cholesterol)

- Hypertriglyceridemia (high triglycerides)
- Inflammatory bowel disease
- Osteoarthritis
- Rheumatoid arthritis
- Weight loss

■ Recommended Dosage

50 milligrams twice a day.

■ Side Effects and Contraindications

Gugulipid has demonstrated anticoagulant activity and may potentiate the effects of anticoagulant drugs. Do not use this supplement if you are taking blood-thinning medications, nutrients, or herbal therapies. If you have a bleeding disorder, do not take this herb. If you are planning to have surgery, discontinue this herbal therapy two weeks before the procedure. Speak to your healthcare provider or pharmacist to learn if any other drugs you're taking might make it unwise to use gugulipid.

In clinical studies, this supplement has not resulted in any significant side effects, but possible side effects can include the following:

- Headache
- Hiccups
- Nausea
- Rash

GYMNEMA SYLVESTRE

Gymnema sylvestre is a plant native to India whose leaves have long been used in Ayurvedic medicine. Containing a number of beneficial components, this plant is best known for its ability to lower blood sugar levels.

■ Functions of Gymnema in Your Body

- Blocks the tongue's ability to taste sweets, possibly curbing sugar cravings
- Is an anti-inflammatory
- Is antimicrobial
- Is protective of the liver
- Lowers blood sugar levels by delaying glucose absorption
- Lowers cholesterol levels
- Scavenges free radicals

■ Conditions That Can Benefit from Gymnema

- Asthma
- Hypercholesterolemia (high cholesterol)
- Infection
- Insulin resistance/diabetes
- Metabolic syndrome
- Obesity

■ Recommended Dosage

200 milligrams twice a day of an extract that is 24 percent gymnemic acid.

■ Side Effects and Contraindications

Gymnema can lower blood sugar levels, so if you are on a medication to lower blood glucose, speak to your healthcare provider before using this supplement. Stop taking this supplement two weeks before surgery, as it can interfere with blood sugar control during and after surgical procedures.

At high doses, gymnema can cause gastric irritation. One case report showed liver toxicity with the use of this supplement.

HAWTHORN

Hawthorn (*Crataegus laevigata*), a dense bush that grows in the northern hemisphere, has long been valued for its medicinal uses. Every above-ground part of the hawthorn plant—including the flowers, berries, leaves, stems, and even the bark—has been found helpful in the treatment of cardio-vascular illnesses.

■ Functions of Hawthorn in Your Body

- Dilates blood vessels and improves blood flow
- Has collagen-stabilizing properties
- Improves heart rate variability (variation in the time interval between heart beats)
- Is an anti-inflammatory
- Is an antioxidant
- Keeps heart rhythm regular
- Lowers cholesterol levels
- Normalizes blood pressure
- Prevents heart from racing
- Protects against myocardial damage
- Protects the liver

■ Conditions That Can Benefit from Hawthorn

- Anemia
- Arthritis
- Congestive heart failure
- Coronary heart disease
- Hypercholesterolemia (high cholesterol)
- Hypertension (high blood pressure)
- Irregular heartbeat (arrhythmia)

■ Recommended Dosage

900 to 1,200 milligrams daily of dried standardized extract.

■ Side Effects and Contraindications

Hawthorn can interact with a number of medications, from digoxin to blood pressure medications. Speak to your healthcare provider or pharmacist to learn if any drugs you're taking might make it unwise to take hawthorn.

Hawthorn can cause the following side effects:

- Dizziness/vertigo
- Fatigue

- Gastrointestinal symptoms
- Headache, including migraine

- Heart palpitations
- Nausea

HORSE CHESTNUT

Horse chestnut trees (*Aesculus hippocastanum*) are native to the Balkan Peninsula and are grown worldwide. In the United States, the trees are generally known as "buckeyes."

The seeds of the horse chestnut tree have medicinal purposes, the most widespread use being the treatment of venous insufficiency, in which the blood vessels are unable to send the blood back to the heart. The symptoms of this common problem—which can include leg pain, swelling (edema), and itching—are greatly helped by the horse chestnut.

■ Functions of Horse Chestnut in Your Body

- Controls blood vessel growth that feeds tumors
- Has anti-aging properties
- Is an anti-inflammatory
- Is an antioxidant

- Normalizes vascular permeability—the ability of molecules to pass through blood vessels and reach tissues
- Relieves edema (tissue swelling)

■ Conditions That Can Benefit from Horse Chestnut

- Bruising
- Cancer
- Chronic venous insufficiency
- Hemorrhoids

- Swelling after surgery
- Venous leg ulceration
- Wrinkles (topical gel)

■ Recommended Dosage

Horse chestnut supplements can be taken orally or applied to the skin and absorbed transdermally. The raw horse chestnut contains a toxic substance called esculin. Look for a product from which esculin has been removed.

- Oral supplements: 50 to 100 milligrams standardized to 16 to 20 percent of the active ingredient, escin, once or twice daily.

- Topical gel: 3 percent horse chestnut extract in gel form, applied once or twice daily.

■ Side Effects and Contraindications

Do not take horse chestnut supplements if you are pregnant or breastfeeding. Also avoid this supplement if you are allergic to latex. Do not eat raw horse chestnut seeds, bark, flowers or leaves. They can cause death when taken by mouth.

Horse chestnut can slow blood clotting. If you have a bleeding disorder or are taking a medication or supplement that may thin your blood, do not take this herb. If you are planning to have surgery, discontinue this herbal therapy two weeks before the procedure.

This supplement can interact with some medications. Speak to your healthcare provider or pharmacist to learn if any drugs you're taking might make it wise to avoid horse chestnut.

Generally, horse chestnut is well tolerated, but the following side effects can occur:

- Dizziness
- Headache
- Pruritus (itchy skin)
- Gastric irritation
- Nausea
- Skin irritation

There have been reports of the following symptoms with overdose. If any of these symptoms occur, seek medical attention.

- Depression
- Muscle weakness
- Redness of the face
- Diarrhea
- Paralysis, stupor, and loss of consciousness
- Severe thirst
- Enlarged pupils
- Vomiting

IVY GOURD

Ivy gourd (*Coccinia grandis*) is a common vegetable in India, and is now available worldwide. Extracts of the plant's roots, fruit, and leaves offer a range of health benefits, including the regulation of blood sugar levels.

■ Functions of Ivy Gourd in Your Body

- Has a glucose-lowering effect
- Has a laxative effect
- Is a demulcent, which forms a soothing protective film over mucous membranes
- Is an anti-inflammatory
- Is choleretic, increasing the secretion of bile
- Suppresses adipocyte differentiation, helping to decrease fat cell formation

◼ Conditions That Can Benefit from Ivy Gourd

- Insulin resistance/diabetes
- Weight gain (prevention)

◼ Recommended Dosage

250 milligrams twice a day.

◼ Side Effects and Contraindications

Ivy gourd has no know side effects.

JUJUBE

Jujube (*Ziziphus jujuba*) is a small tree, native to Asia, with fruits about the size of dates. This plant is rich in polyphenols, cyclopeptide alkaloids, dammarane saponins, vitamins, minerals, amino acids, and polyunsaturated fatty acids. In Chinese medicine, the "Chinese date," as it is sometimes called, is the most commonly used herb to treat insomnia because it both induces sleep and improves sleep quality. However, the fruit's powerful antioxidants and other compounds provide a range of benefits beyond help for sleeplessness.

◼ Functions of Jujube in Your Body

- Anti-proliferative and apoptotic (kills cancer cells)
- Boosts immune system
- Has anti-ulcer effects
- Helps prevent and treat atherosclerosis
- Improves bowel function
- Improves digestion
- Improves memory
- Improves sleep quality
- Is an antioxidant
- Lowers blood sugar
- Lowers cholesterol
- Protects the liver
- Reduces anxiety

◼ Conditions That Can Benefit from Jujube

- Atherosclerosis
- Cancer
- Cognitive problems
- Constipation
- Convulsions
- Indigestion
- Insomnia
- Insulin resistance/ diabetes
- Irregular heartbeat (arrhythmia)
- Poor appetite
- Ulcers

■ Recommended Dosage

Currently, there is not enough evidence in humans to establish an optimally effective oral dose of jujube supplements. Please follow the manufacturer's directions on the supplement container and speak to your healthcare provider.

■ Side Effects and Contraindications

No safety studies have been performed regarding the use of jujube in pregnant or breastfeeding women, so it should be avoided. Jujube may interfere with the medication venlafaxine and may also cross-react with latex. Therefore, if you have a latex allergy, you should not take this herb. Anaphylactic reactions have been seen.

LICORICE

Licorice (*Glycyrrhiza glabra*) is native to Europe and Asia. The root has been used for thousands of years as a medicinal in China and other parts of the world.

Licorice is packed with nutrients, including glycyrrhizin, the main active constituent; B vitamins; the minerals manganese and phosphorus; amino acids; isoflavones; saponins; flavonoids; essential oils; and more, all of which contribute to the root's healing powers.

There are two types of licorice available. Deglycyrrhizinated licorice (DGL) has had the glycyrrhizin removed, thus preventing certain side effects. It is often used to treat stomach problems. Whole licorice, which still contains the root's active ingredient, is used to treat other medical problems.

■ Functions of Licorice in Your Body

- Acts as an expectorant
- Fights cancer
- Has a protective effect on the gut
- Has antidepressant actions (functions as a serotonin reuptake inhibitor)
- Has antitussive effects
- Has sedative effects
- Is a phytoestrogen
- Is an anti-allergic agent
- Is an antibacterial
- Is an antifungal
- In anti-inflammatory
- Is an antioxidant
- Is an antiparasitic
- Is an anti-ulcer agent

- Is antiviral
- Lowers blood sugar levels
- Lowers cholesterol levels
- Maintains cognition
- Promotes weight loss

- Protects against cisplatin-induced side effects
- Protects nerve cells from damage
- Protects the liver
- Protects the mucous membranes

■ Conditions That Can Benefit from Licorice

Glycyrrhizin-Containing Licorice

- Allergies
- Canker sores
- Chronic fatigue syndrome
- Depression
- Dermatitis (use topically)
- Epstein-Barr virus
- Hepatitis B and C
- HIV infection
- Hypercholesterolemia (high cholesterol)

- Hyperprolactinemia (high prolactin)
- Hypocortisolism (low cortisol)
- Metabolic syndrome
- Oral lichen planus
- Peptic ulcer
- Polycystic ovary disease (PCOS)
- Psoriasis
- Respiratory tract infection
- Seasonal influenza

Deglycyrrhizinated Licorice (DGL)

- Canker sores
- Dysbiosis (microbial imbalance in the gut)
- GI bleeding caused by NSAIDs, such as aspirin

- Indigestion
- Irritable bowel syndrome (IBS)
- Leaky gut syndrome
- Peptic ulcer

■ Recommended Dosage

200 to 300 milligrams twice a day.

■ Side Effects and Contraindications

Do not use licorice if you have severe kidney disease or if you are pregnant or breastfeeding. Also avoid it if you have hypertonia (too much muscle tone), since it may decrease the level of potassium in the body and worsen this condition.

Licorice has a mild estrogenic effect. Therefore, do not use if you have a hormonally related cancer: breast, prostate, uterine, or ovarian. Use licorice with caution if you have fibroids.

Do not use the whole (glycyrrhiza) form of licorice if you have high blood pressure. If you develop hypertension while taking the glycyrrhiza form, discontinue use. Do not use licorice for two weeks before surgery since it may interfere with blood pressure control.

Licorice can interact with many medications. Speak to your healthcare provider or pharmacist to learn if any drugs you're taking might make it unwise to take licorice.

Consuming licorice for several weeks or longer can have serious side effects, including the following:

- Carpal tunnel syndrome
- Contact dermatitis (with topical use)
- Hypokalemia (low potassium level)
- Increased sodium retention
- Rhabdomyolysis
- Thrombocytopenia (low platelet count)
- Visual disturbance (with high dose use)

MILK THISTLE

Milk thistle extract is derived from the seeds of the milk thistle plant (*Silybum marianum*), and has been used as a medicinal for over 2,000 years. The plant's active ingredient, silymarin, is known to have antioxidant, antiviral, and anti-inflammatory properties, and traditionally, it has been used to treat kidney and liver disease.

■ Functions of Milk Thistle in Your Body

- Decreases blood sugar levels
- Helps protect kidneys from the effects of the chemotherapy drug cisplatin
- Increases growth of new tissue to repair damaged areas
- Increases HDL (good) cholesterol
- Increases the production of glutathione, an important antioxidant
- Is an anti-inflammatory
- Is an antioxidant
- Is an antiviral
- Lowers LDL (bad) cholesterol

- Maintains bile flow
- Protects the liver from damage due to toxins, iron, and alcohol

◼ Conditions That Can Benefit from Milk Thistle

- Cirrhosis
- Constipation
- Diarrhea
- Gall bladder disease
- Hepatitis
- Hypercholesterolemia (high cholesterol)

- Inflammation
- Insulin resistance/diabetes
- Kidney disease
- Liver disease
- Prostate disease

◼ Recommended Dosage

Capsules are usually more effective than tea because milk thistle does not dissolve well in water.

- For diabetes: 250 milligrams daily, split into two doses.
- For liver disease: 400 milligrams daily, split into two doses.
- To increase glutathione levels: 150 to 300 milligrams daily, split into two doses.

◼ Side Effects and Contraindications

Do not take milk thistle if you are allergic to ragweed, chrysanthemums, marigolds, chamomile, yarrow, or daisies. Also avoid if you have a history of hormone-related cancers, including breast, uterine, ovarian, and prostate cancer. Use with caution if you have fibroids or endometriosis.

Some drugs, such as birth control pills, can interact with milk thistle. Speak to your healthcare provider or pharmacist to learn if any drugs you're taking might make it unwise to take milk thistle.

The following are possible side effects of milk thistle:

- Diarrhea
- Nausea
- Stomach pain

OLIVE LEAF EXTRACT

Extracted from the leaves of the olive tree (*Olea europaea*), olive leaf extract is rich in the plant chemical oleuropein, which is thought to contribute to the anti-inflammatory and antioxidant properties of this medicinal. In fact, the extract contains a number of bioactive components—secoiridoids, flavonoids, and triterpenes being a few—that make it highly valued throughout the world.

■ Functions of Olive Leaf Extract in Your Body

- Decreases endothelial dysfunction—a pathological state of the endothelium that increases the risk of heart disease

- Decreases the risk of cancer through several mechanisms

- Fights viral and bacterial infections

- Functions as an ACE inhibitor

- Helps prevent tissue-damaging glycation

- Is an anti-inflammatory

- Is an antioxidant

- Lowers blood pressure

- Lowers blood sugar levels by slowing the digestion of starches and increasing the absorption of glucose into the tissues

- Prevents the buildup of uric acid, helping to prevent gout

- Protects the nervous system

■ Conditions That Can Benefit from Olive Leaf Extract

- Cancer prevention

- Gout

- Hypercholesterolemia (high cholesterol)

- Hypertension (high blood pressure)

- Insulin resistance/diabetes

- Osteoarthritis

- Problems with cognitive function

- Rheumatoid arthritis

■ Recommended Dosage

500 milligrams daily. Always take with food to prevent stomach irritation.

■ Side Effects and Contraindications

Since this herb can have blood pressure-lowering and blood glucose-lowering effects, use with caution if you are taking medications to treat these conditions.

Speak to your healthcare provider or pharmacist to learn if any drugs you're using might make it wise to avoid olive leaf extract.

Side effects from olive leaf extract use are typically mild and last for only a few days. They may include:

- Diarrhea
- Dizziness
- Heartburn
- Stomach irritation

PASSION FLOWER

The passion flower (*Passiflora incarnata*) is native to South America but is now popular all over the world because of its value as both an herbal tea and a medicinal. Rich in phytonutrients such as the flavonoid chrysin, it is known for its ability to lower anxiety, treat insomnia, and provide other health benefits.

■ Functions of Passion Flower in Your Body

- Antiepileptic
- Antitussive
- Has a sedative effect without producing confusion on awakening
- Lowers blood sugar
- Reduces anxiety

■ Conditions That Can Benefit from Passion Flower

- Anxiety (use alone or with an anti-anxiety medication)
- Epilepsy
- Insomnia
- Insulin resistance/diabetes
- Narcotic drug withdrawal, used in combination with medication clonidine
- Nicotine addiction or opiate withdrawal

■ Recommended Dosage

Passion flower is available in several forms. The following doses are generally recommended:

- Liquid extract: 45 drops daily.
- Tablet: 90 milligrams daily.

■ Side Effects and Contraindications

Do not use passion flower if you are pregnant or breastfeeding. Also avoid this herb if you are taking an MAO inhibitor or sedative medication.

Passion flower can have blood-thinning effects. If you have a bleeding disorder or are taking a medication or supplement that may thin your blood, do not take this herb. If you are planning to have surgery, discontinue this herbal therapy two weeks before the procedure. Speak to your healthcare provider or pharmacist to learn if any drugs you're taking might make it unwise to use passion flower.

Side effects of passion flower use can include:

- Altered consciousness
- Confusion
- Dizziness
- Drowsiness
- Irregular heartbeat (arrhythmia)
- Nausea

PERILLA SEED EXTRACT

A member of the mint family, perilla (*Perilla frutescens*) is both a food and a medicine in Asia, especially in China and Japan. A unique herb, perilla reduces allergic reactions by inhibiting the synthesis of leukotrienes, which cause inflammation, and the release of histamines, which are responsible for the body's reactions to allergens.

■ Functions of Perilla Seed Extract in Your Body

- Has antimicrobial activity
- Inhibits histamine release from mast cells
- Inhibits the synthesis of leukotrienes
- Is a mild blood thinner
- Is an anti-inflammatory
- Is an antioxidant
- Protects the liver

■ Conditions That Can Benefit from Perilla Seed Extract

- Allergies
- Allergy-induced asthma
- Respiratory diseases
- Rhinoconjunctivitis
- Tooth decay and periodontal disease (inhibits oral microbes)

■ Recommended Dosage

50 to 200 milligrams daily of extract containing a minimum of 3 percent polyphenols.

■ Side Effects and Contraindications

Use with caution if you are taking aspirin, nonsteroidal anti-inflammatory drugs (NSAIDs), ginkgo, or garlic.

RHODIOLA

Rhodiola (*Rhodiola rosea*) grows in cold, mountainous regions of Asia and Eastern Europe. Traditionally, this herb—which is known to contain more than 140 active ingredients—is used to treat anxiety, fatigue, and depression. It belongs to a group of plants known as adaptogens, which can help your body adapt to physical and environmental stress. Active compounds like salidroside and rosavin are able to balance the stress hormone cortisol.

■ Functions of Rhodiola in Your Body

- Decreases depression
- Has antibacterial properties
- Improves mental function
- Improves physical performance
- Is an adaptogen that helps the body manage stress
- Is an anti-inflammatory

- Is an antioxidant
- Is protective of the heart
- Is protective of the liver
- Is protective of the nervous system
- Lowers blood sugar levels
- Reduces anxiety

■ Conditions That Can Benefit from Rhodiola

- Altitude sickness
- Anxiety
- Cognitive problems
- Depression
- Insulin resistance/ diabetes
- Nicotine dependence
- Physical and mental stress

■ Recommended Dosage

200 to 600 milligrams a day in divided doses of standardized 3-percent rosavin and 1-percent salidroside.

■ Side Effects and Contraindications

Rhodiola decreases the possible liver side effects associated with Adriamycin use. It has a synergistic effect with cyclophosphamide's anti-tumor effect and decreases the risk of developing liver toxicity. Speak to your healthcare provider or pharmacist to learn if any drugs you're taking might be affected by rhodiola.

The side effects of rhodiola use are usually mild. At high doses, they may include the following:

- Allergic symptoms
- Fatigue
- Insomnia
- Irritability

ROSEMARY

Rosemary (*Rosmarinus officinalis*) is a woody evergreen shrub that is native to the Mediterranean region but is now grown around the world for its culinary uses. This herb is high in many nutrients, including vitamins A, C, B$_6$, thiamine, and folate; minerals such as magnesium, calcium, copper, iron, and manganese; antioxidant compounds such as diterpene, carnosol, and rosmarinic acid; and essential oils. These components combine to make rosemary a powerful medicinal.

■ Functions of Rosemary in Your Body

- Has anti-cancer properties
- Has anti-ulcer activity
- Improves digestion
- Improves estrogen breakdown
- Improves mood
- Increases bile flow
- Inhibits the bone breakdown associated with osteoporosis
- Inhibits weight gain
- Is an anti-inflammatory
- Is an antioxidant
- Is an antispasmodic
- Is antibacterial
- Is antifungal
- Is antiviral
- Lowers blood sugar
- Protects the liver
- Protects the neurons and brain from ischemic injury (diminished blood flow)
- Reduces oxidative stress

■ Conditions That Can Benefit from Rosemary

- Acne
- Alopecia (hair loss)
- Anxiety disorder
- Asthma
- Cancer
- Cardiovascular disease
- Cataracts
- Constipation
- Dandruff

- Depression
- Herpes simplex infection
- Hypercholesterolemia (high cholesterol)
- Insulin resistance/diabetes
- Irritable bowel syndrome (IBS)
- Macular degeneration
- Memory loss (prevention and treatment)

■ Recommended Dosage

Rosemary is available in several forms:

- Liquid extract (45 percent rosemarinic acid): 1 to 4 milliliters, three times a day.
- Topical preparations (6 to 10 percent essential oil): Apply to the skin once or twice daily.
- Standardized extract: (6 percent carnosic acid, 1.5 percent ursolic acid, 1 percent rosmarinic acid): 200 to 800 milligrams daily.

■ Side Effects and Contraindications

Do not use rosemary if you have epilepsy, since this herb can induce seizures. Also avoid if you are trying to get pregnant, since rosemary can decrease fertility.

Rosemary can interact with a number of medications, from Lasix to lithium. Rosemary can also affect the ability of the blood to clot. If you have a bleeding disorder or are taking a medication or supplement that may thin your blood, do not take this herb. If you are planning to have surgery, discontinue this herbal therapy two weeks before the procedure. Speak to your healthcare provider or pharmacist to learn if any drugs you're taking might make it unwise to use rosemary.

Rosemary may decrease the absorption of iron, so use iron supplements at least two hours after taking rosemary.

If you are allergic to other members of the mint family, you may experience discomfort if you consume or topically apply rosemary to the skin. Reactions are typically mild.

Rosemary can cause side effects, including the following:

- Itchy scalp
- Muscle spasms
- Skin irritation
- Vomiting

SAGE

A member of the mint family, sage (*Salvia officinalis*) is native to the Mediterranean. Commonly used in cooking, the gray-green leaves of the sage plant are packed with chemical compounds that have a wide range of medicinal benefits.

■ Functions of Sage in Your Body

- Calms the gastrointestinal tract
- Has anticancer action
- Has astringent properties
- Inhibits anxiety
- Is an antibacterial
- Is an antifungal
- Is an anti-inflammatory
- Is an antioxidant
- Is antiseptic
- Is antiviral
- Lowers blood sugar levels
- Lowers lipid levels
- Regulates the immune system

■ Conditions That Can Benefit from Sage

- Anxiety disorder
- Asthma
- Bronchitis
- Cancer (treatment and prevention)
- Cough
- Dementia
- Depression
- Diabetes
- Digestive complaints, including bloating, gas, gastritis, diarrhea, and indigestion
- Heart disease
- Hypercholesterolemia (high cholesterol)
- Lupus
- Menstrual symptoms
- Obesity
- Pharyngitis

■ Recommended Dosage

300 milligrams (capsule or tablet) once or twice daily.

■ Side Effects and Contraindications

Sage has a mild estrogenic effect. Therefore, do not use if you have a hormonally related cancer: breast, prostate, uterine, or ovarian. Use sage with caution if you have fibroids.

The tannins in sage can decrease the absorption of iron, magnesium, and calcium. Therefore, do not use sage for two hours before or two hours after eating or taking mineral supplements.

Sage can become toxic if used for long periods of time or at high doses. Possible adverse reactions can include the following:

- Dry mouth
- Seizures
- Vertigo
- Rapid heartbeat
- Tremors
- Vomiting
- Restlessness

SAW PALMETTO

Saw palmetto (*Serenoa repens*) is a small palm tree that grows in the warm climate of the southeastern United States. The fruit of the tree was used medicinally by the Seminole tribe of Florida, and both extracts of the fruit and the ground fruit are used now, usually for urinary problems associated with an enlarged prostate gland.

■ Functions of Saw Palmetto in Your Body

- Helps maintain healthy levels of testosterone
- Inhibits production of the enzyme 5-alpha reductase, which converts testosterone into dihydrotestosterone
- May reduce androgens and prolactin in women with PCOS (polycystic ovary syndrome)
- Reduces an enlarged prostate gland
- Reduces urinary frequency in men with an enlarged prostate gland (BPH)
- Strengthens the immune system
- Works as an anti-inflammatory

■ Conditions That Can Benefit from Saw Palmetto

- Asthma
- Bronchitis
- Chronic pelvic pain syndrome
- Colds and sore throat
- Enlarged prostate
- Hair loss (androgenetic alopecia)

- Hormone imbalance
- Migraine headaches
- Polycystic ovary syndrome (PCOS)
- Symptoms of benign prostatic hyperplasia (BPH)

■ Recommended Dosage

- For enlarged prostate: 150 milligrams twice daily.
- For women who want to decrease testosterone: 250 milligrams twice daily.

■ Side Effects and Contraindications

Because saw palmetto affects hormonal activity in the body, be sure to speak to your healthcare provider before using this supplement if you have a sex hormone-related disorder or if you are taking birth control pills. Do not take saw palmetto if you are having radiotherapy for prostate cancer.

The following are possible side effects of saw palmetto use:

- Altered hormonal activity
- Constipation

- Cramping
- Decreased sexual drive

- Diarrhea
- Headache
- Nausea

Although saw palmetto use is generally safe, the following symptoms and disorders have been associated with the supplement in case reports:

- Acute liver damage
- Coagulopathy (a clotting disorder characterized by prolonged bleeding after injury)

- Intraoperative hemorrhage
- Pancreatitis

SKULLCAP

A member of the mint family, skullcap usually grows in partially shaded, wet-land areas. There are two types of this herb: American skullcap and Chinese skullcap. These forms are not interchangeable and are used to treat different conditions.

AMERICAN SKULLCAP

American skullcap (*Scutellaria lateriflora*) is native to North America, but is now also cultivated in Europe and other parts of the world. Perhaps best known for its calming effects, it is valued for other health benefits, as well.

Functions of American Skullcap in Your Body

- Has a sedative effect
- Is an antioxidant
- Reduces anxiety
- Is an antidepressant
- Is antispasmodic

Conditions That Can Benefit from American Skullcap

- Allergies
- Anxiety
- Depression
- Insomnia
- Neurological disorders such as Alzheimer's and Parkinson's disease

Recommended Dosage

Currently, there is not enough evidence in humans to establish an optimally effective dose of American skullcap supplements. Please follow the manufacturer's directions on the supplement container and speak to your healthcare provider.

Make sure to purchase pharmaceutical grade American skullcap since in the past, this herb has been contaminated with germander (Teucrium), one of a group of plants that can cause liver dysfunction.

Side Effects and Contraindications

Because American skullcap can have a sedating effect, do not use with other herbs that have a sedating effect, such as valerian, catnip, and kava. Also avoid taking it with any medications that have this action. Speak to your healthcare provider or pharmacist to learn if any medications you're using might make it unwise to use skullcap.

High doses of American skullcap can cause any of the following symptoms:

- Giddiness
- Irregular heartbeat (arrhythmia)

- Mental confusion
- Seizures

- Stupor
- Twitching

CHINESE SKULLCAP

Chinese skullcap (*Scutellaria baicalensis*), also known as Baikal skullcap, has been used in China for many years to treat a number of health problems. Chief among them is arthritis as well as other disorders that can benefit from the plant's anti-inflammatory properties. Chinese skullcap also has many healing properties beyond its ability to fight inflammation.

■ Functions of Chinese Skullcap in Your Body

- Balances the immune system
- Can have a sedative effect
- Decreases inflammation by inhibiting COX-2, a hormone that is part of the inflammatory response
- Has antifungal and antiviral properties

- Helps relieve anxiety
- Inhibits the histamine response
- Lowers blood pressure
- Lowers blood sugar levels
- Lowers cholesterol levels
- Lowers triglyceride levels
- Protects the liver

■ Conditions That Can Benefit from Chinese Skullcap

- Allergies
- Anxiety
- Cancer (adjunct to chemotherapy)
- Chronic active hepatitis (combined with other herbal therapies)
- Epilepsy (combined with other herbal therapies)
- Fungal and viral infections
- Gingivitis

- Inflammation
- Headache
- Hypertension (high blood pressure)
- Hypercholesterolemia (high cholesterol)
- Hypertriglyceridemia (high triglycerides)
- Insulin resistance
- Noise-induced hearing loss
- Ulcers

■ Recommended Dosage

Currently, there is not enough evidence in humans to establish an optimally effective dose of Chinese skullcap supplements. Please follow the manufacturer's directions on the supplement container and speak to your healthcare provider.

■ Side Effects and Contraindications

Do not use Chinese skullcap if you have stomach problems or dysfunction of your spleen.

Because Chinese skullcap can have a sedating effect, do not use it with other herbs that have a sedating effect, such as valerian, catnip, and kava. Also avoid taking it with medications that have this action, and be cautious if you are using drugs that lower blood sugar levels. Speak to your healthcare provider or pharmacist to learn if any medications you're using might make it unwise to use skullcap.

Although Chinese skullcap is generally considered safe, there have been reported cases of interstitial pneumonia and acute respiratory failure in people taking this supplement. This risk is increased in the elderly, in those taking the supplement for a long time, and in those who take the drug interferon.

ST. JOHN'S WORT

St. John's wort (*Hypericum perforatum*), a flowering shrub native to Europe, has been used for centuries to treat mental health conditions and other health disorders. It is important to note that this herb is not effective for cases of major depression, which should always be treated with the help of a healthcare professional, but it can contribute to the management of milder mental health problems.

■ Functions of St. John's Wort in Your Body

- Has antibacterial properties
- Increases the body's levels of dopamine, gamma-aminobutyric acid (GABA), glutamate, noradrenaline, and serotonin, helping to improve mood
- Is an anti-inflammatory
- May inhibit viral infections

■ Conditions That Can Benefit from St. John's Wort

- Alcoholism (may reduce cravings by treating depression)
- Anxiety
- Atopic dermatitis
- Burns
- Herpes
- Hot flashes
- Hypercholesterolemia (high cholesterol)
- Inflammation
- Mild to moderate depression
- Nerve pain
- Obsessive-compulsive disorder (OCD)
- Opiate withdrawal (reduces symptoms)
- Premenstrual syndrome (PMS)
- Psoriasis
- Seasonal affective disorder (SAD)
- Wounds

■ Recommended Dosage

900 to 1,200 milligrams, split into two or three doses daily. It takes an average of two to six weeks of daily consumption to begin working effectively. St. John's wort is also available as a topical cream for burns and sores.

■ Side Effects and Contraindications

St. John's wort interacts with many drugs. Speak to your healthcare provider or pharmacist to learn if any drugs you're taking might make it unwise to use this supplement.

St. John's wort can cause any of the following side effects:

- Anxiety
- Dizziness
- Dry mouth
- Headache
- Mild palpitations
- Sexual dysfunction
- Stomachache
- Photosensitivity (rash develops when you go out in the sun)

STINGING NETTLE

Stinging nettle (*Urtica dioica*) is a perennial wild plant that originally came from Europe and Asia. Its name is derived from the tiny sharp hairs that encompass the plant and can irritate or sting the skin when the plant is touched.

For hundreds of years, the stinging nettle has been used to treat painful muscles and joints, eczema, and other disorders that can be relieved by the herb's anti-inflammatory, antioxidant, and anti-histamine actions. Today, this herb is also used to treat urinary problems during the early stages of enlarged prostate (benign prostatic hyperplasia, or BPH).

■ Functions of Stinging Nettle in Your Body

- Balances the immune system
- Decreases joint pain
- Has analgesic properties
- Has anti-histamine qualities that alleviate allergic reactions
- Has anti-inflammatory properties
- Has antiviral properties
- Helps slow or stop the spread of prostate cancer cells
- Is a diuretic
- May lower blood sugar
- May lower blood pressure
- Protects the liver

■ Conditions That Can Benefit from Stinging Nettle

- Allergic rhinitis
- Arthritis
- Benign prostatic hyperplasia (BPH)
- Eczema

■ Recommended Dosage

120 milligrams stinging nettle root, three times a day.

■ Side Effects and Contraindications

Stinging nettle can interfere with numerous medications, from blood-thinning drugs to diuretics and blood pressure medications. Speak to your health-care provider or pharmacist to learn if any drugs you're taking might make it unwise to use stinging nettle, or if any medication doses may have to be adjusted. Do not take if you are pregnant.

Stinging nettle rarely causes allergic reactions. Avoid this supplement if you are allergic or sensitive to nettle or plants in the same family.

Occasional side effects can include the following:

- Diarrhea and other gastrointestinal problems
- Hives or rash (mainly from contact with plant)
- Sweating

THYME

Because of its distinctive taste, thyme (*Thymus vulgaris*) has long been a culinary staple. In recent years, thyme has also gained a reputation for its medicinal properties. This herb is packed with vitamins and minerals, including vitamin C, vitamin A, riboflavin, iron, copper, manganese, and more. It also contains phenolic antioxidants like zeaxanthin, lutein, and thymonin. But the most important substance responsible for the biological activity of thyme is thymol. Thyme essential oil contains 20 percent to 54 percent thymol, as well as the oils carvacrol, borneol, and geraniol. Together, these components give thyme important medicinal properties.

■ Functions of Thyme in Your Body

- Has antibacterial properties
- Has anticancer properties
- Has astringent properties
- Is an analgesic
- Is an antifungal
- Is an anti-inflammatory
- Is an antioxidant

- Is an antiparasitic
- Is an antispasmodic
- Is an antitussive
- Is an antiviral
- Is an expectorant
- Promotes good digestion

■ Conditions That Can Benefit from Thyme

- Build-up of dental plaque
- Common cold, bronchitis, laryngitis, and tonsillitis
- Candida vaginitis (vaginal yeast infection)
- Cough/bronchitis

- Diarrhea
- Gastritis
- Indigestion
- Rheumatological disorders such as arthritis
- Skin infections

■ Recommended Dosage

Currently, there is not enough evidence in humans to establish an optimally effective dose of thyme supplements. Please follow the manufacturer's directions on the tea, liquid extract, oil, and ointment containers, and speak to your healthcare provider.

■ Side Effects and Contraindications

Do not use thyme if you are allergic to the mint family. Also avoid during pregnancy.

Thyme can affect the ability of the blood to clot. If you have a bleeding disorder or are taking a medication or supplement that may thin your blood, do not take this herb. If you are planning to have surgery, discontinue this herbal therapy two weeks before the procedure. Speak to your healthcare provider or pharmacist to learn if any drugs you're taking might make it unwise to use thyme.

Thyme oil is usually safe when applied to the skin. Since there have been some reports of skin irritation, you should always test the thyme preparation on a small area of skin before applying it to a larger area.

The ingestion of thyme can lead to a number of possible side effects, including the following:

- Convulsions
- Dizziness
- Headache
- Nausea
- Vomiting

VALERIAN

Valerian (*Valeriana officinalis*) is a native of Europe that has a very long history of use. For centuries, the dried root has been valued for its calming and sedative effects. It has been shown to reduce the time it takes to fall asleep and to decrease the number of nighttime awakenings. Valerian has also been shown to improve mood, calm fear and restlessness, and even curb aggression.

■ Functions of Valerian in Your Body

- Alleviates pain
- Calms fear and restlessness
- Curbs aggression
- Has a sedative effect
- Improves sleep quality and mood
- Lowers blood pressure
- Reduces anxiety
- Relaxes smooth muscles

■ Conditions That Can Benefit from Valerian

- Hypertension (high blood pressure)
- Insomnia
- Intestinal cramps
- Menstrual cramps
- Migraines

- Neuralgia
- Premenstrual syndrome (PMS)

- Restless leg syndrome
- Rheumatoid arthritis

■ Recommended Dosage

100 to 600 milligrams standardized extract (1.0 percent to 1.5 percent valtrate or 0.5 percent valerenic acid).

■ Side Effects and Contraindications

Do not take valerian if you have liver disease or if you abuse alcohol. Because valerian can cause sedation, be sure to use it with caution if you are taking other sedatives, antihistamines, antidepressants, or anti-anxiety agents. Do not use before surgery, since its use may cause a valerian-anesthetic interaction. Speak to your healthcare provider or pharmacist to learn if any drugs you're taking might make it unwise to use valerian.

In addition to sedation, the following side effects have been rarely reported:

- Liver toxicity
- Paradoxical stimulating effects
- Vivid dreams

WHITE WILLOW BARK EXTRACT

Derived from the bark of the white willow tree (*Salix alba*), white willow bark extract has been used for thousands of years as a medicinal. Chiefly, it is valued for its analgesic, anti-inflammatory, and fever-reducing effects. It is worth noting that aspirin owes its effectiveness to substances (salicylates) found in willow tree bark.

■ Functions of White Willow Bark Extract in Your Body

- Is an anti-inflammatory
- Is an antioxidant
- Prevents platelets from sticking together and forming blood clots

- Reduces fever
- Relieves pain

■ Conditions That Can Benefit from White Willow Bark Extract

- Fever
- Headache

- Low back pain
- Menstrual cramps

- Musculoskeletal pain
- Osteoarthritis

- Rheumatoid arthritis

■ Recommended Dosage

120 to 240 milligrams daily in divided doses.

■ Side Effects and Contraindications

If you are allergic to salicylates, do not use white willow bark extract. Since higher doses of white willow have blood-thinning effects, do not take this herb if you have a bleeding disorder or are taking a medication or supplement that may thin your blood. If you are planning to have surgery, discontinue this herbal therapy two weeks before the procedure. Speak to your healthcare provider or pharmacist to learn if any drugs you're taking might make it unwise to use white willow bark.

The possible side effects of this supplement include:

- Dizziness
- Nausea

- Rash
- Stomachache

6

Other Nutrients

This chapter will look at certain nutrients that have not yet been discussed. Although they may not fit into the categories of the previous chapters, they are all important to your nutritional health and overall well-being. Please consult your physician before taking any supplement if you have kidney or liver disease, are pregnant, or are nursing.

ALPHA LIPOIC ACID (ALA)

A powerful antioxidant, alpha lipoic acid (ALA) is sometimes called the "universal antioxidant" because it is soluble in both fat and water. This compound is made by the body in small amounts, with the quantities produced getting smaller as you age. ALA has a number of functions, which include protecting the body's tissues from oxidative stress, helping the body use glucose, and much more.

■ Functions of ALA in Your Body

- Acts as a metal chelator, rendering cadmium, copper, and iron inactive

- Crosses the blood-brain barrier to protect the brain and nerve tissue

- Enhances the immune system

- Helps insulin work more effectively

- Helps lower blood sugar by improving glucose transport and utilization

- Helps prevent cataracts

- Improves function of the endothelium, which lines the heart and blood vessels

- Increases glutathione, another powerful antioxidant, by 30 to 70 percent

- Increases the synthesis of nitric oxide, which helps regulate blood flow, platelet function, and energy production
- Is a cofactor for mitochondrial enzymes, needed for energy production
- Is a powerful antioxidant that neutralizes damaging free radicals
- Lowers blood pressure
- Lowers levels of calcium when they are elevated
- Protects collagen from cross-linking, thus combating sagging and wrinkles
- Protects the liver
- Recycles coenzyme Q_{10}, glutathione, vitamin C, and vitamin E
- Slows brain aging
- Stimulates the sprouting of new nerve fibers on nerve cells
- Stops the activation of NF-kappa B, helping prevent cancer, heart disease, and other disorders
- Stops the adhesion of macrophages (large white blood cells that can cause heart disease) to your artery wall

■ Symptoms of ALA Deficiency

- ☐ Cataracts
- ☐ Cognitive decline
- ☐ Fatigue
- ☐ Insulin resistance/diabetes
- ☐ Skin wrinkling

■ Causes of ALA Deficiency

- Aging process
- Nutritional deficiencies

Food Sources of ALA

- Broccoli
- Brussels sprouts
- Green peas
- Kidney
- Liver
- Potatoes
- Spinach
- Tomatoes
- Yeast

■ Conditions That Can Benefit from ALA

- Alcoholic liver disease
- Alzheimer's disease

- Amyotrophic lateral sclerosis (ALS)
- Burning mouth syndrome
- Burns
- Carpal tunnel syndrome
- Cataracts
- Circulatory disorders
- Diabetes mellitus
- Diabetic neuropathy (numbness and tingling of the extremities due to diabetes)
- Eczema
- Erectile dysfunction
- Glaucoma
- Heart disease
- Hepatitis C
- HIV/AIDS
- Hypertension (high blood pressure)
- Lupus
- Lyme disease
- Macular degeneration
- Memory disorders
- Migraine headache (prevention)
- Multiple sclerosis (MS)
- Parkinson's disease
- Photo-aging of the skin
- Polycystic ovary syndrome (PCOS)
- Psoriasis
- Rheumatoid arthritis
- Scleroderma
- Skin cancer
- Stroke
- Vitiligo
- Wound healing

■ Recommended Dosage

50 to 400 milligrams daily.

■ Side Effects and Contraindications

If you take 600 mg a day or more of alpha lipoic acid, you may experience decreased conversion of T4 to T3 and have symptoms of hypothyroidism (low thyroid function). For some conditions, such as hepatitis C, you may need high-dose alpha lipoic acid. Do not use a dose above 500 milligrams a day unless you are under the direction of a healthcare provider who can monitor your thyroid studies on a regular basis.

If you are using insulin or an oral hypoglycemic agent along with alpha lipoic acid, the dose of insulin or oral hypoglycemic agent may need to be lowered. Check your blood sugar on a regular basis. ALA can also interact with thyroid medications. Speak to your healthcare provider or pharmacist to learn if any drugs you're taking might make it unwise to take ALA.

Other possible side effects, most common at doses above 1,200 milligrams a day, include the following:

- Diarrhea
- Fatigue
- Headaches
- Insomnia

- Itching sensations
- Nausea
- Skin rash
- Vomiting

ALPHA-GPC (ALPHA-GLYCERYLPHOSPHORYLCHOLINE)

Alpha-GPC, which is produced in the brain, is a direct precursor to choline. This compound, in turn, is rapidly converted into acetylcholine, an important neurotransmitter involved in communication between brain cells. Because of this conversion, alpha-GPC is believed to improve memory formation and learning and to be a powerful tool against Alzheimer's disease and other types of cognitive decline.

▣ Functions of Alpha-GPC in Your Body

- Enhances attention and focus
- Enhances peak muscle performance
- Helps prevent age-related cognitive decline
- Increases acetylcholine synthesis
- Increases growth hormone production

- Increases pre-synaptic choline transporters
- May help the brain recover from traumatic injury
- May improve memory
- Supports cell membrane synthesis and fluidity

▣ Symptoms of Alpha-GPC Deficiency

☐ Cognitive decline

▣ Causes of Alpha-GPC Deficiency

None known.

Food Sources of Alpha-GPC

There are no direct food sources, but alpha-GPC is produced after the breakdown of soy and other plants.

■ Conditions That Can Benefit from Alpha-GPC

- Alzheimer's disease and other forms of dementia
- CVA/TIA (stroke/mini-stroke)
- Traumatic brain injury (TBI)

■ Recommended Dosage

1,000 milligrams daily.

■ Side Effects and Contraindications

Alpha-GPC supplements are considered safe. However, they may interfere with scopolamine, since this medication blocks acetylcholine in the body. Speak to your healthcare provider or pharmacist to learn if any drugs you're taking might make it unwise to use alpha-GPC.

Possible side effects of this supplement include:

- Confusion
- Headache
- Insomnia
- Dizziness
- Heartburn
- Skin rash

BERBERINE

Berberine is a chemical compound found in several plants, including goldenseal, Oregon grape, European barberry, and goldthread. This substance, although unknown to most people, has been found to lower blood sugar levels, improve heart health, and provide a broad range of other health benefits.

■ Functions of Berberine in Your Body

- Boosts fat burning in the mitochondria
- Dilates the blood vessels
- Enhances the immune system
- Increases blood flow
- Increases noradrenaline, a neurotransmitter
- Increases serotonin, a neurotransmitter
- Is an antibacterial

- Is an antifungal
- Is an anti-inflammatory
- Is an antiparasitic
- Is an antiviral
- Lowers blood pressure
- Lowers blood sugar through numerous mechanisms
- Lowers cholesterol and triglycerides
- Regulates lipid metabolism
- Stimulates the release of nitric oxide, which helps regulate blood flow, platelet function, and energy production
- Works as an antiarrhythmic to normalize heart rhythms

■ Conditions That Can Benefit from Berberine

- Alzheimer's disease
- Burns
- Cancer
- Cardiovascular disease
- Cerebral ischemia
- Congestive heart failure
- Depression
- Diarrhea (due to antibacterial effects)
- Hypercholesterolemia (high cholesterol)
- Hypertension (high blood pressure)
- Hypertriglyceridemia (high triglycerides)
- Infections
- Inflammation
- Insulin resistance/diabetes
- Metabolic syndrome
- Nonalcoholic fatty liver disease
- Osteoporosis
- Polycystic ovary syndrome (PCOS)
- Thrombocytopenia (low platelet count)

■ Recommended Dosage

For candidiasis: 50 mg three times a day.

For high cholesterol and other disorders: 200 to 500 milligrams two to three times a day.

■ Side Effects and Contraindications

Berberine can cause uterine contractions, so it should be avoided in pregnancy. Also avoid this supplement if you are breastfeeding.

Some drugs, such as cyclosporine, can interact with berberine. Speak to your healthcare provider or pharmacist to learn if any drugs you're taking might make it unwise to take this supplement.

Berberine is generally safe to take. The following digestion-related side effects may occur:

- Constipation
- Diarrhea
- Stomach pain
- Cramping
- Gas

BETA-SITOSTEROL

Beta-sitosterol, a sterol found in various plants, is usually extracted from South African star grass. This extract has been found in studies to relieve the symptoms of benign prostatic hyperplasia (BPH), lower cholesterol, and have anti-inflammatory effects. Some scientists believe that beta-sitosterol may inhibit the growth of prostate and breast cancer cells. As of this time, more research is needed to confirm this theory.

■ Functions of Beta-Sitosterol in Your Body

- Is an anti-inflammatory
- Lowers cholesterol by inhibiting the intestinal absorption of cholesterol
- May help prevent and treat cancer
- Relieves the symptoms of benign prostatic hyperplasia (BPH)

Food Sources of Beta-Sitosterol

- Avocados
- Nuts, including almonds, macadamia nuts, and peanuts
- Oils, including olive, rice bran, sesame, corn, and canola
- Wheat germ

■ Conditions That Can Benefit from Beta-Sitosterol

- Allergies
- Asthma
- Benign prostatic hyperplasia (BPH)
- Bronchitis
- Cancer
- Chronic fatigue syndrome
- Fibromyalgia
- Hair loss

- Hypercholesterolemia (high cholesterol)
- Lupus
- Migraine headaches

- Psoriasis
- Rheumatoid arthritis
- Tuberculosis

■ Recommended Dosage

20 mg two times a day.

■ Side Effects and Contraindications

Do not use plant sterols, including beta-sitosterol, if you have a rare autosomal recessive genetic disorder called *phytosterolemia,* which causes over-absorption of phytosterols. Beta-sitosterol is not recommended for women who are pregnant or breastfeeding since the safety has not been studied.

Beta-sitosterol may increase the effectiveness of cholesterol-lowering statin drugs if taken together. Speak to your healthcare provider or pharmacist to learn if any drugs you're taking might make it unwise to use this supplement.

Few side effects have been reported with beta-sitosterol use. Some men taking it for BPH have reported problems with digestion.

CARNITINE

Naturally produced in the body, carnitine is derived from the essential amino acids lysine and methionine. This substance is involved in many processes in the body and is best known for the critical role it plays in energy production.

■ Functions of Carnitine in Your Body

- Can be converted to acetylcholine, which functions as a neurotransmitter (a chemical "messenger" in the brain)
- Energizes the heart
- Enhances short- and long-term memory
- Has antioxidant properties
- Helps convert stored body fat into energy

- Improves mental focus and energy
- Increases oxygen availability and respiratory efficiency
- Lowers LDL (bad) cholesterol
- May slow the progression of Alzheimer's disease
- Needed for the transport of long-chain fatty acids into the cells
- Prevents the degeneration of DNA

- Promotes DNA repair from mutations that occur due to free radical damage
- Raises HDL (good) cholesterol
- Reduces the build-up of acids and metabolic waste
- Reduces triglycerides

■ Symptoms of Carnitine Deficiency

Carnitine deficiency can cause no symptoms, or it can cause symptoms that are quite severe. These deficiency signs can include the following:

- ☐ Decreased or floppy muscle tone
- ☐ Edema (swelling of tissues)
- ☐ Fatigue
- ☐ Irritability
- ☐ Muscle weakness
- ☐ Shortness of breath

■ Causes of Carnitine Deficiency

- Certain medications, from Abacavir to Zidovudine, can cause a carnitine deficiency. Speak to your healthcare provider or pharmacist to learn if any of the drugs you're taking might be causing carnitine loss.
- Deficiency of folic acid
- Deficiency of S-adenosylmethionine (SAMe)
- Deficiency of vitamins B_6, B_{12}, or C
- Digestive disorder that prevents adequate absorption of nutrients
- Iron deficiency
- Kidney disease
- Liver disease
- Lysine deficiency
- Malnutrition
- Mitochondrial disease
- Use of Ipecac syrup
- Vegetarian diet

■ Conditions That Can Benefit from Carnitine

- Alzheimer's disease
- Angina pectoris
- Attention deficit disorder (ADD)
- Brain injuries
- Cognitive impairment not related to Alzheimer's disease
- Congestive heart failure
- Depression
- Diabetic neuropathy
- Erectile dysfunction
- Hypercholesterolemia (high cholesterol)
- Hyperthyroidism (overactive thyroid)

- Increased triglycerides
- Infertility, with low sperm count and motility
- Kidney disease
- Memory problems
- Mitral valve prolapse

- Narcolepsy
- Nerve injury
- Parkinson's disease
- Peyronie's disease
- Stroke
- Weight loss

Food Sources of Carnitine

- Apricots
- Artichokes
- Asparagus
- Avocados
- Bananas
- Beans
- Broccoli
- Brussels sprouts
- Buckwheat

- Collard greens
- Corn
- Kale
- Lentils
- Millet
- Mustard greens
- Oatmeal
- Okra
- Parsley

- Peanuts
- Peas
- Pumpkin, sunflower, and sesame seeds
- Red meat
- Rice
- Whole wheat

■ Recommended Dosage

500 to 4,000 milligrams daily. Three forms of carnitine are recommended for use:

- L-carnitine: the most widely available
- Acetyl-L-carnitine: often used in studies of Alzheimer's disease and other brain disorders
- Propionyl-L-carnitine: often used in studies for heart disease and peripheral vascular disease

Avoid D-carnitine supplements, as they interfere with the natural form of L-carnitine and may produce side effects.

Nutrients that Increase Carnitine's Effectiveness

- Alpha lipoic acid
- B vitamins

- Docosahexaenoic acid (DHA, an omega-3 fatty acid)

- Eicosapentaenoic acid (EPA, an omega-3 fatty acid)
- Phosphatidylcholine (PC)
- Phosphatidylserine (PS)

▊ Side Effects and Contraindications

Check with your doctor before starting an amino acid regimen if you have diabetes, hypertension, kidney disease, or liver disease. Also discuss carnitine with your doctor if you have heart disease.

Some people experience body odor when taking carnitine supplements. This can be prevented by taking riboflavin along with the carnitine.

Taking carnitine may increase the risk of seizures in individuals with a history of seizure disorder. Carnitine may also increase the risk of bleeding in people taking blood-thinning medications. If you have elevated TMAO levels, you may not be able to take carnitine. Therefore, it is always best to check with your healthcare provider before taking this important amino acid.

Although side effects of carnitine supplementation are rare, they can include:

- Agitation
- Increased appetite
- Skin rash
- Dizziness
- Nausea
- Vomiting
- Headache

CBD OIL (HEMP OIL)

The plant species *Cannabis sativa* has been used in folk medicine for thousands of years. Most people know of the marijuana plant—one varietal of this species—and its psychoactive component tetrahydrocannabinol (THC), which causes the sensation of getting "high." But until recently, few people have been aware of the species' non-psychoactive component cannabidiol (CBD), which has been found to have remarkable healing effects. While CBD is present in all types of cannabis, it is present in largest amounts in the *Cannabis sativa* varietal known as hemp, which is also notable for containing only minute amounts of THC (approximately 0.3%). This is what makes hemp oil an appealing option for people who want symptom relief without the mind-altering effects of marijuana.

It's important to understand that while THC (chiefly found in marijuana) continues to be a class 1 drug, making it illegal in many states, hemp-derived CBD oil is legal and available in all fifty states. And because hemp oil has such low levels of THC, you can enjoy its health benefits with few or no side effects.

■ Functions of CBD in Your Body

- Balances the immune system
- Decreases inflammation
- Decreases muscle spasms
- Decreases nausea and vomiting
- Decreases pain by modulating receptors in the brain
- Decreases seizure activity in people with epilepsy
- Is a potent antioxidant
- Kills or slows bacterial growth
- May help prevent Alzheimer's disease
- May reduce blood sugar levels
- Modulates neurotransmission
- Reduces anxiety

■ Conditions That Can Benefit from CBD

- Alzheimer's disease
- Amyotrophic lateral sclerosis (ALS)
- Anxiety
- Arthritis
- Autism
- Bipolar disorder
- Cancer
- Chronic fatigue syndrome
- Colitis
- Crohn's disease
- Depression
- Diabetes
- Epilepsy
- Fibromyalgia
- Huntington's disease
- Insomnia
- Irritable bowel syndrome (IBS)
- Migraine headaches
- Multiple sclerosis (MS)
- Nausea
- Obsessive compulsive disorder (OCD)
- Pain
- Parkinson's disease
- Post-traumatic stress disorder (PTSD)
- Psoriasis
- Rheumatoid arthritis
- Schizophrenia
- Substance abuse disorders
- Ulcerative colitis

■ Recommended Dosage

5 to 500 milligrams daily. The best way to find the proper dose is to start taking 5 milligrams once or twice a day, and increase the amount slowly until you

find relief from your symptoms. To maintain adequate blood levels, divide the dose rather than taking one large dose daily. Do not exceed 500 milligrams a day without consulting your healthcare provider. Be aware that it can take thirty to ninety minutes after use to notice any benefits. If treating inflammatory conditions of the skin, use topical balms or creams as needed in addition to the oral supplements.

When taking CBD oil orally, choose sublingual drops, which deliver CBD in a relatively *bioavailable* form—a form that is able to have an active effect when introduced into the body. (Sublingual drops are absorbed into the bloodstream via the sublingual gland.) About 20 to 30 percent of the CBD in sublingual drops is bioavailable, while only 5 percent of CBD in oral capsules and gummies is bioavailable. So, for example, 25 milligrams of CBD in sublingual drops will deliver an estimated four to six times the amount of CBD to the body than will an equal amount of CBD in a capsule. Sublingual consumption also affects the body more quickly, because it is more direct.

When choosing a product, check the Supplement Facts panel to make sure that the bottle reads "hemp oil (aerial parts)." The term "aerial parts," refers to the parts of the hemp plant that grow above ground. Ideally, the plant should be 100-percent organically grown to minimize exposure to pesticides. Request a third-party certificate of analysis to show if there are any unwanted contaminants such as heavy metals and to show the levels of CBD and THC. You want a product that contains less than 0.3 percent THC.

◼ Side Effects and Contraindications

Studies have shown that CBD is generally well tolerated and safe for consumption, even in high doses and with continuous use. However, it has also been shown that CBD can inhibit the body system that processes roughly 60 percent of all prescribed medications. This means that it has the potential to interfere with the actions of certain drugs. Speak to your healthcare provider or pharmacist to learn if any drugs you're taking might make it unwise to take CBD or if the dosage of your medications should be adjusted.

Some research has suggested that high doses of CBD may worsen tremors and muscle movement in people with Parkinson's disease. Until more information is available, it is prudent to avoid use.

Although side effects of CBD oil are rare, they can include the following:

- Diarrhea
- Dizziness
- Drowsiness
- Dry mouth
- Lightheadedness
- Low blood pressure
- Nausea

CHLORELLA

Chlorella is a green freshwater algae that packs a big nutritional punch. It is high in protein; a good source of fiber; contains vitamins A, B$_2$, B$_6$, C, E, and K; and offers minerals such as calcium, magnesium, iron, zinc, phosphorus, and iodine. Also included in this algae's impressive nutritional profile are a wide range of antioxidants, omega-3 fatty acids, and the green plant pigment chlorophyll.

■ Functions of Chlorella in Your Body

- Acts as an antioxidant
- Binds to heavy metals and other harmful compounds, helping detoxify the body
- Decreases body fat
- Enhances the immune system
- Helps keep blood pressure in check
- May improve blood sugar levels
- May lower cholesterol and triglycerides

■ Conditions That Can Benefit from Chlorella

- Allergies
- Arterial stiffness that can lead to heart disease
- Body odor
- Cognitive decline
- Constipation
- Digestive problems
- Fatigue
- Fibromyalgia
- Hypertension (high blood pressure)
- Hypercholesterolemia (high cholesterol)
- Hypertriglyceridemia (high triglycerides)
- Insulin resistance
- Premenstrual syndrome (PMS)
- Problems due to accumulation of toxic metals and pollutants in body
- Skin ulcers (use topically)
- Weight gain
- Wounds (treatment)

■ Recommended Dosage

Currently, there is not enough evidence to establish an optimally effective oral dose of chlorella. Also, chlorella supplements differ from one manufacturer to another. Please follow the manufacturer's directions on the supplement container and speak to your healthcare adviser.

■ Side Effects and Contraindications

Avoid chlorella during pregnancy and breastfeeding, as no studies have been performed to support its safety. Also avoid it if you are allergic to iodine, as chlorella can contain this substance; or if you have high iron levels or the disease process hemochromatosis. Because some individuals have allergies to chlorella, begin supplement therapy with caution. Note, too, that this supplement can cause photosensitivity (sensitivity to sunlight) in some people. If you experience this, discontinue use of the product.

Chlorella contains a high amount of vitamin K, which is used by the body to help blood clot. Thus, this supplement could interfere with the actions of blood-thinning medications. Chlorella can also have interactions with immunosuppressant drugs. Speak to your healthcare provider or pharmacist to learn if any drugs you're taking might make it unwise to use chlorella.

The following are possible side effects of chlorella use:

- Diarrhea
- Gas (flatulence)
- Nausea
- Skin rash due to photosensitivity
- Stomach cramping

CHOLINE

Choline is an important vitamin-like nutrient that plays a role in almost every body system. Several essential compounds—including acetylcholine, lecithin, and phosphatidylcholine—are derived from choline. As such, this nutrient is believed to protect against certain types of age-related dementia, to be vital for membrane stabilization, and to perform many other functions.

■ Functions of Choline in Your Body

- Aids in the metabolism of fats

- Allows movement and coordination

- Enhances attention, memory, and focus

- Increases the release of neurotransmitters made from tyrosine (norepinephrine, epinephrine, and dopamine)

- Is a component of every cell membrane

- Is a precursor of acetylcholine, lecithin, and phosphatidylcholine
- Is essential for the transport of cholesterol from the liver
- Is needed for VLDL (very low-density lipoprotein) assembly and excretion
- Is required for normal brain function
- Protects against age-related dementia

■ Symptoms of Choline Deficiency

☐ Cognitive decline   ☐ High cholesterol levels

☐ High blood pressure   ☐ Nervous system disorders

■ Causes of Choline Deficiency

- Folic acid deficiency   - Nicotine use
- Genetics   - Use of fibrate drugs
- High alcohol consumption   - Use of the drug methotrexate
- High sugar intake   - Vegetarian/vegan diet

Food Sources of Choline

- Beef   - Fish   - Oats
- Chicken   - Liver   - Peanut butter
- Egg yolks   - Nuts   - Soy

■ Conditions That Can Benefit from Choline

- Alzheimer's disease
- Bipolar disorder
- Coronary heart disease (prevention)
- Glaucoma
- Hepatitis
- Hypercholesterolemia (high cholesterol)
- Liver disease
- Nonalcoholic fatty liver disease (prevention)
- Peripheral artery disease (prevention)
- Stroke (prevention)

■ Recommended Dosage

500 to 1,000 milligrams daily in divided doses. Therefore, you should take 250 to 500 milligrams twice a day. Never take more than 3 grams (3,000 milligrams) a day unless you are under the supervision of a healthcare provider.

■ Side Effects and Contraindications

Take choline only under your doctor's direction when you are pregnant. High-dose supplementation (over 3,000 milligrams a day) increases the risk of neural tube defects.

The following side effects can occur with high doses of choline:

- Excessive sweating
- Fishy body odor
- Hypotension (low blood pressure)
- Liver toxicity
- Vomiting

CHONDROITIN SULFATE

Chondroitin sulfate is a major constituent of cartilage, where it provides structure, holds water and nutrients, and permits other molecules to move through cartilage. This is important, as cartilage has no blood supply. Chondroitin is also found in bone.

High levels of the amino acid homocysteine can negatively affect the formation of chondroitin sulfate in the body. Although it is commonly sold as a supplement, it is usually less effective than the similar glucosamine (also found in cartilage and discussed on page 297), because its large size doesn't allow it to be easily absorbed and utilized. Yet, its sulfur molecules are able to be absorbed. As a result, sufferers of osteoarthritis often report pain relief after taking chondroitin sulfate, although it can take several months to become effective. Chondroitin sulfate sold as a supplement either comes from shark and bovine cartilage or is synthesized in a laboratory.

■ Functions of Chondroitin Sulfate in Your Body

- Delays the progression of osteoarthritis
- Helps keep cartilage healthy by absorbing fluid (particularly water) into the connective tissue
- Improves joint function
- May block the enzymes that break down cartilage
- Provides the building blocks for the production of new cartilage
- Reduces pain and inflammation

■ Conditions That Can Benefit from Chondroitin Sulfate

- Breast and colorectal cancer (prevention)
- Interstitial cystitis
- Joint pain
- Osteoarthritis
- Overactive bladder (the bladder is irrigated with chondroitin)

■ Recommended Dosage

400 milligrams three times a day or 600 milligrams twice a day.

■ Side Effects and Contraindications

If you have asthma, have prostate cancer or a history of it, or are pregnant or breastfeeding, do not use chondroitin. Also avoid this supplement if you are taking blood-thinning medication. Speak to your healthcare provider or pharmacist to learn if any drugs you're taking might make it unwise to take chondroitin.

The following side effects can occur with chondroitin sulfate:

- Allergic reactions such as skin rash
- Diarrhea
- Drowsiness
- Headache
- Upset stomach

COCOA

Cocoa powder is made by fermenting, drying, roasting, and crushing cocoa beans. Much of the natural fat of the beans is removed during this process.

For centuries, cocoa was valued for its many culinary uses. More recently, it has come to be valued for its many health benefits. Studies have shown that cocoa flavanols, the beneficial phytonutrients found naturally in the beans, help the body in numerous ways. The cardiovascular system and the brain seem to profit the most from cocoa flavanols, but these mighty nutrients boost a variety of physiological functions.

It's useful to know that the bitterness of cocoa comes mostly from its flavanols. Traditional cocoa processing methods—especially "dutching"—mellow the flavor of cocoa by destroying these compounds. That's why when you choose cocoa for health reasons, you'll want to purchase a product in which the flavanols have been preserved. Fortunately, now that the benefits of flavanols have been recognized, cocoa is often processed using techniques that maintain a high flavanol content.

■ Functions of Cocoa in Your Body

- Aids in the release of neurotransmitters like serotonin, anandamide, and phenylethylamine
- Contains antioxidants
- Helps the skin look more youthful
- Improves blood flow to the brain and brain function
- Improves memory
- Improves mood and symptoms of depression
- Improves the elasticity of arterial walls
- Is an anti-inflammatory
- Lowers blood pressure by improving nitric oxide levels
- Lowers blood sugar levels
- Lowers cholesterol
- May have cancer-protective properties
- May lower your risk of heart attack and stroke
- Reduces oxidative stress
- Relaxes the bronchioles of the lungs, making breathing easier
- Improves function of the endothelium, the thin membrane that lines the heart and blood vessels

■ Conditions That Can Benefit from Cocoa

- Alzheimer's disease and other forms of cognitive decline
- Asthma
- Cancer (prevention)
- Cardiovascular disease (prevention)
- Chronic fatigue syndrome
- Depression
- Diabetes
- Huntington's disease
- Hypercholesterolemia (high cholesterol)
- Hypertension (high blood pressure)
- Metabolic syndrome
- Multiple sclerosis (MS)
- Parkinson's disease
- Traumatic brain injury

■ Recommended Dosage

Studies have not yet shown the exact amount of cocoa that should be included in the diet on a daily basis to achieve health benefits. However, the European Food Safety Authority and many nutritionists recommend 2.5 grams (0.1 ounce) of unsweetened high-flavanol cocoa powder per day to enhance heart health. (This is about half a teaspoon.) It's best to avoid chocolate, since even dark chocolate includes sugar and fat and is high in calories compared with an unsweetened product. Instead, buy unsweetened cocoa powder—avoid dutched cocoa, which has reduced flavanols—and incorporate the cocoa in your diet. For an even healthier product, choose *cacao*, unprocessed cocoa that retains all of the cocoa bean's nutrients. Remember that the less processed the cocoa is, the greater will be the benefits.

Here are a few suggestions for including cocoa (or cacao) in your meals:

- Add the powder to your favorite healthy smoothie recipe for rich taste.

- Sprinkle the powder over fresh or cooked fruit. The natural sweetness of fruit tames the bitterness of the cocoa.

- Include the powder in baked goods.

- Add the powder to your favorite granola bar or trail mix. Or, to add crunch to your snacks, use cacao nibs (gently crushed cacao) instead of cocoa powder.

- Stir the powder into coffee for an intense mocha taste.

- Stir the powder into chili for greater depth of flavor.

■ Side Effects and Contraindications

Cocoa can interact with certain medications including anticoagulants, stimulant drugs, estrogens, antidiabetes drugs, and more. Speak to your healthcare provider or pharmacist to learn if any drugs you're taking might make it unwise to increase your cocoa consumption.

Although an allergy to cocoa is rare, symptoms such as skin rashes, headaches, and other allergic reactions have been reported. More often, people have allergic responses to the non-cocoa ingredients in chocolate, such as soy or milk. If you have food allergies or sensitivities, be sure to check the ingredients in your cocoa product before purchasing it.

Cocoa contains caffeine and related chemicals. It is recommended that large amounts of cocoa be avoided during pregnancy, as they could be associated with premature delivery, low birth weight, and miscarriage. Consuming large amounts of cocoa can also cause caffeine-related side effects such as the following:

- Anxiety
- Fast heartbeat
- Insomnia
- Diarrhea
- Increased urination
- Nervousness

COENZYME Q₁₀

Coenzyme Q_{10} (CoQ_{10}) is a fat-soluble nutrient that is made in nearly all of the body's tissues. It is sometimes called *ubiquinone* because it is ubiquitous. It is well known for the part it plays in generating energy in cells by boosting mitochondrial function, and is also a free radical scavenger that reduces oxidative damage. Studies have also shown that it helps prevent breast cancer. In fact, this essential substance performs a range of important functions in the body. Unfortunately, the body makes less CoQ_{10} as you get beyond fifty years of age. Because this nutrient is so vital to health, it is highly recommended that both men and women take it in supplemental form after age fifty.

■ Functions of Coenzyme Q₁₀ in Your Body

- Enhances the regeneration of vitamin E
- Has a positive effects on endothelial function
- Helps prevent breast cancer
- Is a coenzyme in the energy-producing metabolic pathways
- Is an antioxidant
- Is associated with a reduction of peripheral neuropathy and other diabetes-related problems
- Lowers blood pressure
- Protects the heart
- Protects the nerves
- Reduces platelet stickiness, decreasing the risk of heart disease
- Regulates genomic expression
- Stimulates the immune system

■ Symptoms of CoQ₁₀ Deficiency

- ☐ Breast cancer
- ☐ Cardiomyopathy
- ☐ Congestive heart failure
- ☐ Cystic fibrosis
- ☐ Decreased exercise tolerance
- ☐ Depression
- ☐ Fibromyalgia
- ☐ General fatigue/chronic fatigue syndrome
- ☐ Hypertension (high blood pressure)
- ☐ Hyperthyroidism (overproduction of thyroid hormones)
- ☐ Ischemic heart disease
- ☐ Muscle weakness/mitochondrial myopathy

■ Causes of CoQ$_{10}$ Deficiency

- Aging process
- Deficiency of taurine
- Deficiency of vitamins B$_1$, B$_5$, B$_6$, and B$_{12}$
- Excess exercise
- Folic acid deficiency
- Genetic mutations/genetic defects
- Hyperthyroidism (overproduction of thyroid hormones)

- Malabsorption due to celiac disease/sprue or steatorrhea (excessive fat in stools)
- Medications are a major cause of CoQ$_{10}$ deficiency. Drugs from antibiotics to over-the-counter supplements used for weight loss can cause a deficiency of this nutrient. Speak to your healthcare provider or pharmacist to learn if any drugs you're taking might be causing CoQ$_{10}$ loss.

Food Sources of CoQ$_{10}$

- Anchovies
- Beef
- Broccoli
- Cauliflower
- Chicken
- Liver
- Mackerel
- Nuts
- Oranges
- Peanuts
- Pork
- Salmon
- Sardines
- Sesame seeds
- Soybeans
- Spinach
- Strawberries
- Trout

■ Conditions That Can Benefit from CoQ$_{10}$

- Alzheimer's disease
- Angina pectoris
- Arrhythmia (irregular heart rhythm)
- Asthma
- Breast cancer
- Cardiomyopathy
- Chronic fatigue syndrome (CFS)
- Chronic obstructive pulmonary disease (COPD)

- Congestive heart failure
- Coronary heart disease
- Cystic fibrosis
- Depression
- Diabetes
- Dilated cardiomyopathy
- Fibromyalgia
- Hearing loss
- Huntington's disease

- Hypercholesterolemia (high cholesterol)
- Hypertension (high blood pressure)
- Hyperthyroidism (overproduction of thyroid hormones)
- Lyme disease
- Macular degeneration
- Male infertility
- Migraine headaches

- Mitral valve prolapse
- Muscular dystrophy
- Parkinson's disease
- Periodontal disease
- Peyronie's disease
- Pulmonary fibrosis
- Sun-damaged skin (use orally or topically)
- Tinnitus (ringing in ears)
- Weight loss

◼ Recommended Dosage

30 to 1,600 milligrams daily, depending on the diagnosis. For the dosage specific to your disease process, see your healthcare provider. If you are over the age of fifty, 100 milligrams a day is a great starting dose. If you want to take a larger dose, increase the dosage slowly over a one-month period to help prevent side effects.

Some individuals may better absorb *ubiquinol*—the more active form of CoQ_{10}—than *ubiquinone*. When young, the body can readily convert ubiquinone to ubiquinol. With age, the body is less able to produce the active form.

◼ Side Effects and Contraindications

Do not use CoQ_{10} if you are pregnant or breastfeeding. If you take a blood-thinning medication, consult your doctor before using. Speak to your healthcare provider or pharmacist to learn if any drugs you're taking might make it unwise to use CoQ_{10}.

The following side effects can occur from taking CoQ_{10} supplementation. However, they are usually less severe if you take the supplement after meals.

- Abdominal discomfort
- Appetite loss
- Diarrhea (when doses are greater than 100 milligrams)
- Heartburn

- Increase in liver enzymes (when doses are greater than 300 milligrams)
- Insomnia (when doses are greater than 100 milligrams)
- Irritability

- Palpitations
- Photophobia (extreme sensitivity to light)

CORDYCEPS

Cordyceps (*Cordyceps sinsensis* and *Cordyceps militaris*) is a fungus that has long been used in traditional Chinese and Tibetan medicine. Because natural cordyceps is difficult to obtain and is expensive when available, most supplements are made with cordyceps that has been created in a laboratory (Cordyceps CS-4).

Cordyceps is nutritionally rich, containing various types of essential amino acids; vitamins B_1, B_2, B_{12}, and K; carbohydrates; and trace elements. Studies have indicated that cordyceps can boost energy and oxygen during exercise; improve heart health; and combat inflammation, cancer, diabetes, and aging.

■ Functions of Cordyceps in Your Body

- Has antibacterial properties
- Has anticancer properties
- Has anti-inflammatory properties
- Has antimicrobial properties
- Has antioxidant properties
- Improves cardiac output
- Improves heart rhythm
- Improves kidney function
- Improves lung capacity
- Increases energy levels
- Lowers blood sugar levels
- Lowers cholesterol levels
- Lowers fibrinogen (a clotting factor)
- Modulates the immune system
- Protects the nervous system
- Provides adrenal support for stress

■ Conditions That Can Benefit from Cordyceps

- Asthma
- Bronchitis
- Cancer
- Cardiac arrhythmia (irregular heartbeat)
- Chronic kidney disease (use only under a healthcare provider's direction)
- Congestive heart failure
- Coughs
- Diabetes
- Hepatic cirrhosis
- Hepatitis B
- High cholesterol
- Infection

- Sexual dysfunction
- Stress due to adrenal fatigue

▉ Recommended Dosage

400 milligrams twice a day. Be sure to use a pharmaceutical grade product, as some lower-grade products have been found to contain lead.

▉ Side Effects and Contraindications

Cordyceps can cause problems when taken with medications such as prednisolone, antiviral drugs, and diabetic medications. Speak to your healthcare provider or pharmacist to see if it is safe to take this supplement with your medications and if any cautions should be exercised.

Taking cordyceps may increase the risk of bleeding if you have a bleeding disorder or are taking medications that change bleeding time. Use with caution. Because cordyceps might increase the risk of bleeding during surgery, discontinue use two weeks before surgery.

Do not take cordyceps if you are allergic to mold, if you have an autoimmune disease, or if you are pregnant or breastfeeding.

DIGESTIVE ENZYMES

Digestive enzymes help the body properly digest proteins, fats, and carbohydrates. There are three principal kinds of digestive enzymes: amylase, lipase, and protease.

- *Amylase* breaks down starches into simple sugars. Produced in the pancreas and salivary glands, it can also be ingested in certain foods, such as raw fruits and vegetables, nuts, and whole grains.

- *Lipase* breaks down fats, particularly triglycerides. It is secreted by the pancreas and can also be found in certain foods, such as avocados, walnuts, pine nuts, lentils, and oats.

- *Protease* breaks down proteins into smaller proteins or amino acids so they can be absorbed by the intestine. Some forms of this enzyme are synthesized by the pancreas and some are found in foods. For instance, pineapple contains the protease bromelain, while papaya contains papain.

Even if you don't have symptoms of indigestion, digestive enzymes are valuable because when your gut isn't processing your food fully, a chain reaction of imbalances can occur in the body. This can lead to health problems that are seemingly unrelated to digestion, from chronic fatigue to a dysfunctional immune system.

■ Functions of Digestive Enzymes in Your Body

- Are anti-inflammatory
- Balance the immune system
- Enhance digestive health
- Enhance the absorption of nutrients
- Increase fibrinolysis—the breakdown of the fibrin in blood clots—to prevent harmful clots
- Reduce autoimmunity—the attack of the body by its own immune system
- Speed up the breakdown of food molecules into their "building block" components, such as amino acids

■ Symptoms of Digestive Enzyme Deficiency

- ☐ Allergies
- ☐ Arthritis
- ☐ Celiac disease
- ☐ Food intolerances
- ☐ Increased risk of heart disease
- ☐ Lactose intolerance
- ☐ Malabsorption
- ☐ Maldigestion
- ☐ Pancreatic insufficiency
- ☐ Steatorrhea (abnormal amounts of fat in feces)

■ Causes of Digestive Enzyme Deficiency

- Aging process
- Bovine growth hormone used in livestock
- Cooking at temperatures over 117°F
- Fluoridation of water
- Heavy metal toxicity
- Hybridization and genetic engineering of plants
- Irradiation of food
- Large intake of unsaturated and hydrogenated fats
- Mercury dental fillings
- Microwaving
- Not chewing food properly
- Parasitic or tapeworm infection
- Pasteurization
- Pesticides

- Radiation and electromagnetic fields
- Root canals and hidden dental infections

- Small intestinal bowel overgrowth
- Stress
- Surgery that removes part of the small intestine

Food Sources of Digestive Enzymes

- Avocados
- Bananas
- Broccoli
- Brussels sprouts

- Cabbage
- Mangos
- Nuts
- Oats

- Papaya
- Pineapple
- Wheat grass
- Whole grains

■ Conditions That Can Benefit from Digestive Enzymes

- Allergies
- Angina
- Arterial obstruction
- Atherosclerotic plaques and arterial obstruction, which lead to heart disease
- Autism
- Casein and gluten intolerance
- Celiac disease
- Cerebrovascular disease
- Chronic candidiasis
- Chronic pancreatitis
- Cystic fibrosis
- Diabetes
- Diarrhea
- Effects of radiation and chemotherapy in cancer patients
- Food sensitivities

- Heart disease (prevention)
- Hypercholesterolemia (high cholesterol)
- Hypertension (high blood pressure)
- Ischemic disease
- Lactose intolerance
- Leaky gut syndrome
- Malabsorption
- Maldigestion
- Osteoarthritis
- Pancreatic cancer
- Pancreatic insufficiency
- Post-surgical recovery (relieves pain and reduces edema)
- Rheumatic heart disease
- Rheumatoid arthritis
- Rosacea

- Sprains
- Steatorrhea (abnormal amounts of fat in feces)
- Tendonitis
- Thrombotic disease

■ Recommended Dosage

Look for a digestive enzyme product that includes at least protease, amylase, and lipase. Together, they should aid the digestion of most foods. If you have a specific digestive intolerance, such as lactose intolerance, you may want to add additional enzymes—in this case, lactase. Follow the manufacturer's instructions regarding dosage. In most cases, digestive enzymes should be taken right before eating or with your food. However, digestive enzymes taken on an empty stomach have a greater anti-inflammatory action.

■ Side Effects and Contraindications

Do not take digestive enzymes if you have any kind of active inflammatory bowel disease. Avoid digestive enzymes that contain papain if you are taking Coumadin. Speak to your healthcare provider or pharmacist to learn if any drugs you're taking might make it unwise to use digestive enzymes.

Do not use digestive enzymes that contain papain if you are allergic to papaya. Avoid enzymes with bromelain if you are allergic to pineapple, latex, wheat, celery, carrot, fennel, cypress pollen, or grass pollen.

High doses of digestive enzymes can negatively impact uric acid levels. Therefore, be sure to follow dosage recommendations.

Although relatively rare, the side effects of digestive enzymes can include the following:

- Constipation
- Cough
- Diarrhea
- Gas
- Heartburn
- Nausea
- Sore throat
- Upset stomach

D-RIBOSE

A sugar molecule, D-ribose is used by the body to make adenosine triphosphate, or ATP, the body's most basic form of energy. ATP stores energy that is obtained from the metabolism of food and transports it to areas within the cell when energy-consuming activities take place. D-ribose is also a key component of ribonucleic acid, or RNA, which is essential for life.

The body's cells naturally produce D-ribose, but the process is slow, and different organs produce different amounts of this important chemical. While some organs, such as the liver, produce relatively high amounts of D-ribose, the heart, brain, nerve tissues, and muscles produce only enough to meet their daily needs. With some diseases, such as cardiovascular disease, and with aging, D-ribose production slows. This, in turn, slows ATP production. Without sufficient energy, cells cannot maintain integrity and function. Supplementing with D-ribose has been shown to improve cellular processes when there is dysfunction of the mitochondria—the cellular powerhouses where ATP is produced.

■ Function of D-Ribose in Your Body

- Is a key component of RNA, a molecule involved in protein synthesis and other cellular activities

- Plays a major role in the synthesis of adenosine triphosphate (ATP)

Food Sources of D-Ribose

• Anchovies	• Cream cheese	• Poultry
• Asparagus	• Eggs	• Sardines
• Beef	• Herring	• Spinach
• Broccoli	• Milk	• Whole grains
• Caviar	• Mushrooms	• Yogurt
• Cheddar cheese	• Nuts	

■ Conditions That Can Benefit from D-Ribose

- Alzheimer's disease
- Amyotrophic lateral sclerosis (ALS)
- Autism spectrum disorder
- Bipolar mood disorders
- Chronic fatigue syndrome
- Congestive heart failure
- Coronary artery disease
- Diabetes
- Fibromyalgia
- Friedreich's ataxia
- Gastrointestinal motility disorders
- Huntington's disease
- Lyme disease
- Metabolic syndrome
- Multiple sclerosis (MS)
- Muscle fatigue
- Parkinson's disease
- Schizophrenia
- Systemic lupus erythematosus

■ Recommended Dosage

15,000 milligrams three times a day. Choose D-ribose, the natural form of this nutrient, rather than N-ribose, the synthetic form.

■ Side Effects and Contraindications

D-ribose is considered safe for short-term use. However, this supplement can lower blood sugar levels, so check with your healthcare provider or pharmacist before taking ribose with any diabetes medication, especially insulin. Supplementation with D-ribose can also cause the following symptoms: diarrhea, headache, nausea, and stomach discomfort.

FIBER

Fiber is a type of carbohydrate that passes through the body undigested. It occurs in two forms. *Soluble fiber*, which dissolves in water, helps lower levels of both glucose and cholesterol. *Insoluble fiber*, which does not dissolve in water, helps food move through the digestive system, supporting regularity and helping to prevent constipation. Most plant-based foods contain both types of fiber, although the amount of each type varies in different foods.

■ Functions of Fiber in Your Body

- Helps control blood sugar levels
- Increases stool bulk
- Lowers cholesterol levels
- Maintains optimal pH in the intestines to prevent microbes from producing cancerous products
- May contribute to healthy weight by making you feel fuller

- May help prevent diseases of the colon
- May lower the risk of hemorrhoids and diverticular disease
- Promotes the movement of food through the digestive system
- Promotes the regular elimination of stool from the body
- Removes toxic waste from the colon

■ Symptoms of Insufficient Fiber Intake

☐ Abdominal pain

☐ Constipation

- ☐ Diet-related nausea
- ☐ Excessive gas
- ☐ Fatigue or weakness
- ☐ Frequent hunger
- ☐ Hemorrhoids
- ☐ Hypercholesterolemia (high cholesterol)
- ☐ Hyperglycemia (high blood sugar)
- ☐ Increased risk of developing gallstones
- ☐ Irritable bowel syndrome (IBS)
- ☐ Loss of appetite
- ☐ Overeating
- ☐ Upset stomach
- ☐ Varicose veins

Food Sources of Soluble Fiber

- Apples
- Apricots
- Bananas
- Barley
- Beans
- Blackberries
- Broccoli
- Brussels sprouts
- Cabbage
- Carrots
- Flaxseed
- Nuts
- Oat bran
- Okra
- Oranges
- Pears
- Prunes
- Psyllium
- Sweet potatoes

Food Sources of Insoluble Fiber

- Bananas
- Beans
- Broccoli
- Brown rice
- Brussels sprouts
- Cauliflower
- Celery
- Corn
- Grains
- Lentils
- Pasta
- Potato (with skin)
- Prunes
- Spinach
- Wheat bran

■ Conditions That Can Benefit from Fiber

Soluble Fiber

- Cancer (prevention)
- Excess weight
- Hypercholesterolemia (high cholesterol)
- Hyperglycemia (high blood sugar)

- Hypertension (high blood pressure)
- Irritable bowel syndrome (IBS)

- Metabolic syndrome
- Overweight or obesity

Insoluble Fiber

- Constipation

- Loose stools

■ Recommended Dosage

The suggested daily intake for fiber is 25 grams for adult women and 38 grams for adult men. For adults over fifty years of age, the recommendation is 21 grams for women and 30 grams for men. It is always best to eat your way to adequate fiber intake rather than relying on supplemental fiber. If you choose to take a commercial fiber supplement, be sure to select one that contains no added sugar.

■ Side Effects and Contraindications

Adding too much fiber or adding fiber too quickly to your diet may cause gas, bloating, cramps, and diarrhea. Therefore, add 5 grams of fiber to your eating program daily at two-week intervals. Drink a lot of water when you ingest a large amount of fiber so that you do not become constipated.

If you are taking a fiber supplement, remember that fiber can decrease the absorption of many drugs as well as vitamin and mineral supplements. Take medications at least one hour before or two hours after a high-fiber meal or fiber supplement, and take nutritional supplements at least two hours before or two hours after a high fiber-meal or fiber supplement.

GAMMA-AMINOBUTYRIC ACID (GABA)

Gamma-aminobutyric acid (GABA) is a *neurotransmitter*—a chemical that helps send messages between the brain and the nervous system. Specifically, GABA is the chief inhibitory neurotransmitter, which means that it reduces the activity of the nerve cells by controlling the action of epinephrine, norepinephrine, dopamine, and serotonin. For this reason, it is thought to help relieve feelings of anxiety and fear and to promote calm. Its high concentration in the hypothalamus suggests that it plays an important role in hypothalamic-pituitary function.

GABA is derived from the amino acid glutamate via glutamic acid decarboxylase (GAD). Decreased GAD activity leads to lower GABA function and is also associated with the development of disorders such as schizophrenia, epilepsy, and bipolar disorder. Vitamin B_6, inositol, and magnesium are all needed for GABA to do its work.

■ Functions of GABA in Your Body

- Aids with pain control
- Burns fat
- Enhances immune function
- Helps control hypoglycemia (low blood sugar)
- Helps prevent anxiety
- Improves gastrointestinal function by enhancing motility, stomach emptying, stomach acid secretions, and esophageal sphincter relaxation

- Increases exercise endurance
- Increases focus
- Increases growth hormone secretion
- Is a muscle relaxant
- Lowers blood pressure
- Produces a calming effect
- Promotes sleep
- Regulates the neurotransmitters norepinephrine, epinephrine, dopamine, and serotonin

■ Symptoms of GABA Deficiency

- ☐ Anxiety
- ☐ Depression
- ☐ Fretfulness
- ☐ Impulsivity
- ☐ Inability to handle stress
- ☐ Irritability
- ☐ Racing mind
- ☐ Rapid heart rate
- ☐ Restlessness
- ☐ Sleep disturbances/ insomnia

■ Causes of GABA Deficiency

- Alcohol withdrawal
- Chronic pain
- Chronic stress and adrenal fatigue
- Excessive caffeine intake
- Imbalance of gut microbiome
- Lack of glutamine

- Low levels of progesterone
- Non-restorative sleep
- Nutritional deficiencies of vitamin B_6, inositol, and magnesium
- Poor blood sugar stability
- Toxic levels of lead or mercury

Food Sources of GABA

- Almonds
- Bananas
- Beans
- Broccoli
- Dairy products
- Eggs
- Fish
- Legumes
- Lentils
- Meat
- Nuts
- Oranges
- Seafood
- Seeds
- Spinach
- Walnuts
- Whole grains
- Red wine

■ Conditions That Can Benefit from GABA

- Anxiety disorder/panic attacks
- Attention-deficit/hyperactivity disorder (ADHD)
- Depression
- Insomnia
- Irritable bowel syndrome (IBS)
- Pain control
- Premenstrual disorder (PMS)
- Weight loss

■ Recommended Dosage

250 to 500 milligrams twice a day. Use the lower dose if you weigh less than 125 pounds. Always take a multivitamin to supply the nutrients that are needed to use GABA. Take before going to bed, as GABA may make you drowsy.

■ Side Effects and Contraindications

Check with your doctor before using GABA if you have diabetes, hypertension, kidney disease, liver disease, psychiatric illness, or ADHD.

Some people experience a tingling sensation in their face and a slight shortness of breath after taking GABA. Typically, however, this lasts only for a few minutes. For some people, GABA is best taken at night since it may cause drowsiness.

The following are possible symptoms of an increased level of GABA. If you experience any of these symptoms, contact your healthcare provider before taking further supplements.

- Anxiety
- Facial flushing
- Facial numbness
- Hypertension (high blood pressure)
- Inability to sit still
- Increased levels of prolactin

- Nausea and vomiting
- Sensation of tingling and itching
- Tachypnea (abnormally rapid breathing)

GLUCOSAMINE SULFATE

Glucosamine occurs naturally in the human body and is used by the body to produce chemicals that are involved in the building of tendons, ligaments, cartilage, and synovial fluid—the thick fluid that lubricates the joints, allowing for ease of movement. Many researchers believe that glucosamine sulfate supplements increase the cartilage and fluid surrounding the joints, help prevent the breakdown of these substances, or perform both of these functions.

■ Functions of Glucosamine Sulfate in Your Body

- Aids bone structure development
- Aids skin hydration
- Delays the deterioration of cartilage
- Has cartilage-, ligament-, and tendon-building properties
- Is anti-inflammatory
- Is needed for the synthesis of synovial fluid
- Protects the gastrointestinal tract and enhances digestion
- Reduces joint pain and tenderness

■ Symptoms of Glucosamine Sulfate Deficiency

☐ Aches and pains in joints ☐ Arthritis ☐ Stiffness in joints

■ Causes of Glucosamine Sulfate Deficiency

- Aging. As people get older, they often gradually lose their ability to produce adequate levels of glucosamine.

Food Sources of Glucosamine Sulfate

There are no natural food sources of glucosamine, but some nutrition drinks are fortified with glucosamine as well as other joint-supporting compounds.

■ Conditions That Can Benefit from Glucosamine Sulfate

- Aging skin
- Chronic back pain
- Inflammatory bowel disease
- May be helpful for osteoporosis

- Osteoarthritis
- Rheumatoid arthritis
- Wounds (treatment)

■ Recommended Dosage

500 milligrams capsule or tablet three times a day for a total of 1,500 milligrams. If you are overweight, you may need a higher dose. It may take two to three months for the glucosamine to take full effect.

Glucosamine sulfate is the most effective of the different types of glucosamine on the market. Most of these supplements are processed from shellfish, but if you have a shellfish allergy, you can find a product that has another source. Glucosamine sulfate can also be made in a laboratory. This compound is often found in supplements that also contain other substances, like chondroitin and MSM, to increase effectiveness.

Water pills (diuretics) reduce the effectiveness of glucosamine supplements. If you take water pills, speak to your healthcare provider about the best glucosamine dosage for you.

■ Side Effects and Contraindications

Avoid shellfish-derived supplements if you have a shellfish allergy.

Some studies show—and some studies refute—that glucosamine can alter blood sugar levels. If you have prediabetes or diabetes, consult your healthcare provider before using this supplement.

Glucosamine can have a blood-thinning effect. If you have a bleeding disorder or are taking a medication or supplement that may thin your blood, do not take glucosamine. Discontinue use two weeks before surgery.

When glucosamine is combined with a nonsteroidal medication, the dosage of the nonsteroidal may be able to be decreased, which decreases the risk of side effects. Speak to your healthcare provider about the possible need to adjust your prescription. Also speak to your healthcare provider or pharmacist to learn if any other drugs you're taking might interact with glucosamine.

Although glucosamine is usually well tolerated, the following side effects may occur:

- Constipation
- Diarrhea

- Epigastric pain (pain below your ribs in the area of your upper abdomen)

- Heartburn

- Nausea

GRAPE SEED EXTRACT

See OPCs (Oligomeric Proanthocyanidins).

INDOLE-3-CARBINOL (I-3-C)

Indole-3-carbinol (I-3-C) is developed from the breakdown of glucobrassicin, a compound that occurs when cruciferous vegetables (those in the cabbage family) are broken down or cooked. These vegetables are known for their health benefits, and indole-3-carbinol is one of the chief reasons why. It appears to reduce the risk for estrogen-dependent cancers and enhance health in other ways, as well.

■ Functions of Indole-3-Carbinol in Your Body

- Helps prevent the development of estrogen-dependent cancers (such as breast, cervical, and uterine cancers) by supporting healthy estrogen metabolism and hormonal balance

- Inhibits the angiogenesis (development of new blood vessels) associated with tumor cell growth

- Is an anti-inflammatory

- Is an antioxidant

- May help prevent the development of prostate cancer by supporting optimal estrogen metabolism

■ Symptoms of Indole-3-Carbinol Deficiency

☐ Abnormal estrogen metabolism (breakdown)

■ Causes of Indole-3-Carbinol Deficiency

- Low dietary intake of cruciferous vegetables.

Food Sources of Indole-3-Carbinol

Consume the following vegetables lightly steamed when possible. Boiling these foods leads to the loss of nutrients.

- Broccoli
- Brussels sprouts
- Cabbage
- Cauliflower
- Collard greens
- Mustard greens
- Radish
- Kale
- Kohlrabi
- Mustard greens
- Rutabaga
- Turnips

■ Conditions That Can Benefit from Indole-3-Carbinol

- Breast, colon, cervical, endometrial, pancreatic, and prostate cancer (prevention and therapy)

- Conditions related to human papilloma virus (HPV), such as cervical intraepithelial neoplasia (CIN)
- Lupus

■ Recommended Dosage

300 to 500 milligrams daily.

■ Side Effects and Contraindications

Possible side effects of low-dose supplementation include a mild elevation of liver enzymes and a skin rash. Possible side effects of high-dose supplementation include dizziness and tremor.

MALIC ACID

Malic acid is found naturally in the body, where it is synthesized every day during the process of converting carbohydrates to energy. This acid can also be consumed in apples, cherries, and most tart fruits.

Malic acid is essential to life, as it is involved in cellular energy production. Despite its importance, healthy people do not usually require malic acid supplementation. However, it should be noted that cisplatin, a chemotherapy medication, and certain other drugs can reduce the level of malic acid in the body. Preliminary evidence also suggests that people with fibromyalgia might have difficulty creating or using this substance. In addition, it has been found that malic acid supplements may benefit certain conditions.

◾ Functions of Malic Acid in Your Body

- Essential for producing cellular energy

- Increases urinary citrate excretion and pH

Food Sources of Malic Acid

Of all the fruits, apples are the highest in malic acid, but the other foods listed below are also good sources of this compound.

- Apple cider vinegar
- Apples
- Apricots
- Bananas
- Blackberries
- Broccoli

- Carrots
- Cherries
- Lychees
- Mangos
- Nectarines
- Peaches
- Pears

- Peas
- Potatoes
- Rhubarb
- Strawberries
- Tomatoes
- Watermelon

◾ Conditions That Can Benefit from Malic Acid

- Calcium oxalate stone disease

- Chronic fatigue syndrome

- Exhaustion

- Fibromyalgia

- Muscle pain

◾ Recommended Dosage

Although malic acid deficiency is rare, as you learned above, this supplement does have therapeutic uses.

- For treatment of calcium oxalate stone disease: 1,200 milligrams daily for one week.

- For treatment of fibromyalgia and other conditions: 600 milligrams malic acid with 200 milligrams magnesium, once daily. After one week, take two doses a day.

◾ Side Effects and Contraindications

Malic acid appears to be safe at recommended doses. Safety has not been established for pregnant and breastfeeding women or people with severe liver and kidney disease. These people should avoid taking malic acid supplements.

In addition, preliminary studies indicate that malic acid may reduce blood pressure. If you have low blood pressure, speak to your healthcare provider before using malic acid.

MELATONIN

Melatonin is a hormone produced in the pineal gland. Production in the brain is associated with the time of day, rising in the evening to promote sleep and falling in the morning to promote wakefulness. Staying in a lighted room at night blocks secretion of the hormone, and aging causes production to decrease.

Aside from its relationship to the sleep-wake cycle, melatonin also has other functions in the body, such as acting as an antioxidant and helping to balance the stress response.

■ Functions of Melatonin in Your Body

- Affects the release of sex hormones
- Blocks estrogen from binding to receptor sites
- Boosts the immune system
- Decreases levels of cortisol, the "stress hormone," helping to balance the stress response
- Decreases platelet stickiness, reducing the risk of heart disease
- Helps prevent cancer and treat some cancers
- Improves mood
- Improves sleep quality
- Is an antioxidant
- Promotes healthy cholesterol levels
- Protects the heart
- Relieves jet lag
- Stimulates the parathyroid gland
- Stimulates the production of the growth hormone

■ Symptoms of Melatonin Deficiency

- ☐ Anxiety
- ☐ Early morning awakening
- ☐ Fatigue
- ☐ Frequent waking at night
- ☐ Heart disease
- ☐ Immunological disorders
- ☐ Increased risk of cancer
- ☐ Insomnia
- ☐ Seasonal affective disorder
- ☐ Stress

■ Causes of Melatonin Deficiency

- Alcohol
- Caffeine
- Some drugs, from acetaminophen to ronidazole, can cause a melatonin deficiency. Speak to your healthcare provider or pharmacist to learn if any drugs you're taking might be affecting your melatonin levels.
- Tobacco
- Too many high glycemic index foods
- Vitamin B_{12} deficiency

Food Sources of Melatonin

- Asparagus
- Barley
- Black olives/green olives
- Black tea/green tea
- Broccoli
- Brussels sprouts
- Corn
- Cucumber
- Oats
- Peanuts
- Pomegranate
- Red grapes
- Rice
- Strawberries
- Tart cherry juice concentrate
- Tart cherries
- Tomatoes
- Walnuts

■ Conditions That Can Benefit from Melatonin

- Alzheimer's disease (prevention and treatment)
- Closed head injury
- Heart disease (prevention and treatment)
- Hypercholesterolemia (high cholesterol)
- Insomnia
- Parkinson's disease
- Some cancers
- Stroke
- Weak immune system

■ Recommended Dosage

1 to 3 milligrams daily. If taken as a sleep aid, melatonin should be taken thirty to sixty minutes before bedtime in a dark room. Start with one milligram.

It is important to measure melatonin levels by saliva testing before taking doses larger than 1 to 3 milligrams. High doses of melatonin can lower serotonin levels and lead to depression. See an anti-aging/functional medicine provider for salivary testing.

Larger doses of melatonin can be used to treat breast cancer along with traditional therapies. Consult your physician regarding melatonin dosage for this purpose.

■ Symptoms of Elevated Levels of Melatonin

- Daytime sleepiness/fatigue
- Depression
- Headaches

- Increased cortisol levels
- Intense dreaming/nightmares
- Suppression of serotonin

■ Causes of Elevated Levels of Melatonin

- Certain medications, such as clorgyline, desipramine, fluvoxamine, thorazine, and tranylcypromine, can increase levels of this hormone. Speak to your healthcare provider or pharmacist to learn if any drugs you're taking might be elevating your melatonin levels
- High intake of foods containing melatonin
- Melatonin supplementation
- St. John's wort supplementation

■ Side Effects and Contraindications

Melatonin is an immune stimulator. Therefore, if you have an autoimmune disease, you should see your doctor before taking this supplement. Avoid taking melatonin if you are pregnant or breastfeeding; if you are on prescription steroids; or if you are suffering from depression or other mental illness, leukemia, or lymphoma. Speak to your healthcare provider or pharmacist to learn if any drugs you're taking might make it unwise to use melatonin.

MSM (METHYLSULFONYLMETHANE)

Methylsulfonylmethane (MSM) is a substance that is produced in the body and is also found in a number of vegetables. MSM supplies the mineral sulfur—an important compound that is vital to life. Note that sulfur is not related to sulfa drugs, so if you are allergic to sulfa, you can still take MSM.

MSM is formed from the oxidation of the sulfur compound dimethyl sulfoxide (DMSO). Although DMSO has pain-relieving attributes similar to those of MSM, DMSO can cause side effects that range from nasal congestion to shortness of breath to body odor. Therefore, MSM is a better way to get sulfur.

■ Functions of MSM in Your Body

- Eliminates toxins from the body
- Increases blood supply
- Inhibits histamine
- Inhibits pain impulses along nerve fibers
- Is an anti-inflammatory
- May control GI hyperacidity (high acid)
- Needed to make antibodies

- Needed to make connective tissue such as cartilage and collagen
- Needed to make enzymes
- Needed to make glutathione
- Reduces muscle spasms
- Reduces oxidative stress
- Softens scar tissue
- Supports the immune system

■ Symptoms of MSM Deficiency

- ☐ Allergies/allergic rhinitis
- ☐ Joint pain
- ☐ Muscle spasms/pain

■ Causes of MSM Deficiency

- Insufficient dietary intake of foods high in MSM (MSM is rapidly used by the body, so you may not get enough in the diet alone.)

Food Sources of MSM

- Alfalfa sprouts
- Brussels sprouts
- Cabbage
- Cauliflower
- Coffee
- Corn
- Garlic
- Horseradish
- Kale
- Leeks
- Milk
- Mustard greens
- Onions
- Peppers
- Radishes
- Tea
- Tomatoes
- Watercress

■ Conditions That Can Benefit from MSM

- Acne
- Allergies
- Cancer (breast and liver)
- Bursitis
- Carpal tunnel syndrome
- Chronic back pain
- Chronic headaches
- Cognitive decline
- Diverticulosis
- Emphysema

- Fibromyalgia
- Hair loss
- Heartburn
- Hemorrhoids
- Inflammation after an injury
- Joint pain

- Muscle pain
- Osteoarthritis
- Psoriasis
- Rheumatoid arthritis
- Rosacea
- Scleroderma

- Stretch marks
- Temporomandibular joint (TMJ) disorder
- Tendonitis
- Wound healing
- Wrinkles

▪ Recommended Dosage

Start with 500 milligrams, three times a day. You may increase the dose to 3,000 milligrams, three times a day, usually without side effects. Take with a meal when you first start supplementing to avoid possible heartburn. MSM can be taken as a capsule, powder, or tablet, or applied as a lotion or gel. You will need to take MSM for at least one month before you see results.

▪ Side Effects and Contraindications

Do not take MSM during pregnancy or while breastfeeding.

If you apply a lotion that contains MSM to the lower extremities, it can increase swelling and pain if you have circulatory problems or varicose veins. Therefore, do not use MSM topically if you have circulatory issues or varicosities.

Low-dose oral MSM supplementation usually does not cause side effects. Larger doses, particularly over 15 grams (15,000 milligrams), may cause the following:

- Abdominal discomfort
- Bloating
- Diarrhea

- Difficulty concentrating
- Fatigue
- Headache

- Insomnia
- Itching
- Nausea

OPCs (OLIGOMERIC PROANTHOCYANIDINS)

Oligomeric proanthocyanidins (OPCs) are a class of flavonoids that are found in grape seeds, pine bark, red wine, and a few other plant parts. The body cannot make OPCs. A powerful antioxidant, this supplement can relieve a number of medical conditions.

■ Functions of OPCs in Your Body

All forms of OPCs have some similarities. They all have anti-carcinogenic properties and act as anti-inflammatories. However, extracts from different sources can also have different effects on the body.

Grape Seed Extract

- Boosts immune system
- Has anti-cancer properties
- Is a natural antihistamine
- In an anti-inflammatory
- Is an antioxidant
- Lowers LDL (bad) cholesterol
- Prevents damage to DNA

Pine Bark Extract

- Boosts immune system
- Has anti-cancer properties
- Helps treat venous inadequacies
- Is an anti-inflammatory
- Is an antioxidant
- Protects the cells from oxidative damage
- Treats certain skin conditions

Red Wine Extract

- Decreases cholesterol
- Has anti-cancer properties
- Is an anti-inflammatory
- Is an antioxidant
- Lowers apolipoprotein B, thereby lowering the risk of heart disease
- Prevents platelet stickiness, reducing the risk of heart disease
- Reduces triglycerides

■ Conditions That Can Benefit from OPCs

- Allergies
- Alzheimer's disease and cognitive decline
- Arthritis
- Asthma
- Attention-deficit/hyperactivity disorder (ADHD)
- Cancer
- Certain skin disorders
- Chronic fatigue syndrome
- Glaucoma
- Heart disease
- Hypercholesterolemia (high cholesterol)
- Hypertension (high blood pressure)

- Insulin resistance/diabetes
- Lupus
- Lymphedema
- Melasma
- Pancreatitis
- Varicose veins/vascular insufficiency
- Weight problems

■ Recommended Dosage

50 to 200 milligrams daily. If using Pycnogenol, a trade name for an extract of French maritime tree bark, follow the manufacturer's instructions.

■ Side Effects and Contraindications

OPCs may have some anticoagulant properties when taken in high doses. Speak to your healthcare provider or pharmacist to learn if any drugs you're taking might make it unwise to use these supplements.

Side effects are rare, but when they do occur, they are limited to occasional allergic reactions and mild digestive distress.

PHOSPHATIDYLCHOLINE (PC)

Phosphatidylcholine (PC) is a phospholipid and a major component of lecithin. Often, the word "lecithin" is used as a synonym for "phosphatidylcholine," but they are not the same and cannot be used interchangeably.

PC is the major lipid (fat) of cell membranes and blood proteins and is found in every cell of the body. It is also the body's main source of choline, the precursor to the neurotransmitter acetylcholine, and is critical for many vital body functions. Levels of PC generally decrease as we age.

■ Functions of Phosphatidylcholine in Your Body

- Aids in the breakdown of fats
- Enhances liver health
- Is a vital component of pulmonary surfactant, which makes it possible to breathe
- Is one of the chief components of the mucus that lines and protects the gut
- Maintains cell structure
- Needed for production of the neurotransmitter acetylcholine, which plays an important role in memory and cognition
- Required for VLDL (very low-density lipoprotein) assembly and subsequent secretion by the liver

■ Symptoms of Phosphatidylcholine Deficiency

☐ Cognitive decline

☐ Hypercholesterolemia (high cholesterol)

☐ Muscle damage

☐ Nonalcoholic fatty liver disease

☐ Ulcerative colitis

■ Causes of Phosphatidylcholine Deficiency

- Genetic changes involved in the manufacture of choline or folate

- Low intake of foods that contain this nutrient

- Pregnancy

- Some drugs, such as methotrexate, can cause a PC deficiency. Speak to your healthcare provider or pharmacist to learn if any drugs you're taking might be causing loss of this nutrient.

Food Sources of Phosphatidylcholine

- Cruciferous vegetables such as cauliflower and broccoli
- Dairy
- Eggs
- Fish
- Meat
- Mustard
- Peanuts
- Poultry
- Soy
- Sunflower seeds

■ Conditions That Can Benefit from Phosphatidylcholine

- Anxiety disorder

- Depression

- Eczema

- Fibrocystic breast disease

- Fibroids

- Hepatitis C (used with interferon)

- Hypercholesterolemia (high cholesterol)

- Hyperhomocysteinemia (high homocysteine)

- Lipomas

- Memory loss, including Alzheimer's disease

- Nonalcoholic fatty liver disease

- Premenstrual syndrome (PMS)

- Stroke

- Ulcerative colitis

- Xanthelasmas (yellowish deposit of cholesterol under the skin around the eyes)

■ Recommended Dosage

600 to 1,200 milligrams daily, most commonly taken as a pill. Phosphatidyl-choline can also be taken subcutaneously or intravenously.

The best way to determine dosage is to have your healthcare provider order a fatty acid analysis test. The dosage may be dependent on your own gut microbiota (gut flora) and how well you are able to absorb phosphatidylcho-line. The need for this supplement may increase if you are pregnant or if you are taking the drug methotrexate. Again, consult your healthcare provider.

■ Side Effects and Contraindications

There are three metabolites of the dietary lipid phosphatidylcholine: choline, trimethylamine N-oxide (TMAO), and betaine. The breakdown of choline into TMAO may increase your risk of developing atherosclerosis. It is suggested that you have your healthcare provider measure your TMAO levels before taking phosphatidylcholine.

Phosphatidylcholine can interact with some medications. Speak to your healthcare provider or pharmacist to learn if any drugs you're taking might make it unwise to use this supplement. Use with caution if you have malab-sorption problems, as this could exacerbate them.

Possible side effects of this nutrient, if taken by mouth, include the following:

- Diarrhea
- Excessive sweating
- Upset stomach

PHOSPHATIDYLSERINE (PS)

Phosphatidylserine (PS), a phospholipid, is a key building block for every cell in the brain and is present in every cell in the body. Although it is made in the body from L-serine, glycerophosphate, and two fatty acids, we obtain most of what we require from food.

■ Functions of Phosphatidylserine in Your Body

- Combats depression
- Critical for neurotransmission
- Directly affects the hormones norepinephrine, serotonin, and dopamine
- Enhances immune function
- Increases the number of membrane receptor sites for receiving messages

- Influences the fluidity of nerve-cell membranes

- Needed for the electrical activity of the brain

- Needed for the formation and functioning of cell membranes

- Reduces levels of cortisol, a stress hormone

- Restores the supply of acetylcholine, the main neurotransmitter involved in memory

- Used in bone formation

Symptoms of Phosphatidylserine Deficiency

☐ Cognitive decline   ☐ Depression

☐ Decreased focus   ☐ Stress

Causes of Phosphatidylserine Deficiency

- Low intake of nutrients needed for synthesis

Food Sources of Phosphatidylserine

- Barley
- Fish, particularly cod, mackerel, tuna, anchovies, trout, herring
- Meat
- Soy lecithin
- White beans

Conditions That Can Benefit from Phosphatidylserine

- Alzheimer's disease and other forms of memory decline

- Anxiety

- Attention-deficit/hyperactivity disorder (ADHD)

- Depression

- Exercise-induced stress (prevention)

- Parkinson's disease

- Poor learning and concentration

- Stress

- Stroke (recovery)

Recommended Daily Dosage

100 to 500 milligrams daily. The most common dose is 300 milligrams a day.

■ Side Effects and Contraindications

Phosphatidylserine interacts with a number of drugs. Speak to your health-care provider or pharmacist to learn if any drugs you're taking might make it unwise to use this nutrient.

Side effects are very rare but can include insomnia and stomach upset.

POLICOSANOL

Policosanol is a mixture of fatty alcohols that is usually isolated from the wax of sugar cane but can also be derived from wheat, yams, or beeswax. The policosanol used in studies is sugar cane-based. This supplement is most commonly used to lower cholesterol, to prevent platelets from forming dangerous clots, and to treat leg pain due to poor blood circulation (intermittent claudication).

■ Functions of Policosanol in Your Body

- Decreases platelet clumping, reducing the risk of heart disease

- Increases the excretion of bile acids in the stool, helping prevent the development of gallstones

- Inhibits the development of atherosclerosis (narrowing of the arteries due to plaque build-up)

- Inhibits the production of cholesterol by the liver

- Lowers LDL (bad) cholesterol

- Raises HDL (good) cholesterol

■ Conditions That Can Benefit from Policosanol

- Atherosclerosis (prevention and treatment)

- Hypercholesterolemia (high cholesterol)

- Intermittent claudication (leg pain typically caused by obstruction of the arteries)

■ Recommended Dosage

5 to 10 milligrams twice a day. Choose a policosanol supplement made from sugar cane, as cane sugar-derived supplements have been used in medical trials with positive results.

■ Side Effects and Contraindications

Because of policosanol's effects on platelet aggregation, do not take this supplement if you have a bleeding disorder or are taking a medication or supplement that may thin your blood. If you are planning to have surgery, discontinue taking this product two weeks before the procedure. Policosanol may also increase the effects and side effects of levodopa. Speak to your healthcare provider or pharmacist to learn if any drugs you're taking might make it unwise to use policosanol.

This supplement is generally well tolerated, but the following side effects may occur:

- Dizziness
- Drowsiness
- Indigestion

- Insomnia
- Irritability
- Migraine headache

- Nose and gum bleeds
- Skin rash
- Weight loss

PROBIOTICS

The human digestive system is full of friendly microorganisms that benefit your health by helping digest your food, destroying disease-causing microorganisms, and producing vitamins. They enable your body to function properly and increase your defenses against disease. Collectively, these microorganisms are known as the *gut microbiome*. Although many types of microbes live inside you—including bacteria, virus, and fungi—most studies have focused on bacteria.

A poor diet and the overuse of antibiotics—which kill both good and bad bacteria—can create an overgrowth in the bowel of unhealthy bacteria while destroying beneficial bacteria. This can cause a range of problems, including infection, insulin resistance, diabetes, high cholesterol, high triglycerides, high blood pressure, heart disease, food allergies or sensitivities, sugar cravings, decline of immune system function, skin problems such as eczema, and weight gain. If during and after a course of antibiotics, you take probiotic supplements—which contain healthy bacteria—you will limit the negative effects of antibiotics by decreasing the unhealthy bacteria and encouraging the repopulation of your gut with healthy microorganisms. To reap the benefits of probiotics, however, it is important to take them on a daily basis even if you are not on antibiotics. This will help keep your body in balance, your gut healthy, and your immune system strong.

■ Functions of Probiotics in Your Body

- Aids in the metabolism of medications
- Enhances GI motility
- Enhances the immune system
- Has anti-cancer properties
- Improves central nervous system activity
- Improves digestion
- Increases nutrient absorption
- Inhibits the growth of pathogens
- Is an antioxidant

- Is involved in the production of polyamines and short-chain fatty acids (SCFAs)
- Is needed for the synthesis of the B vitamins and vitamin K
- Lowers blood sugar
- Makes lactase, an enzyme needed to help the digestion of milk products
- Promotes weight loss
- Relieves abdominal distention due to gas

Food Sources of Probiotics and Prebiotics

Some foods, such as yogurt, contain *probiotics*—healthy bacteria. Some foods are known as *prebiotics* because they feed beneficial bacteria. The list below includes both types of food. To differentiate between the two, prebiotics are marked with an asterisk (*).

- Asparagus*
- Bananas*
- Chicory*
- Garlic*

- Kefir
- Kimchi
- Miso
- Onions*

- Sauerkraut (not pasteurized)
- Tempeh
- Yogurt

■ Conditions That Can Benefit from Probiotics

- Acne
- Allergies
- Autism
- Autoimmune diseases
- Cancer (prevention)
- Chronic constipation
- Chronic yeast infection

- *Clostridium difficile* infection
- Decrease of beneficial bacteria due to antibiotic use
- Diabetes
- Digestive problems
- Eczema (prevention)
- Gas

- Gastrointestinal infection (prevention)

- *H. pylori* infection (prevention)

- Heart disease

- Hepatic encephalopathy

- Hypercholesterolemia (high cholesterol)

- Hyperhomocysteinemia (high homocysteine)

- Hypertension (high blood pressure)

- Immune dysfunction

- Inflammatory bowel disease (IBD)

- Intestinal hyperpermeability (leaky gut syndrome)

- Irritable bowel syndrome (IBS)

- Kidney stone formation

- Lactose intolerance

- Necrotizing enterocolitis (NEC)

- Neurological diseases

- Obesity

- Oxidative stress

- Peptic ulcer

- Psychiatric disorders

- Tooth decay (prevention)

- Urinary tract infection (prevention and treatment)

- Vaginal infection (prevention and treatment)

- Weight gain and obesity

■ Recommended Dosage

The proper dose of probiotics partly depends on the specific probiotics being used. However, in most cases, you should take approximately 20 billion units once a day.

Lactobacillus acidophilus (L. acidophilus) is the most commonly used probiotic. Other common products include several different species, such as *Lactobacillus bulgaricus, Lactobacillus casei, Lactobacillus reuteri, Lactobacillus GG, Bifidobacterium longum, Bifidobacterium bifidum, Streptococcus thermophiles,* and *Saccharaomyces boulardii.* Unless otherwise directed by your healthcare provider, take a general probiotic that contains several strains with a total of at least 20 billion units per dose.

If you are taking probiotics to aid in weight loss, it is important to choose *Lactobacillus gasseri* and/or *Lactobacillus plantarum.* Avoid *Lactobacillus acidophilus, Lactobacillus fermentum,* and *Lactobacillus ingluviei,* which in studies have been associated with weight gain.

Do not take probiotics at the same time of day that you take an antibiotic, antiviral, or antifungal agent. There should be at least a two-hour period both before and after usage of the medication when taking probiotics.

Read the label of your probiotics to see if they need refrigeration. Change the brand every six months, rotating products from three to four companies to provide comprehensive therapy. Note that the need for probiotics increases when you are stressed.

■ Side Effects and Contraindications

Do not use live strains of probiotics if you have a compromised immune system or are receiving chemotherapy or immunosuppressive drugs. You should also avoid live probiotics if you have an artificial heart valve.

Although most people do not experience side effects when taking probiotics, the following reactions may occur. To avoid side effects, begin with a low dose of probiotics and slowly increase the dose over several weeks.

- Bloating
- Constipation
- Diarrhea
- Gas
- Gastrointestinal upset
- Increased thirst

PYCNOGENOL

See OPCs (Oligomeric Proanthocyanidins).

QUERCETIN

Quercetin is a flavonoid—a plant pigment—that is found in a number of different fruits, vegetables, grains, and other plants, including apples, red onions, purple grapes (and red wine), tea, and berries. It is also present in ginkgo biloba, St. John's wort, and American elder. One of the most studied of all flavonoids, quercetin is known to be a powerful and highly versatile antioxidant that has a wide range of important biological functions.

■ Functions of Quercetin in Your Body

- Enhances memory
- Improves sperm quality
- Inhibits the release of histamine, reducing the allergic response
- Is an anti-inflammatory
- Is an antioxidant
- Lowers blood pressure
- Lowers blood sugar
- Modulates the immune system
- Protects the gastrointestinal tract
- Protects the heart
- Protects the kidneys
- Protects the nervous system

Food Sources of Quercetin

- Apples
- Asparagus
- Bell peppers
- Black currants
- Black tea
- Blueberries
- Broccoli
- Buckwheat
- Capers

- Cherries
- Cocoa powder
- Concord grapes
- Green chili peppers
- Green tea
- Kale and other leafy green vegetables

- Nectarines
- Purple grapes
- Radicchio
- Raspberries
- Red onion
- Red wine
- Tomatoes

■ Conditions That Can Benefit from Quercetin

- Allergies
- Asthma
- Bone loss (prevention)
- Cancer (prevention)
- Canker sores
- Cataracts
- Chronic fatigue syndrome
- Cognitive impairment
- Coronary heart disease
- Diabetes/insulin resistance
- Hypercholesterolemia (high cholesterol)

- Hypertension (high blood pressure)
- Interstitial cystitis (painful bladder syndrome)
- Male infertility
- Osteoarthritis
- Peptic ulcer
- Prostatitis
- Rheumatoid arthritis
- Sarcoidosis
- Upper respiratory infection (prevention)

■ Recommended Dosage

300 to 1,000 milligrams three times a day. For best results, always take quercetin with bromelain and vitamin C.

■ Side Effects and Contraindications

If you have a bleeding disorder or are taking a medication or supplement that may thin your blood, do not take quercetin, as this supplement may enhance the drugs' effects. If you are planning to have surgery, discontinue this therapy two weeks before the procedure. Be aware that quercetin can interact with other medications, as well. Speak to your healthcare provider or pharmacist to learn if any of the drugs you are taking might make it unwise to use this supplement.

Quercetin may inhibit thyroid function. If you have thyroid problems, do not take this supplement without speaking to your healthcare provider.

Quercetin is an iron chelator and therefore inhibits the body's absorption of iron. Therefore, do not take quercetin at the same time that you take an iron supplement or eat a food that is high in iron. Wait at least two hours before or after taking iron to take a quercetin supplement.

RED YEAST RICE

Red yeast rice (RYR) is made by fermenting a type of yeast called *Monascus purpureus* with rice. The resulting rice is bright red-purple in color and contains a natural statin drug known as monacolin K. This is why RYR is most often used to control cholesterol.

Scientists aren't sure whether RYR lowers cholesterol because of monacolin K or because of naturally occurring plant compounds that may also have cholesterol-lowering effects. Currently, FDA regulations make it illegal for the product to contain more than trace amounts of monacolin K. Nevertheless, some products may still contain substantial amounts.

Like a statin drug, red yeast rice can inhibit the body's synthesis of coenzyme Q_{10} (CoQ$_{10}$). Therefore, if you are taking red yeast rice, also take supplemental CoQ$_{10}$.

■ Functions of Red Yeast Rice in Your Body

- Has anti-cancer properties
- Is anti-inflammatory
- Lowers blood pressure
- Lowers blood sugar
- Lowers cholesterol
- Lowers triglycerides

■ Conditions That Can Benefit from Red Yeast Rice

- Hypercholesterolemia (high cholesterol)
- Hypertriglyceridemia (high triglycerides)
- Hypertension (high blood pressure)
- Insulin resistance/diabetes
- Osteopenia/osteoporosis (bone loss)

- Prostate cancer
- Ventricular arrhythmias (irregular heart rhythms)

■ Recommended Dosage

600 mg twice a day. When taking red yeast rice, always be sure to take 100 milligrams a day of pharmaceutical grade CoQ_{10}.

■ Side Effects and Contraindications

Do not use red yeast rice if you are pregnant or breastfeeding. Also avoid this supplement if you have had an organ transplant.

Be aware that red yeast rice may interact with many other medications, including blood thinners and statins. Speak to your healthcare provider or pharmacist to learn if any drugs you're taking might make it unwise to take this supplement. Never use red yeast rice with a statin drug.

Grapefruit and grapefruit juice can increase the level of statin in the body, including the statin-like substance in red yeast rice. Do not consume grapefruits or their juice when using this supplement.

Some red yeast rice contains a contaminant called citrinin, which can cause kidney failure. Make sure you are taking pharmaceutical grade red yeast rice.

Monacolin K, found in some red yeast rice products, has been associated with adverse effects such as myopathy, rhabdomyolysis (destruction of skeletal muscle), and liver toxicity. Consult your pharmacist or healthcare provider before starting this supplement. If you experience muscle aches when taking this supplement, stop taking it immediately and call your healthcare provider.

Side effects of red yeast rice are rare but can include the following:

- Bloating
- Gas
- Heartburn

- Dizziness
- Headache
- Stomachache

RESVERATROL

Resveratrol is part of a group known as polyphenols—plant compounds that act as antioxidants. Because one of the sources of resveratrol is red wine, in the past, it was thought that this substance explained the "French paradox"—the contradiction between the low occurrence of cardiovascular disease in the French people and their relatively high-fat diets. However, most experts now agree that there is not enough resveratrol in wine to account for this phenomenon. Whether or not it is involved in the French paradox, we know that resveratrol has numerous important functions in the body, including activities that support cardiovascular health.

■ Functions of Resveratrol in Your Body

- Decreases platelet stickiness, reducing the risk of heart disease
- Dilates (opens) the arteries by increasing nitric oxide
- Has anticancer actions
- Improves bone health
- Improves mitochondrial function
- Increases HDL (good) cholesterol
- Induces phase II liver detoxification enzymes
- Inhibits oxidation of LDL (bad) cholesterol
- Is a phytoestrogen
- Is an antioxidant
- Is anti-inflammatory
- Is antimicrobial
- Is antiviral
- Lowers blood sugar and regulates high insulin levels
- Protects endothelial function, lowering the risk of heart disease
- Stops the proliferation of cells that narrow arteries

■ Symptoms of Resveratrol Deficiency

- ☐ Elevated blood sugar
- ☐ Hypercholesterolemia (high cholesterol)
- ☐ Hypertension (high blood pressure)
- ☐ Memory loss

■ Causes of Resveratrol Deficiency

- Low dietary intake of foods containing resveratrol

Food Sources of Resveratrol

- Bilberries
- Blueberries
- Cocoa
- Cranberries
- Grape juice
- Grape skins
- Mulberries
- Peanuts
- Red wine

■ Conditions That Can Benefit from Resveratrol

- Cognitive decline/Alzheimer's disease

- Colon, pancreatic, prostate, stomach, and thyroid cancer (prevention and treatment)
- Coronary heart disease
- Hypertension (high blood pressure)
- Insulin resistance/diabetes
- Weight loss

■ Recommended Dosage

20 to 1,000 milligrams daily. Because resveratrol oxidizes easily, you should store the supplements in a cool, dry place.

■ Side Effects and Contraindications

Do not use resveratrol if you have or have had an estrogen-related cancer until more is known about the estrogenic activity of resveratrol. When used in high doses, resveratrol may cause any of the following symptoms:

- Abdominal pain
- Diarrhea
- Gas
- Nausea

TEA TREE OIL

Tea tree oil is made from the leaves of the *Melaleuca alternifolia*, a small tree that grows in Australia. Used as traditional medicine for centuries, it is valued for its ability to kill certain bacteria, viruses, and fungi, and is often used topically to improve skin, scalp, and oral health. At least some of its benefits are due to a high concentration of terpinen-4-ol, a compound with anti-inflammatory properties.

■ Functions of Tea Tree Oil in Your Body

- Is antifungal
- Is anti-inflammatory
- Is antimicrobial
- Is antiviral
- Is antiseptic

■ Conditions That Can Benefit from Tea Tree Oil

- Acne
- Athlete's foot
- *Candida albicans* (treatment should be by prescription from a healthcare provider)
- Cervicitis (treatment should be by prescription from a healthcare provider)
- Cold sores
- Contact dermatitis

- Cystitis (treatment should be by prescription from a healthcare provider)
- Dandruff
- Gingivitis (gum disease)
- Methicillin-resistant *Staphylococcus aureus* (MRSA) infections

- Nail fungus
- Psoriasis
- Vaginitis (treatment should be by prescription from a healthcare provider)

■ Recommended Dosage

Skin Conditions

Acne: Apply tea tree gel twice daily, and leave on skin for twenty minutes. Wash off.

Athlete's foot: Apply tea tree oil in cream base to affected area twice daily for at least one month.

Contact dermatitis: Apply tea tree oil in cream base to affected area twice daily until the condition clears.

Nail fungus: Apply 100-percent tea tree oil directly to nails twice a day for six months.

Other Applications

Cold sores: Apply tea tree oil gel directly to cold sores for five to seven days.

Dandruff: Use tea tree oil shampoo daily for at least one month.

Gingivitis: Use 2.5-percent tea tree gel toothpaste. (Have it compounded with natural toothpaste as a prescription by your healthcare provider.) Brush your teeth with this preparation twice daily for eight weeks. Be careful not to swallow the toothpaste!

Methicillin-resistant *Staphylococcus aureus* infection: Use tea tree oil nasal cream three times a day for five days, and tea tree oil body wash for five days.

■ Side Effects and Contraindications

Tea tree oil should never be swallowed. Doing so can lead to serious side effects, including the inability to walk, confusion, and coma. A diluted gel can be used to treat gingivitis, but it should be used by prescription only and should not be swallowed.

When applied to the skin, tea tree oil may cause any of the following side effects:

- Burning and stinging
- Itching
- Redness
- Skin dryness
- Skin irritation and swelling

THEANINE

Theanine is a unique amino acid that is found not in protein but in tea leaves, both green and black. This substance, which has been shown to cross the blood-brain barrier, is valued for its calming qualities as well as for other health benefits.

■ Functions of Theanine in Your Body

- Augments dopamine in the brain
- Helps reduce mind chatter
- Improves blood vessel function by increasing nitric oxide production
- Improves cognition
- Improves sleep quality
- Increases GABA
- Increases serotonin
- Lowers blood pressure
- May enhance the immune system
- May help relieve sinuses by promoting the movement of mucus-clearing cilia
- May help with weight loss
- May reduce symptoms of depression
- Promotes relaxation
- Reduces plasma norepinephrine
- Reduces stress and anxiety
- Supports focus and attention

■ Conditions That Can Benefit from Theanine

- Anxiety
- Attention-deficit/hyperactivity disorder (ADHD)
- Bipolar disorder
- Depression
- Hypertension (high blood pressure)
- Mind chatter
- Obsessive compulsive disorder (OCD)
- Panic disorder
- Poor cognitive function
- Schizophrenia
- Stress
- Overweight/obesity

■ Recommended Dosage

100 to 200 mg twice a day.

■ Side Effects and Contraindications

Because theanine lowers blood pressure, you should use with caution if you have low blood pressure. Generally, though, there are no confirmed side effects of taking this supplement.

VINPOCETINE

Vinpocetine is a synthetic derivative of the periwinkle plant. Widely used in Europe and Japan, it is valued for its ability to help maintain and improve brain health and cognition.

■ Functions of Vinpocetine in Your Body

- Decreases the deformity of red blood cells

- Helps prevent hair loss

- Improves the brain's utilization of oxygen

- Increases memory by enhancing blood flow to the brain, improving the rate at which the brain cells create energy, and speeding up the brain's use of its main fueling source, glucose

- Increases the level of serotonin (a neurotransmitter that affects behavior and emotions)

- Prevents platelets from sticking together and forming blood clots

■ Conditions That Can Benefit from Vinpocetine

- Chronic fatigue syndrome

- Dementia

- Depression

- Headache

- Macular degeneration

- Memory loss

- Meniere's disease

- Menopause

- Migraine headaches

- Mood changes

- Seizure disorder

- Sensorineural hearing loss

- Sleep disorders

- Stroke

- Tinnitus (ringing in the ears)

- Vertigo

■ Recommended Dosage

10 to 20 milligrams twice a day.

■ Side Effects and Contraindications

If you are taking blood thinners, do not take vinpocetine. If you are having a dental or surgical procedure, discontinue use of this supplement for two weeks before and after the procedure.

The following side effects have been reported:

- Decrease of immune system function
- Dizziness
- Dry mouth
- Headaches
- Nausea
- Skin problems such as hives, itchiness, or rashes
- Stomach pain
- Tightness in chest

ZINC CARNOSINE

Zinc carnosine (ZnC) is a one-to-one combination of the mineral zinc and the amino acid carnosine. The process of bonding the two nutrients makes a highly potent supplement that has antioxidant and anti-inflammatory properties, improves cell function, enhances digestion, and provides the body with many other benefits. (For information on zinc, see page 115. For information on carnosine, see page 150.)

■ Functions of Zinc Carnosine in Your Body

- Adheres to stomach ulcer sores, acting as a barrier between the sores and gastric juices
- Increases the growth and development of endothelial and fibroblast cells
- Inhibits the effect of *H. pylori* bacteria
- Is an antioxidant
- Is anti-inflammatory
- Promotes genomic stability
- Protects the membranes of epithelial cells in the stomach
- Stimulates gut repair processes
- Stimulates small bowel integrity
- Stimulates the production of IGF-1 (growth hormone)

■ Conditions That Can Benefit from Zinc Carnosine

- Duodenal ulcers
- Gastric cancer (prevention)
- Gastric ulcers
- Low-dose aspirin-induced small-bowel injury
- Peptic ulcers
- Stomatitis (mouth ulcers) in people receiving chemotherapy (prevention)

■ Recommended Dosage

50 to 75 milligrams twice daily for all uses except duodenal and peptic ulcers. To treat duodenal and peptic ulcers, take 75 milligrams twice a day, between meals, for eight weeks. Use in conjunction with the "triple therapy" prescribed by your healthcare provider. (This will include a proton pump inhibitor plus antibiotics.)

■ Side Effects and Contraindications

When taken at the recommended dosage, zinc carnosine supplements are safe and do not cause side effects. Do not exceed 75 milligrams twice a day.

PART 2

Health Conditions

Your body's complex inner workings have the ability to heal many ailments. Today, however, pharmaceuticals are often prescribed frequently and indiscriminately. While these conventional treatments may provide quick relief, they usually do not treat the cause of the problem.

The natural products discussed in Part 1 can not only help you achieve optimal health, but also help your body fight various diseases and disorders. Unlike many pharmaceuticals, nutrients boost your immune system while also balancing your other bodily systems and helping them work more effectively and efficiently. Part 2 of this book explores many common—and some less common—health problems and the appropriate natural remedies.

There are times—such as most emergency situations and acute conditions—at which pharmaceuticals are the best option. Unfortunately, their prescription is not reserved for those times only. The following pages provide powerful and competent alternatives to the conventional therapies. However, my intention is not to have the natural ways completely replace the pharmaceuticals. Sometimes, the natural and the conventional must be combined to achieve the best results. With the help of your healthcare provider, you will need to determine—and possibly experiment with—your personalized treatment plan. But when at all possible, I strongly encourage the use of natural healing over pharmaceuticals to avoid unhealthy and far-reaching side effects. In addition, prescribed medication almost always causes the depletion of nutrients. It is therefore paramount that you also work with your healthcare provider to replenish the nutrients that may be diminished by your traditional medication.

Each discussion begins with an explanation of the disease or disorder, including symptoms and causes. This is followed by a table which lists suggested supplements that can help you avoid or recover from the problem. The table includes recommended adult doses and, in many instances, important considerations when taking each supplement. Be aware that the doses recommended in Part 2 may be different (lower or higher) than the doses recommended in Part 1 for those nutrients. This is because in Part 2, we're looking at the amounts that have been found to work best for specific health disorders. If you want more detailed information on any of the recommended supplements, see the relevant entries in Part 1. It's a good idea to learn all you can about the supplements you take.

There are a number of different therapeutic options given for most of the following conditions. You may find that some treatments are most effective when combined. However, they do not all have to be used simultaneously. One size does not fit all when it comes to your medical treatment. If a supplement is of interest to you, read the Part 1"Side Effects and Contraindications" section on that nutrient, and, if possible, work with an anti-aging/personalized medicine healthcare provider trained in nutrition to select the best supplements for you and determine the appropriate dosage. (Information on locating an appropriate healthcare provider is found on page 483 of Resources.)

Many herbs and other supplements—sometimes several that are recommended in a single table—have blood-thinning properties. Current research is unclear regarding whether it is problematic to take more of than one of these nutrients at a time. Until more research is available, do not incorporate more than one potentially blood-thinning supplement into your regimen, and do not take any of these nutrients with a prescription drug, such as Coumadin, that also affects blood clotting. (In the following tables, we have marked potentially blood-thinning nutrients with asterisks.)

Supplements should always be taken with a full glass of water. It is also important that, in addition to the considerations stated in the table, you note the following precautions. The dosages given are intended for adults without kidney or liver disease. If you have kidney or liver disease, you may need to take lower doses of most supplements, and should consult your doctor before embarking on a nutritional program. Similarly, if you are pregnant or nursing, consult your doctor before following any of these protocols. If you are having surgery, do not take any nutrients (except for the protocol that your doctor gives you) for one week before and one week after your surgery date.

The following section on conditions covers a wide range of disorders, but it by no means includes everything that can be treated through nutritional supplements. Your healthcare provider should be able to help you with information regarding disorders that are not discussed here.

ACNE

An inflammatory skin condition, acne is characterized by clogged pores, blackheads, and pimples. It is caused by a problem with the oil-secreting sebaceous glands, which lubricate the skin and are found in large numbers on the face, chest, and back. When the sebaceous glands produce too much oil (called *sebum*) and combine with dead skin cells, the pores become clogged, bacteria multiply, and the skin becomes inflamed and forms pimples. A blackhead forms when the sebum combines with skin pigments and is trapped in the pores.

The exact cause of acne is not known, but there are a number of factors that can contribute to this condition. One major factor is hormonal imbalance, which is why so many teenagers, who experience increased hormone production during puberty, suffer from acne. Because hormonal changes also occur before and after menstruation—as well as before, during, and after pregnancy and menopause—some women experience outbreaks (usually short-lived) during these times. Other factors can include a family history of acne; emotional or physical stress; allergies; an overconsumption of junk food, saturated fats, and hydrogenated fats; a high iodine intake; weather changes; exercise; skin care products that contain vitamin C, alcohol, hazel, peppermint, eucalyptus oil, or menthol; or even fluorescent lighting. The use of certain drugs, such as steroids, oral contraceptives, and lithium, can also contribute to this skin condition.

Some foods have been known to trigger acne. Common culprits include the following:

- Avocados
- Bananas
- Canned tuna
- Chocolate
- Citrus fruit
- Hot soup
- Lima beans, navy beans, and peas
- Liver
- Marinades
- Milk, cheese, and other dairy products
- Nuts
- Oranges
- Pork
- Smoked foods
- Soy sauce
- Spicy foods, especially hot peppers and black pepper
- Tomatoes
- Vinegar
- Wheat

Along with treating acne by following the supplement program presented below, wash your skin once or twice a day with a mild cleanser. Avoid scrubbing the skin or washing more frequently, as this can worsen the condition.

Use oil-free skin products and cosmetics that are labeled "water-based" or "non-comedogenic," which means that they do not contain mineral oil, which can clog pores and aggravate acne.

SUPPLEMENTS TO TREAT ACNE		
Supplements	Dosage	Considerations
B-complex vitamins	50 mg twice a day	I suggest taking a multivitamin along with your B-complex vitamins.
Copper	2 to 3 mg once a day	Your copper-to-zinc ratio is very important for your health. (See page 119 for details.) Also, do not take copper supplement cupric oxide, which has a very low bioavailability.
Dandelion*	100 mg once or twice a day	If you have gallstones or obstructed bile ducts, consult your healthcare practitioner before taking. Do not use dandelion if you are taking a blood-thinning drug or supplement. Avoid if you are allergic to plants such as ragweed, chrysanthemums, marigolds, or daisies.
EPA/DHA (fish oil)	1,000 to 3,000 mg once a day	Choose a source that contains vitamin E to prevent oxidation.
Gamma-linolenic acid (GLA) as evening primrose oil (EPO)*	500 to 1,000 mg once a day	It is important to maintain the proper ratio of omega-6 fatty acids to omega-3 fatty acids. (See page 129.) Evening primrose oil may interfere with some medications, such as nonsteroidal anti-inflammatories; can act as a blood thinner; and can lower the seizure threshold. Consult your healthcare provider or pharmacist before taking this supplement.
Glucosamine sulfate	1,000 mg once a day	If you are allergic to shellfish, be sure to choose a supplement that is not shellfish based. Consult use with your healthcare provider if you have diabetes, because glucosamine can alter blood sugar levels.
Milk thistle	200 mg once a day	Do not take if you are allergic to ragweed, chrysanthemums, marigolds, chamomile, or daisies. This supplement reduces the efficiency of certain blood pressure medication and other drugs. Speak to your healthcare provider or pharmacist before taking.
Probiotics	20 billion units once a day	If taking an antibiotic, take the probiotics at least two hours before or two hours after using the antibiotics. Do not take them at the same time.
Selenium	Have your blood levels measured by your healthcare provider, who will then determine proper dosage	Do not exceed 200 mcg a day without consulting your healthcare provider.

Taurine	1,000 to 2,000 mg once a day	Take between meals. Discontinue use if you suddenly have feelings of chest or throat tightness or if you break out in hives. Do not take with aspirin. Have your healthcare provider measure your taurine levels before starting therapy.
Tea tree oil gel	Apply the gel directly to blemishes twice a day, leaving it on for 20 minutes and then rinsing it off.	Do not ingest or use in ears.
Vitamin A and mixed carotenoids	5,000 to 10,000 IU—half vitamin A and half mixed carotenoids—once a day	Use caution when taking vitamin A supplements because they have the potential to be toxic. Do not take for extended periods of time. Do not take more than 8,000 IU a day if you have liver disease, are a smoker, or have been exposed to asbestos.
Vitamin C	500 to 1,500 mg twice a day	Do not take high doses if you are prone to kidney stones or gout. High doses can also cause diarrhea.
Vitamin D_3	Have your blood levels measured by your healthcare provider, who will determine proper dosage.	
Vitamin E*	400 IU once a day	Take mixed tocopherols, the more active type of vitamin E. Consult your healthcare provider first if you are taking a blood thinner.
Zinc	25 to 75 mg once a day as zinc picolinate or zinc citrate	Your copper-to-zinc ratio is very important for your health. (See page 119 for details.) If you are taking zinc and iron supplements, take one in the morning and one in the evening. (Taking them together reduces the efficiency of both.)

*This supplement can have a blood-thinning action. See page 328 for more information.

ADHD

See Attention-Deficit/Hyperactivity Disorder (ADHD).

ADRENAL FATIGUE AND EXHAUSTION

The adrenal glands—triangle-shaped glands that sit on top of the kidneys—are chiefly responsible for regulating the body's short-term stress response through the production of hormones such as cortisol and dehydroepiandros-terone (DHEA). Many believe that under long-term stress, the adrenal glands become overworked, begin to function improperly, and eventually become unable to respond to stress. This condition—referred to as *adrenal fatigue, adrenal exhaustion,* and *hypoadrenia*—can lead to a wide range of symptoms, including weakness, fatigue, depression, muscle and bone loss, suppression of the immune system, hormonal imbalance, autoimmune disorders, and many other problems. (See the inset below for more possible symptoms of adrenal fatigue.)

Symptoms of Adrenal Fatigue and Exhaustion

As explained on page 331, stress that continues for a long period of time can lead to fatigue and exhaustion of the adrenal glands. This, in turn, can cause the following symptoms and disorders.

- Absent-mindedness
- Allergies
- Autoimmune disorders
- Bone loss
- Cravings for salt
- Cravings for spices
- Cravings for sugar
- Depression
- Dizziness
- Fatigue that worsens in evenings and with stress
- Frustration
- Headaches
- Hormone imbalance
- Hypoglycemia
- Immune system suppression
- Inability to concentrate
- Insomnia
- Irritability
- Lightheadedness
- Moodiness
- Muscle loss
- Nervousness
- Pale, cold, clammy skin
- Restlessness
- Tachycardia (fast heart rate) and/or palpitations
- Weakness

It is believed that adrenal fatigue is largely a disorder of the modern world. The adrenal glands are designed to handle only short-term stress, but today's world creates constant stress through job problems; lack of sleep; poor diet, including dieting, skipped meals, and high caffeine intake; chemical toxins; and widespread use of prescription drugs without supplementation of the nutrients that become depleted. This continuous stress taxes the adrenal glands until they become first fatigued, and then exhausted. The end result is often an inability to produce DHEA, a precursor hormone to estrogen and testosterone; and destructively high levels of cortisol. If the stress continues for a long enough period of time, the body will also have a decreased ability to produce sufficient levels of cortisol.

Prayer, meditation, yoga, qigong, relaxation therapies, adequate sleep, regular exercise, acupuncture, and a sound diet are all vital to repair of the adrenal glands and normal adrenal function. There are also a number of supplements that can help relieve the symptoms of adrenal fatigue, as well as restore healthy function of the glands.

SUPPLEMENTS FOR ADRENAL SUPPORT

Supplements	Dosage	Considerations
Ashwagandha root	1,000 mg twice a day	High doses can cause gastrointestinal problems.
Asian ginseng*	200 mg twice a day	Always take with food. Use with caution if you have high blood pressure. Do not use if you are taking a blood thinner or if you have a hormonally related cancer such as breast, prostate, uterine, or ovarian.
Cordyceps	400 mg twice a day	Be sure to use a pharmaceutical grade product to avoid lead contamination. Do not take if you have an autoimmune disorder. Cordyceps can interact with many drugs. Speak to your healthcare provider before taking it.
DHEA	As prescribed by your doctor.	
Rhodiola	100 mg twice a day of 3-percent rosavin and 1-percent salidroside	Rhodiola can interact with many drugs. Speak to your healthcare provider before taking it.
Vitamin B$_6$ (pyridoxine)	50 mg twice a day	Do not take more than 500 mg a day. If you are taking levodopa for Parkinson's disease, do not take B$_6$ without first consulting your doctor. High doses can deplete your body of other vitamins in the B complex, so take a B-complex vitamin twice a day.
Vitamin C	250 mg to 500 mg twice a day	Do not take high doses if you are prone to kidney stones or gout. High doses can also cause diarrhea.

*This supplement can have a blood-thinning action. See page 328 for more information.

SUPPLEMENTS FOR STRESS ACCOMPANIED BY ANXIETY AND JITTERINESS

Supplements	Dosage	Considerations
Ashwagandha root	1,000 mg twice a day	High doses can cause gastrointestinal problems.
B-complex vitamins	50 mg twice a day	I suggest taking a multivitamin along with your B-complex vitamins.
Chamomile*	400 to 1,000 mg daily in capsule form, or 3 cups of tea daily	Consult your healthcare practitioner before taking if you are on a blood thinner. Do not take if you are allergic to plants such as ragweed, aster, daisies, and, chrysanthemums. Also avoid if you have a hormonally related cancer, such as breast or prostate.
Chromium	300 mcg once a day as chromium picolinate	Combining with the protein picolinate allows your body to absorb chromium more efficiently. However, some chromium picolinate supplements contain more chromium than necessary. Ask your healthcare provider for a recommendation on chromium consumption.

EPA/DHA (fish oil)*	2,000 mg once a day	Choose a source that contains vitamin E to prevent oxidation.
Gamma-aminobutyric acid (GABA)	300 to 1,200 mg once a day	Always take with a multivitamin to supply the nutrients that are needed to metabolize GABA. This supplement may make you drowsy, so take before going to bed.
Inositol	50 to 100 mg once a day	May stimulate uterine contractions. Women who wish to become pregnant should consult their doctor regarding its use. Doses larger than 200 mg should be taken only under physician supervision.
Magnesium	400 to 600 mg once a day	Consult your healthcare provider for dosage if you have kidney disease. Discontinue use and see your doctor if you experience abdominal pain. Take a lower dose if it causes diarrhea.
Taurine	1,000 to 2,000 mg once a day	Take between meals. Discontinue use if you have feelings of chest or throat tightness or if you break out in hives. Do not take with aspirin. Have your healthcare provider measure levels before starting.

*This supplement can have a blood-thinning action. See page 328 for more information.

SUPPLEMENTS FOR STRESS ACCOMPANIED BY FATIGUE

Supplements	Dosage	Considerations
Ashwagandha root	1,000 mg twice a day	High doses can cause gastrointestinal problems.
Asian ginseng*	200 mg twice a day	Always take with food. Use with caution if you have high blood pressure. Do not take if you are taking a blood thinner or if you have a hormonally related cancer such as breast, prostate, uterine, or ovarian.
B-complex vitamins	50 mg twice a day	I recommend taking a multivitamin along with your B-complex vitamins.
Cordyceps	400 mg twice a day	Use a pharmaceutical grade product to avoid lead contamination. Do not take if you have an autoimmune disorder. Cordyceps can interact with many drugs. Speak to your healthcare provider before taking it.
Licorice (glycyrrhiza)	300 mg twice a day	Do not use if you have high blood pressure, and discontinue use if you develop high blood pressure while taking supplements.
Rhodiola	100 mg twice a day of 3-percent rosavin and 1-percent salidroside	Rhodiola can interact with many drugs. Speak to your healthcare provider before taking it.

*This supplement can have a blood-thinning action. See page 328 for more information.

ALLERGIES

See Food Allergies.

ALOPECIA

See Hair Loss.

ALZHEIMER'S DISEASE

Alzheimer's disease, the most frequent form of dementia, is a progressive deterioration of the brain. The most common symptoms are memory loss, inability to recognize family or friends, difficulty speaking and remembering words, personality changes, and difficulty making decisions. Although the symptoms are usually mild at the onset of the disease, they often progress to such an extent that work and socializing become impossible.

Alzheimer's usually afflicts people who are over the age of sixty. If you fear that you or someone you love may have Alzheimer's, see a doctor for a diagnosis. This disease is incurable, but its progression can often be slowed down. The following supplements can help.

SUPPLEMENTS TO SLOW THE PROGRESSION OF ALZHEIMER'S DISEASE

Supplements	Dosage	Considerations
Alpha lipoic acid	200 to 400 mg once a day	Alpha lipoic acid can interact with medication taken for diabetes and thyroid problems. Speak to your healthcare provider to see if any of the medications you take make it unwise to use this supplement.
B-complex vitamins	50 mg twice a day	I suggest taking a multivitamin along with your B-complex vitamins.
Carnitine*	1,500 to 3,000 mg once a day	The most effective form for this purpose is acetyl-L-carnitine (ALCAR). Have your healthcare provider measure your TMAO levels before starting long-term supplementation with carnitine.
Cocoa	2.5 g (0.1 ounce) unsweetened cocoa powder (about 0.5 teaspoon)	Cocoa can interact with some medications, so speak to your healthcare provider or pharmacist before starting long-term supplementation. Cocoa also contains caffeine, which can cause side effects in some people.

Coenzyme Q$_{10}$*	100 to 300 mg once a day	If you are on blood-thinning medications, speak to your healthcare provider before using CoQ$_{10}$. Since some medications can cause a deficiency of this nutrient, speak to your healthcare provider to determine if you might need a larger dose.
D-ribose	15,000 mg three times a day	D-ribose can lower blood sugar levels, so check with your healthcare provider before taking this supplement with any diabetes medication, especially insulin.
EPA/DHA (fish oil)*	1,000 to 2,000 mg once a day	Choose a source that contains vitamin E to prevent oxidation.
Ginkgo biloba*	120 to 240 mg once a day	Do not use with blood-thinning medications or supplements.
Inositol	500 mg twice a day (under medical supervision)	May stimulate uterine contractions. Women who wish to become pregnant should consult their doctor regarding its use. Doses larger than 200 mg should be taken only under physician supervision.
Magnesium	400 to 600 mg once a day	Consult your healthcare provider for dosage if you have kidney disease. Discontinue use and see your doctor if you experience abdominal pain. Take a lower dose if it causes diarrhea.
Phosphatidylcholine (PC)	200 to 600 mg once a day	Use with caution if you have malabsorption problems, as this could exacerbate them.
Phosphatidylserine (PS)	300 to 500 mg once a day	This product is particularly helpful to prevent Alzheimer's, as well as at the onset of the disease. However, PS can interact with many drugs, so speak to your healthcare provider before taking it.
Selenium	100 to 200 mcg once a day	Do not exceed 200 mcg a day without consulting your healthcare provider.
Vinpocetine*	10 to 40 mg once a day	Do not use with blood-thinning medications or supplements.
Vitamin A and mixed carotenoids	10,000 to 25,000 IU—half vitamin A and half mixed carotenoids—once a day	Use caution when taking vitamin A supplements because they have the potential to be toxic. Do not take for extended periods of time. Do not take more than 8,000 IU a day if you have liver disease, are a smoker, or have been exposed to asbestos.
Vitamin B$_9$ (folic acid)	400 to 500 mcg twice a day	High doses can deplete your body of other vitamins in the B complex, so take a B-complex vitamin twice a day.
Vitamin B$_{12}$ (cobalamin)	2,500 to 5,000 mcg twice a day	High doses can deplete your body of other vitamins in the B complex, so take a B-complex vitamin twice a day.
Vitamin C	1,000 to 2,500 mg twice a day	Do not take high dosages if you are prone to kidney stones or gout. High doses can also cause diarrhea.

Vitamin D$_3$	Have your blood levels measured by your healthcare provider, who will determine proper dosage.	
Vitamin E	400 IU once a day	Take mixed tocopherols, the more active type of vitamin E. Consult your healthcare provider first if you are taking a blood thinner.

*This supplement can have a blood-thinning action. See page 328 for more information.

SUPPLEMENTS TO IMPROVE MEMORY

Supplements	Dosage	Considerations
Alpha lipoic acid	100 to 200 mg once a day	Alpha lipoic acid can interact with medication taken for diabetes and thyroid problems. Speak to your healthcare provider to see if any of the medications you take make it unwise to use this supplement.
B-complex vitamins	50 mg twice a day	I suggest taking a multivitamin along with your B-complex vitamins.
Carnitine*	1,000 to 2,000 mg once a day	The most effective form for this purpose is acetyl-L-carnitine (ALCAR). Have your healthcare provider measure your TMAO levels before starting long-term supplementation with carnitine.
Coenzyme Q$_{10}$*	100 to 200 mg once a day	If you are on blood-thinning medications, speak to your healthcare provider before using CoQ$_{10}$. Since some medications can cause a deficiency of this nutrient, speak to your healthcare provider to determine if you might need a larger dose.
Cysteine	1,000 mg once a day as n-acetylcysteine, or NAC	When taking NAC supplements, also take extra vitamin C, copper, and zinc.
EPA/DHA (fish oil)*	1,000 to 2,000 mg once a day	Choose a source that contains vitamin E to prevent oxidation.
Ginkgo biloba*	100 to 250 mg once a day	Do not use with blood-thinning medications or supplements.
Phosphatidylcholine (PC)	1,000 to 4,000 mg once a day	Use with caution if you have malabsorption problems, as this could exacerbate them.
Phosphatidylserine (PS)	200 to 300 mg once a day	This product is particularly helpful to prevent Alzheimer's, as well as at the onset of the disease. However, PS can interact with many drugs, so speak to your healthcare provider before taking it.
Resveratrol	20 mg a day	Do not use resveratrol if you have or have had a hormonally related cancer until more is known about the estrogenic activity of resveratrol.
Selenium	100 to 200 mcg once a day	Do not exceed 200 mcg a day without consulting your healthcare provider.

Vinpocetine*	5 mg three times a day	Do not use with blood-thinning medications or supplements.
Vitamin A and mixed carotenoids	5,000 IU—half vitamin A and half mixed carotenoids— once a day	Use caution when taking vitamin A supplements because they have the potential to be toxic. Do not take for extended periods of time. Do not take more than 8,000 IU a day if you have liver disease, are a smoker, or have been exposed to asbestos.
Vitamin B$_9$ (folic acid)	400 mcg twice a day	High doses can deplete your body of other B vitamins, so take a B-complex vitamin twice a day.
Vitamin B$_{12}$ (cobalamin)	500 mcg twice a day	High doses can deplete your body of other B vitamins, so take a B-complex vitamin twice a day.
Vitamin C	500 to 1,000 mg twice a day	Do not take high dosages if you are prone to kidney stones or gout. High doses can also cause diarrhea.
Vitamin E*	400 to 800 IU once a day	Take mixed tocopherols, the more active type of vitamin E. Consult your healthcare provider first if you are taking a blood thinner.

*This supplement can have a blood-thinning action. See page 328 for more information.

ANOREXIA NERVOSA

Anorexia nervosa is an eating disorder that arises from a person's intense fear of being overweight. There are many ways that anorexic people control their weight, including starvation, obsessive exercising, purging, and taking diuretics. Although most anorexics have a low—usually unhealthily so—body weight, they often have a distorted self-image. A large majority of anorexics are female, but more and more males are affected each year.

This eating disorder is one of the most dangerous psychiatric disorders. It affects many people and has a variety of serious consequences. Hair can become brittle and fall out; skin can easily bruise; the immune system can weaken; the menstrual cycle can be disrupted; and nerves can deteriorate, causing severe pain during simple movement. There are dozens of other related symptoms that can occur as well. Anorexia can also have devastating effects on the heart and cardiovascular system, and can cause electrolyte imbalances. (The dangers of electrolyte imbalance were discussed in Chapter 2.) Cardiac arrest and even death can occur.

The harm to physical health is very serious, but anorexia can also cause behavioral problems, including withdrawal from friends and activities, self-harming, and suicidal thoughts. In fact, this disorder can affect every part of a person's life. If you or someone you know is anorexic, it is important to seek professional help immediately.

SUPPLEMENTS TO TREAT ANOREXIA NERVOSA

Supplements	Dosage	Considerations
Amino acid supplements	Have your healthcare provider measure your amino acid levels and replace them according to lab results.	Amino acids can interact with some medications. Consult with your healthcare provider before beginning this therapy.
Carnitine*	500 mg once a day	Have your healthcare provider measure your TMAO levels before starting long-term supplementation with carnitine.
Coenzyme Q_{10}*	30 to 50 mg once a day	If you are on blood-thinning medications, speak to your healthcare provider before using CoQ_{10}. Since some medications can cause a deficiency of this nutrient, speak to your healthcare provider to determine if you might need a larger dose.
EPA/DHA (fish oil)*	500 to 1,000 mg once a day	Choose a source that contains vitamin E to prevent oxidation.
Gamma-linolenic acid (GLA) as evening primrose oil (EPO)*	480 to 720 mg once a day	It is important to maintain the proper ratio of omega-6 fatty acids to omega-3 fatty acids. (See page 129.) Evening primrose oil may interfere with some medications, such as nonsteroidal anti-inflammatories; can act as a blood thinner; and can lower the seizure threshold. Consult your healthcare provider or pharmacist before taking this supplement.
Magnesium	400 mg once a day	Consult your healthcare provider for dosage if you have kidney disease. Discontinue use and see your doctor if you experience abdominal pain. Take a lower dose if it causes diarrhea.
Taurine	500 mg once a day	Take between meals. Discontinue use if you suddenly have feelings of chest or throat tightness or if you break out in hives. Do not take with aspirin. Have your healthcare provider measure levels before starting.
Vitamin A and mixed carotenoids	5,000 IU—half vitamin A and half mixed carotenoids—once a day	Use caution when taking vitamin A supplements because they have the potential to be toxic. Do not take for extended periods of time. Do not take more than 8,000 IU a day if you have liver disease, are a smoker, or have been exposed to asbestos.
Vitamin B_1 (thiamine)	50 mg twice a day	High doses can deplete your body of other vitamins in the B complex, so take a B-complex vitamin twice a day.

| Zinc | 25 to 50 mg once a day as zinc picolinate or zinc citrate | Your copper-to-zinc ratio is very important for your health. (See page 119 for details.) If you are taking zinc and iron supplements, take one in the morning and one in the evening. (Taking them together reduces the efficiency of both.) |

*This supplement can have a blood-thinning action. See page 328 for more information.

ANXIETY

Anxiety can be a normal state of mind that allows you to react appropriately to uncomfortable or dangerous situations. However, several million Americans find themselves burdened by excessive apprehension, fear, and stress. When this reaction is disproportionate to the situation, it may be the result of an anxiety disorder. The main causes of these disorders are genetics, life experiences, hormone imbalances, and brain chemistry.

Increased blood pressure, heart rate, and sweating are common ways that feelings of anxiety are exhibited. Anxiety can also manifest itself in chest pains, muscle tension, panic attacks, and shortness of breath, as well as a variety of other symptoms. See a doctor if any of these problems interfere with your daily life or become crippling. If your anxiety is not hindering your normal activities but is causing you discomfort, the supplements listed in the table below may be sufficient in treating the problem.

Dietary changes can also help you manage anxiety. Avoiding alcohol, caffeine, and sugar can be helpful, as can avoiding aspartame. If you have food allergies, be sure to stay away from the foods to which you are sensitive.

Finally, be aware that some health disorders—chronic yeast infection and reactive hypoglycemia, for instance—can trigger anxiety. Consider seeing your healthcare provider, who can determine if you have any underlying conditions that require treatment.

SUPPLEMENTS TO TREAT ANXIETY

Supplements	Dosage	Considerations
B-complex vitamins	50 mg twice a day	I suggest taking a multivitamin along with your B-complex vitamins. Deficiencies of vitamins B_3, B_6, folate, and B_{12} have all been reported to cause anxiety.
Calcium	500 mg twice a day	Although most people are deficient in calcium, there is a danger in taking too much calcium. Do not ingest more than 1,000 to 1,200 mg of calcium a day.

CBD oil (hemp oil)	5 to 500 mg a day in the form of sublingual drops. Start with 5 mg and increase slowly until you find relief.	CBD is generally well tolerated and safe for consumption, even in high doses and with continuous use. However, do not exceed 500 mg a day without consulting your healthcare provider. Make sure to buy a product marked "hemp oil (aerial parts)."
EPA/DHA (fish oil)*	1,000 to 3,000 mg a day	Choose a source that contains vitamin E to prevent oxidation.
Gamma-aminobutyric acid (GABA)	375 to 750 mg three times a day	Always take with a multivitamin to supply the nutrients that are needed to metabolize GABA. This supplement may make you drowsy, so take before going to bed.
Glutamine	1,000 mg once a day	If you have a sensitivity to monosodium glutamate (MSG), use glutamine with caution. If you are taking medications for seizures, take glutamine only under the direction of your doctor.
Glycine	1,000 mg once a day	Glycine can interact with other drugs. Speak to your healthcare provider before taking it.
Inositol	12,000 mg once a day (under medical supervision)	May stimulate uterine contractions. Women who wish to become pregnant should consult their doctor regarding its use. Doses larger than 200 mg should be taken only under physician supervision.
Magnesium	300 to 600 mg once a day	Consult your healthcare provider for dosage if you have kidney disease. Discontinue use and see your doctor if you experience abdominal pain. Take a lower dose if it causes diarrhea.
Passion flower*	45 drops liquid extract once a day, or 90 mg tablet once a day	Avoid this supplement if you are taking an MAO inhibitor or a sedative medication. Also avoid if you have a bleeding disorder or are taking a blood-thinning drug or supplement. Consult your healthcare provider or pharmacist before using this supplement.
Threonine	200 to 400 mg a day	To determine the exact dose that you need, have your healthcare provider measure your amino acid levels.
Tryptophan	1,000 mg a day as L-Tryptophan	Check with your doctor before starting an amino acid regimen if you have diabetes, hypertension, kidney disease, or liver disease. Do not take tryptophan if you are pregnant or breastfeeding. Tryptophan can interact with some medications, so consult with your healthcare provider before beginning supplementation.

*This supplement can have a blood-thinning action. See page 328 for more information.

ARTERIOSCLEROSIS

See Atherosclerosis.

ARTHRITIS

Arthritis occurs when there is damage to the joints. It can cause pain, stiffness, and swelling to the affected area. Sufferers often experience diminished mobility of the affected limb. The type of arthritis is determined by its cause. Conventional forms of treatment include physical therapy and medication. *See also* Gout; Inflammation; Osteoarthritis; Rheumatoid Arthritis.

ASTHMA

Asthma is a condition in which a person's *airways*—the tubes through which air travels to and from the lungs—become periodically inflamed. The inflammation causes the tubes to narrow, restricting the amount of air that can be inhaled. Asthma sufferers exhibit symptoms such as coughing, shortness of breath, and wheezing.

Asthma can have mild to serious—even life-threatening—effects. During an asthma attack, a person cannot inhale the proper amount of air and cannot breathe normally. The degree to which air is restricted and the length of the attacks determines the severity of the illness. In addition to these acute attacks, some people with asthma have permanent respiratory problems that may restrict their daily activities.

Attacks can be triggered by allergens, such as animal dander, chemicals, environmental pollution, or smoke. Treatment should begin by identifying and removing, if possible, any applicable triggers. On the other hand, asthma attacks can also be caused by adrenal disorders, anxiety, changes in temperature, exercise, stress, and other unavoidable factors. When the triggers cannot be removed, treatment usually consists of controlling and monitoring the attacks. A doctor can help the asthma patient prepare for attacks as well as identify when an asthma attack is coming. This can often prevent the more serious symptoms.

SUPPLEMENTS TO TREAT ASTHMA

Supplements	Dosage	Considerations
B-complex vitamins	50 mg twice a day	I suggest taking a multivitamin along with a B-complex vitamin.
Curcumin/Turmeric*	100 to 1,000 mg once a day of a formula that includes piperine or bioperine to boost absorption	Do not take curcumin with blood-thinning medications or supplements. Curcumin can also interact with other medications, so speak to your healthcare specialist before taking this supplement.
Cysteine	1,000 to 2,000 mg once a day as n-acetylcysteine, or NAC	When taking NAC supplements, also take extra vitamin C, copper, and zinc.
EPA/DHA (fish oil)*	2,000 mg once a day	Choose a source that contains vitamin E to prevent oxidation.
Gingko biloba*	80 to 240 mg once a day	Do not use with blood-thinning medications or supplements.
Grape seed extract*	300 mg three times a day	Do not use with blood-thinning medications or supplements.
Magnesium	400 to 600 mg once a day	Consult your healthcare provider for dosage if you have kidney disease. Discontinue use and see your doctor if you experience abdominal pain. Take a lower dose if it causes diarrhea.
Methylsulfonylmethane (MSM)	1,000 to 3,000 mg three times a day	Use with caution if you are allergic to sulfur. Start by taking 500 mg three times a day, and gradually increase dose. Take with meals to avoid possible heartburn. May cause stomach upset in dosages larger than 6,000 mg.
Probiotics	20 billion units once a day	If taking an antibiotic, take the probiotics at least two hours before or two hours after using the antibiotics. Do not take them at the same time.
Quercetin*	500 mg three times a day	For best results, take with bromelain and vitamin C. Do not use with blood-thinning medications or supplements.
Selenium	100 to 200 mcg once a day	Do not exceed 200 micrograms a day without consulting your healthcare provider.
Taurine	1,000 to 3,000 mg once a day	Take between meals. Discontinue use if you suddenly have feelings of chest or throat tightness or if you break out in hives. Do not take with aspirin. Have your healthcare provider measure levels before starting taurine therapy.
Vitamin A and mixed carotenoids	50 to 5,000 IU—half vitamin A and half mixed carotenoids—once a day	Use caution when taking vitamin A supplements because they have the potential to be toxic. Do not take for extended periods of time. Do not take more than 8,000 IU a day if you have liver disease, are a smoker, or have been exposed to asbestos.

Vitamin B₉ (folic acid)	400 to 500 mcg twice a day	High doses can deplete your body of other B vitamins, so take a B-complex vitamin twice a day.
Vitamin B₁₂ (cobalamin)	500 to 1,000 mcg twice a day	High doses can deplete your body of other B vitamins, so take a B-complex vitamin twice a day.
Vitamin C	1,000 mg twice a day	Do not take high doses if you are prone to kidney stones or gout. High doses can also cause diarrhea.
Vitamin E*	400 to 800 IU once a day	Take mixed tocopherols, the more active type of vitamin E. Consult your healthcare provider first if you are taking a blood thinner.
Zinc	25 mg once a day as zinc picolinate or zinc citrate	Your copper-to-zinc ratio is very important for your health. (See page 119 for details.) If you are taking zinc and iron supplements, take one in the morning and one in the evening. (Taking them together reduces the efficiency of both.)

*This supplement can have a blood-thinning action. See page 328 for more information.

ATHEROSCLEROSIS

Atherosclerosis, a type of arteriosclerosis, is a build-up of fat deposits (plaque) on the walls of your arteries. These deposits cause artery walls to lose elasticity and become hard and thick, sometimes restricting blood flow to your organs and tissues. The plaque can also break loose (rupture), triggering a blood clot that can cause a heart attack or stroke.

Doctors may treat severely clogged arteries by performing an angioplasty. This procedure stretches and widens the narrow arteries so that the blood can flow more smoothly through the body.

On the other hand, the fat may not rupture. Instead, an *aneurysm*—a bulge in the wall of an artery—may form to accommodate the growing size of the deposits. Unfortunately, the aneurysm can burst and cause a stroke. There are several treatment options available for people with aneurysms. It is important to take care of the problem with the help of your doctor since both ruptured fat deposits and aneurysms can cause life-threatening problems, such as cardiac arrest, heart attack, stroke, or death.

Risk factors for developing atherosclerosis include family history of heart disease, high cholesterol levels (see page 404), hypertension (see page 398), and smoking. Yet these factors do not apply to a large percentage of people with atherosclerosis. Research is still being performed on the disease so that we can gain a more complete understanding of it. But there are precautions you can take. Along with the nutrients listed below, a diet rich in olive oil and "good" fats may ward off many deaths related to atherosclerosis.

SUPPLEMENTS TO PREVENT ATHEROSCLEROSIS

Supplements	Dosage	Considerations
Carnitine*	1,000 to 4,000 mg once a day	Have your healthcare provider measure your TMAO levels before starting long-term supplementation with carnitine
Chromium	400 mcg once a day as chromium picolinate	Combining with the protein picolinate allows your body to absorb chromium more efficiently. However, some chromium picolinate supplements contain more chromium than necessary. Ask your healthcare provider for a recommendation on chromium consumption.
Coenzyme Q_{10}*	100 to 300 mg a day	If you are on blood-thinning medications, speak to your healthcare provider before using CoQ_{10}. Since some medications can cause a deficiency of this nutrient, speak to your healthcare provider to determine if you might need a larger dose.
Copper	2 to 4 mg once a day	Your copper-to-zinc ratio is very important for your health. (See page 119 for details.) Also, do not take copper supplement cupric oxide, which has a very low bioavailability.
EPA/DHA (fish oil)*	500 to 2,000 mg once a day	Choose a source that contains vitamin E to prevent oxidation.
Fiber, soluble	Suggested daily intake is 25 grams for women and 38 grams for men. Try to get most of your fiber from whole foods.	Choose a fiber supplement with no added sugar, and take with several glasses of water to prevent side effects.
Gamma-linolenic acid (GLA) as evening primrose oil (EPO)*	480 mg once a day	It is important to maintain the proper ratio of omega-6 fatty acids to omega-3 fatty acids. (See page 129.) Evening primrose oil may interfere with some medications, such as nonsteroidal anti-inflammatories; can act as a blood thinner; and can lower the seizure threshold. Consult your healthcare provider or pharmacist before taking this supplement.
Magnesium	500 to 1,000 mg once a day	Consult your healthcare provider for dosage if you have kidney disease. Discontinue use and see your doctor if you experience abdominal pain. Take a lower dose if you experience diarrhea.
Red yeast rice	600 mg twice a day	Be sure to take with 100 mg of pharmaceutical grade CoQ_{10}. Do not take with a statin drug.
Selenium	100 to 200 mcg a day	Do not exceed 200 mcg a day without consulting your healthcare provider.

Taurine	1,000 to 2,000 mg once a day	Take between meals. Discontinue use if you suddenly have feelings of chest or throat tightness or if you break out in hives. Do not take with aspirin. Have your healthcare provider measure levels before starting taurine therapy.
Vitamin B_3 (niacin)	50 mg twice a day	Do not drink alcohol or hot drinks within one hour of taking niacin. High doses can deplete your body of other vitamins in the B complex, so take a B-complex vitamin twice a day.
Vitamin B_6 (pyridoxine)	50 mg twice a day	Do not take more than 500 mg a day. If you are taking levodopa for Parkinson's disease, do not take B_6 without first consulting your doctor. High doses can deplete your body of other vitamins in the B complex, so take a B-complex vitamin twice a day.
Vitamin B_9 (folic acid)	200 to 400 mcg twice a day	High doses can deplete your body of other B vitamins, so take a B-complex vitamin twice a day.
Vitamin B_{12} (cobalamin)	500 mcg twice a day	High doses can deplete your body of other B vitamins, so take a B-complex vitamin twice a day.
Vitamin C	500 to 2,500 mg twice a day	Do not take high doses if you are prone to kidney stones or gout. High doses can also cause diarrhea.
Vitamin D_3	Have your blood levels measured by your healthcare provider, who will determine your proper dosage.	
Vitamin E*	400 IU once a day	Take mixed tocopherols, the more active type of vitamin E. Consult your healthcare provider first if you are taking a blood thinner.
Vitamin K*	500 mcg a day of K_2 or MK-7	If you are on blood-thinning medications, speak to your healthcare provider before using vitamin K.
Zinc	25 to 50 mg once a day as zinc picolinate or zinc citrate	Your copper-to-zinc ratio is very important for your health. (See page 119 for details.) If you are taking zinc and iron supplements, take one in the morning and one in the evening. (Taking them together reduces the efficiency of both.)

*This supplement can have a blood-thinning action. See page 328 for more information.

ATTENTION-DEFICIT/HYPERACTIVITY DISORDER (ADHD)

Attention-deficit/hyperactivity disorder, or ADHD, is usually characterized by an inability to maintain focus or pay attention. People with ADHD may also exhibit uncontrollable hyperactivity.

ADHD is often inherited, but can also be caused by environmental factors such as brain injury, high fever, and toxic exposure. Diet, food allergies, metal toxicities, prenatal fatty acid deficiencies, zinc deficiencies, and zinc-to-copper imbalances can also play a role, as can imbalances in neurotransmitters such as dopamine, serotonin, and norepinephrine. Therefore, ADHD is a multifactorial problem.

Stimulants are the conventional medicinal treatment for ADHD. Unfortunately, these pharmaceuticals reduce the overall blood flow to the brain and disturb glucose metabolism. Moreover, drug use does not produce or increase the production of neurotransmitters. It addresses only the symptoms of the problem—not the cause. On the other hand, a nutritional approach, such as that shown in the following table, can increase academic and social abilities. In addition to using the recommended supplements, try to avoid sugar, food additives, and food colorings. A gluten-free diet may also be beneficial.

SUPPLEMENTS TO TREAT ADHD		
Supplements	Dosage	Considerations
American ginseng*	200 mg once a day	Do not use if you are taking a blood thinner or if you have a hormonally related cancer such as breast, prostate, uterine, or ovarian.
Amino acid supplements	Have your healthcare provider measure your amino acid levels and replace them according to lab results.	Amino acids can interact with some medications. Consult with your healthcare provider before beginning this therapy.
B-complex vitamins	50 mg twice a day	I suggest taking a multivitamin along with your B-complex vitamins.
Boron	5 to 10 mg once a day	
Carnitine*	2,000 to 4,000 mg once a day	Have your healthcare provider measure your TMAO levels before starting long-term supplementation with carnitine.
EPA/DHA (fish oil)*	500 to 1,000 mg once a day	Choose a source that contains vitamin E to prevent oxidation.
Gamma-linolenic acid (GLA) as evening primrose oil (EPO)*	240 to 720 mg once a day	It is important to maintain the proper ratio of omega-6 fatty acids to omega-3 fatty acids. (See page 129.) Evening primrose oil may interfere with some medications, such as nonsteroidal anti-inflammatories; can act as a blood thinner; and can lower the seizure threshold. Consult your healthcare provider or pharmacist before taking this supplement.
Ginkgo biloba*	60 mg twice a day	Do not use with blood-thinning medications or supplements.

Iron	Have your doctor measure your iron levels to determine dosage.	Supplement with iron if needed and repeat the laboratory tests every three months.
Magnesium	250 to 500 mg once a day	Consult your healthcare provider for dosage if you have kidney disease. Discontinue use and see your doctor if you experience abdominal pain. Take a lower dose if it causes diarrhea.
Phosphatidylserine (PS)	100 to 500 mg once a day	PS can interact with many drugs. Speak to your healthcare provider before taking it.
Probiotics	20 billion units once a day	If taking an antibiotic, take the probiotics at least two hours before or two hours after using the antibiotics. Do not take them at the same time.
St. John's wort*	300 to 1,200 mg once a day	St. John's wort can interact with many drugs. Speak to your healthcare provider before taking it. If you are exposed to the sun, it may cause a skin rash.
Selenium	100 mcg once a day	Do not exceed 200 mcg a day without consulting your healthcare provider.
Vitamin B9 (folic acid)	400 mcg twice a day	High doses can deplete your body of other B vitamins, so take a B-complex vitamin twice a day.
Vitamin B12 (cobalamin)	500 mcg twice a day	High doses can deplete your body of other B vitamins, so take a B-complex vitamin twice a day.
Zinc	25 to 50 mg once a day as zinc picolinate or zinc citrate	Your copper-to-zinc ratio is very important for your health. (See page 119 for details.) If you are taking zinc and iron supplements, take one in the morning and one in the evening. (Taking them together reduces the efficiency of both.)

*This supplement can have a blood-thinning action. See page 328 for more information.

BALDING

See Hair Loss.

BENIGN PROSTATIC HYPERPLASIA (BPH)

Benign prostatic hyperplasia (BPH) is a noncancerous condition in which a man's prostate becomes enlarged. The prostate may then push against the urethra and bladder. Symptoms include frequent, difficult, or painful urination. The cause of BPH is not completely known, but it is believed to be related to an increased conversion of testosterone to dihydrotestosterone by an enzyme called 5-alpha-reductase. This occurs more commonly with age. Men fifty-one to sixty years of age have a 40- to 50-percent chance of having benign prostate enlargement. Men over the age of eighty have an 80-percent chance.

Problems with urination usually begin as mild conditions, but if they occur, you should see your doctor, who will perform a rectal exam to determine whether the problem is actually BPH. This is very important, because the symptoms can also be indicative of a more serious problem. Doctors often suggest that BPH patients wait and see if their situations improve without any medical treatment. Many patients have found it helpful to take the nutrients presented in the following table. If the symptoms do not go away or if they become more uncomfortable, there are two conventional options available. The first is medication, of which there are several different kinds. However, some cause (mostly sexual) side effects—and the BPH symptoms tend to come back when the medication is stopped. The most successful treatment is surgery. Yet doctors often consider surgery a last resort because it does pose a small degree of risk to the patient. Your doctor will be able to suggest which option is most appropriate to your situation.

SUPPLEMENTS TO TREAT BPH		
Supplements	Dosage	Considerations
Amino acid supplements	Have your healthcare provider measure your amino acid levels and replace them according to lab results.	Amino acids can interact with some medications. Consult with your healthcare provider before beginning this therapy.
B-complex vitamins	25 to 50 mg twice a day	I suggest taking a multivitamin along with your B-complex vitamins.
Beta-sitosterol	20 mg three times a day	Do not use if you have a rare disorder called phytosterolemia.
Copper	1 to 2 mg once a day	Your copper-to-zinc ratio is very important for your health. (See page 119 for details.) Also, do not take copper supplement cupric oxide, which has a very low bioavailability.
EPA/DHA (fish oil)*	2,000 mg once a day	Choose a source that contains vitamin E to prevent oxidation.
Gamma-linolenic acid (GLA) as evening primrose oil (EPO)*	500 mg once a day	It is important to maintain the proper ratio of omega-6 fatty acids to omega-3 fatty acids. (See page 129.) Evening primrose oil may interfere with some medications, such as nonsteroidal anti-inflammatories; can act as a blood thinner; and can lower the seizure threshold. Consult your healthcare provider or pharmacist before taking this supplement.

Lycopene	10 mg once a day	May cause GI problems such as diarrhea and gas.
Saw palmetto*	150 mg twice a day	Speak to your healthcare provider before using this supplement if you have a sex hormone-related disorder or if you are taking birth control pills.
Selenium	100 to 200 mcg once a day	Do not exceed 200 mcg a day without seeing your doctor.
Stinging nettle*	120 mg three times a day	Stinging nettle can interfere with many medications. Speak to your healthcare provider or pharmacist before taking this supplement.
Vitamin A and mixed carotenoids	5,000 to 10,000 IU—half vitamin A and half mixed carotenoids—once a day	Use caution when taking vitamin A supplements because they have the potential to be toxic. Do not take for extended periods of time. Do not take more than 8,000 IU a day if you have liver disease, are a smoker, or have been exposed to asbestos.
Vitamin C	1,000 mg once a day	Do not take high doses if you are prone to kidney stones or gout. High doses can also cause diarrhea.
Vitamin E*	400 to 800 IU once a day	Take mixed tocopherols, the more active type of vitamin E. Consult your healthcare provider first if you are taking a blood thinner.
Zinc	35 to 50 mg once a day as zinc picolinate or zinc citrate	Your copper-to-zinc ratio is very important for your health. (See page 119 for details.) If you are taking zinc and iron supplements, take one in the morning and one in the evening. (Taking them together reduces the efficiency of both.)

*This supplement can have a blood-thinning action. See page 328 for more information.

BPH

See Benign Prostatic Hyperplasia.

CANCER

Cancer refers to an abnormal and uncontrolled growth of cells. The renegade cells form a mass—or *malignant tumor*—that can disrupt and potentially destroy the surrounding cells and tissue. They can then spread through a process called *metastasis*. This can occur in nearly any part of the body. The type of cancer is usually named after the location in the body where the tumor originated.

Some tumors are *benign.* They are comprised of similarly abnormal cells, but they do not invade the surrounding areas. Benign tumors need to be regularly monitored by a doctor because they can become cancerous. Additionally, they can displace the body's regular tissues, which can be harmful if occurring in an area such as the brain. Your doctor can perform a biopsy to determine whether a tumor is malignant or benign.

The goal of cancer treatment is the complete removal of the malignant cells. Certain types of cancers are more treatable than others. There are many different treatment options, with the most common being surgery, chemotherapy, and radiation therapy (or some combination of these three procedures). Surgery is often the best option if the tumor has not yet begun to spread. However, if metastasis has already occurred, it can be difficult to eliminate all the cancerous cells this way. *Chemotherapy,* the use of one or more drugs to destroy the cancer cells, may be used instead. These drugs can be taken orally or intravenously. *Radiation* concentrates ionizing radiation on the affected area in an attempt to kill the cancer or at least alter the cells so that they can no longer multiply. Your doctor will advise you on the most effective way to treat your cancer.

Naturally, it is preferable to avoid cancer in the first place. Although it may be beyond your control, there are steps you can take to decrease your risk. Try to avoid *carcinogens*—cancer-causing agents such as smoking tobacco, asbestos, and prolonged exposure to the sun. Recent cancer journals suggest that diet plays an important role, as well. In fact, Dr. Bruce Ames stated that diet "is expected to contribute to about one-third of preventable cancers." He then pointed specifically to the harm caused by vitamin and mineral deficiencies. The following list of supplements will help you maintain good health and fight the negative effects of carcinogens.

SUPPLEMENTS TO HELP PREVENT CANCER		
Supplements	Dosage	Considerations
Alpha lipoic acid	100 to 300 mg once a day	Alpha lipoic acid can interact with medication taken for diabetes and thyroid problems. Speak to your healthcare provider to see if any of the medications you take make it unwise to use this supplement.
Chlorella*	1 tbsp once a day	Avoid if you are allergic to iodine, if you have high iron levels, or if you have hemochromatosis. If you are taking a blood-thinning medication, consult your healthcare provider before using.
Coenzyme Q_{10}*	100 to 400 mg a day	If you are on blood-thinning medications, speak to your healthcare provider before using CoQ_{10}. Since some medications can cause a deficiency of this nutrient, speak to your healthcare provider to determine if you might need a larger dose.

Curcumin/Turmeric*	100 to 1,000 mg once a day of a formula that includes piperine or bioperine to boost absorption	Do not take curcumin with blood-thinning medications or supplements. Curcumin can also interact with other medications, so speak to a healthcare provider before taking this supplement.
EGCG (green tea extract)*	1,000 mg twice a day	Green tea extract can interact with a number of drugs. Check with your healthcare provider before taking this supplement.
EPA/DHA (fish oil)*	2,000 mg once a day	Choose a source that contains vitamin E to prevent oxidation.
Indole-3-carbinol (I-3-C)	300 to 500 mg once a day	May cause a mild elevation of liver enzymes and a skin rash.
Iodine	150 mcg once a day	Most table salts contain iodine, but sea salts do not. Before starting iodine supplementation, have your healthcare provider measure your iodine level.
Lycopene	10 to 20 mg once a day	May cause GI problems such as diarrhea, gas, and nausea.
Magnesium	600 mg once a day	Consult your healthcare provider for dosage if you have kidney disease. Discontinue use and see your doctor if you experience abdominal pain. Take a lower dose if it causes diarrhea.
Pycnogenol (OPCs)*	20 mg to 40 mg once a day	Pycnogenol may affect blood sugar levels.
Quercetin*	300 mg three times a day	For best results, take with bromelain and vitamin C. Do not use with blood-thinning medications or supplements.
Selenium	100 to 200 mcg once a day	Do not exceed 200 mcg a day without consulting your healthcare provider.
Vitamin A and mixed carotenoids	5,000 IU—half vitamin A and half mixed carotenoids— once a day	Use caution when taking vitamin A supplements because they have the potential to be toxic. Do not take for extended periods of time. Do not take more than 8,000 IU a day if you have liver disease, are a smoker, or have been exposed to asbestos.
Vitamin B_3 (niacinamide)	50 mg twice a day	High doses can deplete your body of other vitamins in the B complex, so take a B-complex vitamin twice a day.
Vitamin B_9 (folic acid)	50 to 400 mcg twice a day	High doses can deplete your body of other vitamins in the B complex, so take a B-complex vitamin twice a day.
Vitamin C	500 to 1,000 mg twice a day	Do not take high dosages if you are prone to kidney stones or gout. High doses can also cause diarrhea.
Vitamin D_3	Have your blood levels measured by your healthcare provider, who will determine proper dosage.	

| Vitamin E* | 400 IU once a day | Take mixed tocopherols, the more active type of vitamin E. Consult your healthcare provider first if you are taking a blood thinner. |
| Zinc | 25 mg once a day as zinc picolinate or zinc citrate | Your copper-to-zinc ratio is very important for your health. (See page 119 for details.) If you are taking zinc and iron supplements, take one in the morning and one in the evening. (Taking them together reduces the efficiency of both.) |

*This supplement can have a blood-thinning action. See page 328 for more information.

CANDIDIASIS

Candida albicans, a yeast, is part of your *gut flora*—the microorganisms found in your digestive tract. It is found in your genital area, intestines, mouth, throat, and urinary areas, and does not usually have any ill effects. However, under certain conditions—such as having a compromised immune system, using certain detergents, chronic antibiotic use, taking oral birth control, consuming excess sugar, or having diabetes—it can grow uncontrolled, resulting in the infection candidiasis.

There are many symptoms of candidiasis. Men usually get red sores near their penis or foreskin, while women may have vaginal burning, discharge, or itching. Other common symptoms include abdominal pain, anxiety, bloating, constipation, fatigue, insomnia, intestinal gas, muscle aches, and muscle weakness. However, you may also have chronic rashes or itching, food sensitivity, headaches, moodiness, rectal itching, sinusitis, or a white tongue. Men may also have prostate inflammation. If you suspect you have candidiasis, see your healthcare provider, who will test the infected area.

Candidiasis can be treated. Your symptoms—which often mimic the flu—may get worse for a week or two as the yeast die off. Then, about three weeks after beginning treatment, the budding yeast expire. This can cause the flu-like symptoms to resurface.

Diet is a very important part of treating chronic yeast infections. When you are combating an infection, be sure to avoid the following foods:

- Alcoholic beverages
- Apricots
- Cheeses
- Dairy products
- Dried fruits
- Figs
- Melons
- Mushrooms
- Peanuts
- Potatoes
- Raisins
- Sugar
- Winter squash
- Yams

Food allergies can play a role in candidiasis. Ask your healthcare provider to order food allergy testing, and then avoid all of the foods to which you are allergic.

Low stomach acid (hypochlorhydria) can contribute to yeast overgrowth. Have your healthcare provider perform a test to determine if you have low stomach acid, and replace, if necessary, with Betaine HCl. Do not perform this test or use this product if you have an active peptic ulcer.

I recommend CandiBactin-AR and CandiBactin-BR for the treatment of candidiasis. Both products contain a blend of essential oils and herbal extracts that are designed to support intestinal microbial balance and proper digestion. Candibactin-BR, for instance, contains Oregon grape extract, berberine hydrochloride, coptis root extract, and more. Candicid Forte contains many of these nutrients, too. You may also find it helpful to take probiotics (beneficial bacteria) as well as other nutrients listed in the table "Supplements to Treat Candidiasis." Continue the regimen for two to six months. At that point, discontinue your use of glutamine. Continue to take probiotics once a day. When the problem has been resolved, try the supplements in the table "Supplements for Long-Term Management of Yeast Overgrowth."

SUPPLEMENTS TO TREAT CANDIDIASIS

Supplements	Dosage	Considerations
Arginine	1,000 to 5,000 mg once a day	Do not take if you have kidney disease, liver disease, or herpes except under a doctor's supervision. Arginine can interact with some medications. Consult with your healthcare provider before beginning this therapy.
B-complex vitamins	50 mg twice a day	I suggest taking a multivitamin along with your B-complex vitamins.
Berberine*	50 mg three times a day of standardized extract	Do not use this supplement during pregnancy. It can cause uterine contractions.
CandiBactin or Candicid Forte	2 capsules three times a day	These multi-nutrient blends by Metagenics contain many helpful botanical substances, including berberine, ginger, licorice, skullcap, coptis root, and grape seed extract. (See Resources.)
Garlic*	10 mg allicin or a total allicin potential of 4,000 mcg (equal to one clove of garlic) once a day	Garlic is a blood thinner. Do not use if you are taking any kind of blood-thinning medication or supplements.
Glutamine	5,000 to 10,000 mg once a day	If you have a sensitivity to monosodium glutamate (MSG), use glutamine with caution. If you are taking medications for seizures, take glutamine only under the direction of your doctor.

Molybdenum	250 to 500 mcg once a day	Check your copper levels after molybdenum supplementation, because molybdenum can cause a copper deficiency.
Probiotics	20 billion units once a day	If taking an antibiotic, take the probiotics at least two hours before or two hours after using the antibiotics. Do not take them at the same time. Do not start prebiotics, such as fructooligosaccharide (FOS), until you have been treated for yeast overgrowth and have been on probiotics for at least one month. Otherwise, you will feed the yeast and bad bacteria. *S. boulardii* aids in the growth of beneficial bacteria, crowds out yeast, and supports the immune system.
Zinc	25 mg once a day as zinc picolinate or zinc citrate	Your copper-to-zinc ratio is very important for your health. (See page 119 for details.) If you are taking zinc and iron supplements, take one in the morning and one in the evening.

*This supplement can have a blood-thinning action. See page 328 for more information.

SUPPLEMENTS FOR LONG-TERM MANAGEMENT OF YEAST OVERGROWTH

Supplements	Dosage	Considerations
Carnitine*	1,000 to 3,000 mg once a day	Have your doctor measure your TMAO levels before starting long-term supplementation with carnitine.
Chromium	300 mcg once a day as chromium picolinate	Combining with the protein picolinate allows your body to absorb chromium more efficiently. However, some chromium picolinate supplements contain more chromium than necessary. Ask your healthcare provider for a recommendation on chromium consumption.
Gamma-linolenic acid (GLA) as evening primrose oil (EPO)*	240 to 480 mg once a day	It is important to maintain the proper ratio of omega-6 fatty acids to omega-3 fatty acids. (See page 129.) Evening primrose oil may interfere with some medications, such as nonsteroidal anti-inflammatories; can act as a blood thinner; and can lower the seizure threshold. Consult your healthcare provider or pharmacist before taking this supplement.
Magnesium	400 to 800 mg once a day	Consult your healthcare provider for dosage if you have kidney disease. Discontinue use and see your doctor if you experience abdominal pain. Take a lower dose if it causes diarrhea.

Taurine	1,000 to 3,000 mg once a day	Take between meals. Discontinue use if you have chest or throat tightness or if you break out in hives. Do not take with aspirin. Have your healthcare provider measure levels before starting taurine therapy.
Vitamin C	500 mg twice a day	Do not take high doses if you are prone to kidney stones or gout. High doses can also cause diarrhea.
Vitamin E*	400 IU once a day	Take mixed tocopherols, the more active type of vitamin E. Consult your healthcare provider first if you are taking a blood thinner.
Zinc	45 mg a day as zinc picolinate or zinc citrate	Your copper-to-zinc ratio is very important for your health. (See page 119 for details.) If you are taking zinc and iron supplements, take one in the morning and one in the evening. (Taking them together reduces the efficiency of both.)

*This supplement can have a blood-thinning action. See page 328 for more information.

CARDIOVASCULAR DISEASE

See Atherosclerosis; Congestive Heart Failure; High Blood Pressure; Stroke.

CATARACTS

A cataract is a clouding of the eye's natural lens, which lies behind the iris and the pupil. Lenses are composed largely of water and protein, with the protein being arranged in a precise way. When the protein starts to clump together, a cataract begins to form.

Cataracts can develop for a variety of reasons. Simple old age is probably the most common cause, with other causes including diabetes, long-term ultraviolet exposure, exposure to radiation, genetic factors, and eye injury and trauma. Some drugs, such as corticosteroids, can also induce cataract formation.

When cataracts first start to develop, they have little effect on vision. Sometimes, a newly forming cataract can even *improve* close vision, causing near-sightedness. Over time, though, as the cataract grows, vision becomes impaired. Images may become blurred or fuzzy. Night vision may be poor, and street lights may cause glare or appear to be surrounded by halos. Colors may seem to fade or change. Eventually, if the cataract is left untreated, blindness can result. In advanced cases, the lens can even rupture, leading to severe inflammation.

When a cataract has developed to the point where there is a good deal of vision loss, surgery can remove the clouded lens and replace it with a permanent plastic lens. In earlier stages, however, certain nutrients can slow the formation of cataracts and even prevent them from developing in the first place. Studies have also shown that individuals who eat a low-glycemic-index diet that is high in fiber and includes a lot of vegetables have a lower risk of developing cataracts.

SUPPLEMENTS TO TREAT CATARACTS		
Supplements	**Dosage**	**Considerations**
Alpha lipoic acid	100 to 300 mg once a day	Alpha lipoic acid can interact with medication taken for diabetes and thyroid problems. Speak to your healthcare provider to see if any of the medications you take make it unwise to use this supplement.
B-complex vitamins	50 mg twice a day	I suggest taking a multivitamin along with your B-complex vitamins.
Beta-carotene	3 to 6 mg once a day	Do not take for extended periods of time. Do not take high doses if you have liver disease, are a smoker, or have been exposed to asbestos.
Bilberry*	60 to 240 mg once a day	Bilberry may interfere with iron absorption and blood clotting. High doses should be used with caution by people with bleeding disorders.
Carnosine	Oral: 1,000 to 2,000 mg a day Eye drops: Use as directed	Check with your doctor before starting carnosine therapy if you have diabetes, hypertension, kidney disease, or liver disease. Too much carnosine can result in hyperactivity.
Copper	1 mg once a day	Your copper-to-zinc ratio is very important for your health. (See page 119.) Also, do not take copper supplement cupric oxide, which has a very low bioavailability.
Cysteine	500 mg once a day as n-acetylcysteine, or NAC	When taking NAC supplements, also take extra vitamin C, copper, and zinc.
Glutathione	250 to 500 mg once a day as liposomal glutathione.	If you opt to take NAC, there is no need to take glutathione.
Lutein	6 mg to 12 mg once a day	
Manganese	2 mg once a day	Use with caution if you have gallbladder or liver disease.
Quercetin*	500 to 1,000 mg once a day	For best results, take with bromelain and vitamin C. Do not use with blood-thinning medications or supplements.
Selenium	100 to 200 mcg once a day	Do not exceed 200 mcg a day without consulting your healthcare provider.

Taurine	1,000 to 4,000 mg a day	Take between meals. Discontinue use if you have chest or throat tightness or break out in hives. Do not take with aspirin. Have your healthcare provider measure levels before starting taurine therapy.
Vitamin A and mixed carotenoids	5,000 to 10,000 IU—half vitamin A and half mixed carotenoids—once a day	Use caution when taking vitamin A supplements because they have the potential to be toxic. Do not take for extended periods of time. Do not take more than 8,000 IU a day if you have liver disease, are a smoker, or have been exposed to asbestos.
Vitamin C	1,000 mg twice a day	Do not take high doses if you are prone to kidney stones or gout. High doses can also cause diarrhea.
Vitamin E*	400 to 800 IU once a day	Take mixed tocopherols, the more active type of vitamin E. Consult your healthcare provider first if you are taking a blood thinner.
Zinc	25 to 50 mg once a day as zinc picolinate or zinc citrate	Your copper-to-zinc ratio is very important for your health. (See page 119 for details.) If you are taking zinc and iron supplements, take one in the morning and one in the evening.

*This supplement can have a blood-thinning action. See page 328 for more information.

CEREBROVASCULAR ACCIDENT

See Stroke.

CERVICAL CANCER/CERVICAL DYSPLASIA

Cervical cancer occurs when a woman experiences an uncontrolled growth of cells in the cervix (the lower portion of the uterus). Symptoms include vaginal bleeding and discharge and pelvic pain. There are several different treatment options, including chemotherapy and radiation, and 70 percent of infected women are cured of the cancer after treatment.

Nearly all cases are the result of an infection by the human papillomavirus (HPV), a group of sexually transmitted viruses. However, not all cases of HPV lead to cervical cancer. Some strains of the virus manifest into warts, while others will lay dormant and result in no symptoms. (Some strains can also lead to penile cancer in men.) Gardasil is an FDA-approved vaccine that protects against many strains of HPV.

Cervical dysplasia is a precancerous lesion that manifests prior to the cancer's development. Each year, 250,000 to 1 million women in the United States are diagnosed with cervical dysplasia. This condition can occur at any age, with the mean age being twenty-five to thirty-five years. During this early stage, the cells begin to undergo the changes that will result in malignant cells. This is the best time to catch the problem, which can be discovered during a Pap smear or colposcopy (examination of the cervix and vagina). The treatments available for cervical dysplasia—of which there are several—can often cure the disease, and many times, it even resolves on its own. However, there is a 20-percent recurrence rate, so checkups are advised. Because the frequency of these examinations is decided on a case-by-case basis, this should be determined with the help of a healthcare provider.

More than half of patients with cervical cancer have been found to have multiple nutritional deficiencies. A study showed that an increase in the dietary intake of dark green and deep yellow vegetables and fruits is associated with a nearly 50-percent reduction in the risk of developing cervical dysplasia. A diet high in fruits and vegetables is also believed to protect against the development of cancer.

SUPPLEMENTS TO PREVENT AND TREAT CERVICAL DYSPLASIA

Supplements	Dosage	Considerations
Alpha lipoic acid	100 to 300 mg once a day	Alpha lipoic acid can interact with medication taken for diabetes and thyroid problems. Speak to your healthcare provider to see if any of the medications you take make it unwise to use this supplement.
B-complex vitamins	50 mg twice a day	I suggest taking a multivitamin along with your B-complex vitamins.
Bromelain (digestive enzyme)	Use as part of a digestive enzyme product.	Do not take bromelain if you are allergic to pineapple, latex, wheat, celery, carrot, fennel, cypress pollen, or grass pollen.
EGCG (green tea extract)*	200 to 400 mg once a day	Green tea extract can interact with a number of drugs. Check with your healthcare provider before taking this supplement.
EPA/DHA (fish oil)*	1,000 mg once a day	Choose a source that contains vitamin E to prevent oxidation.
Indole-3-carbinol (I-3-C)	200 to 400 mg once a day	May cause a mild elevation of liver enzymes and a skin rash.
Quercetin*	300 to 900 mg once a day	For best results, take with bromelain and vitamin C. Do not use with blood-thinning medications or supplements.
Selenium	200 mcg once a day	Do not exceed 200 mcg a day without consulting your healthcare provider.

Vitamin A and mixed carotenoids	50,000 to 100,000 IU—half vitamin A and half mixed carotenoids—once a day	Use caution when taking vitamin A supplements because they have the potential to be toxic. Do not take for extended periods of time. Do not take more than 8,000 IU a day if you have liver disease, are a smoker, or have been exposed to asbestos.
Vitamin B₉ (folic acid)	400 mcg twice a day	High doses can deplete your body of other B vitamins, so take a B-complex vitamin twice a day.
Vitamin B₁₂ (cobalamin)	500 to 1,000 mcg twice a day	High doses can deplete your body of other B vitamins, so take a B-complex vitamin twice a day.
Vitamin C	250 mg to 500 mg twice a day	Do not take high doses if you are prone to kidney stones or gout. High doses can also cause diarrhea.
Vitamin E*	400 IU once a day	Take mixed tocopherols, the more active type of vitamin E. Consult your healthcare provider first if you are taking a blood thinner.
Zinc	25 mg once a day as zinc picolinate or zinc citrate	Your copper-to-zinc ratio is very important for your health. (See page 119 for details.) If you are taking zinc and iron supplements, take one in the morning and one in the evening. (Taking them together reduces the efficiency of both.)

*This supplement can have a blood-thinning action. See page 328 for more information.

CERVICAL DYSPLASIA

See Cervical Cancer/Cervical Dysplasia.

CHOLESTEROL

See High Cholesterol.

CHRONIC FATIGUE SYNDROME

Approximately 836,000 to 2.5 million Americans have chronic fatigue syndrome, or CFS, a debilitating condition characterized by a profound feeling of fatigue that is not improved by bed rest, and is greatly worsened by activity. In fact, increased fatigue sometimes lasts twenty-four hours after exertion. Other defining symptoms of this condition include substantial impairment in memory and concentration, muscle pain, pain in multiple joints, unusual headaches, sore throat, and tender lymph nodes in the neck or armpit. Less common symptoms include abdominal pain, alcohol intolerance, bloating, chest pain, chronic cough, diarrhea, and dizziness. Generally, to be considered chronic fatigue syndrome, symptoms have to persist for six or more consecutive months. Many patients suffer from both chronic fatigue and fibromyalgia, a disorder that causes muscle pain and fatigue. The overlap between chronic fatigue syndrome and fibromyalgia is believed to be about 70 percent.

There are no physical signs that allow physicians to identify CFS. Instead, physicians must rule out other disorders that have similar symptoms. Moreover, there is no known cause of CFS, and no known cure. However, it is important to avoid substances like alcohol, caffeine, and sugar that can worsen fatigue; to explore the possibility of food allergies; and to use supplements—such as those recommended below—that can foster overall good health and proper energy production. Detoxification can also be helpful.

SUPPLEMENTS TO TREAT CHRONIC FATIGUE SYNDROME

Supplements	Dosage	Considerations
Alpha lipoic acid	50 to 600 mg once a day	Alpha lipoic acid can interact with medication taken for diabetes and thyroid problems. Speak to your healthcare provider to see if any of the medications you take make it unwise to use this supplement.
B-complex vitamins	50 mg twice a day of all B vitamins except those listed below: Folic acid: 400 mcg twice a day; B_{12}: 500 mcg twice a day	I suggest taking a multivitamin along with your B-complex vitamins. Folic acid, B_{12}, B_6, B_2, B_1 have all been shown to be low in patients with CFS.
Bromelain (digestive enzyme)	2,400 mcg three to four times a day	Do not take bromelain if you are allergic to pineapple, latex, wheat, celery, carrot, fennel, cypress pollen, or grass pollen.
Carnitine*	1,000 mg one to three times a day	The most effective form for this purpose is acetyl-L-carnitine (ALCAR). Have your healthcare provider measure your TMAO levels before starting long-term supplementation with carnitine.
CBD oil (hemp oil)	5 to 500 mg a day in the form of sublingual drops. Start with 5 mg and increase slowly until you find relief.	CBD is generally well tolerated and safe for consumption, even in high doses and with continuous use. However, do not exceed 500 mg a day without consulting your healthcare provider. Make sure to buy a product marked "hemp oil (aerial parts)."
Cocoa	2.5 g (0.1 ounce) unsweetened cocoa powder (about 0.5 teaspoon)	Cocoa can interact with some medications, so speak to your healthcare provider or pharmacist before starting long-term supplementation. Cocoa also contains caffeine, which can cause side effects in some people.

Coenzyme Q_{10}*	200 to 300 mg once a day	If you are on blood-thinning medications, speak to your healthcare provider before using CoQ_{10}. Since some medications can cause a deficiency of this nutrient, speak to your healthcare provider to determine if you might need a larger dose.
Copper	1 to 3 mg once a day	Your copper-to-zinc ratio is very important for your health. (See page 119.) Also, do not take copper supplement cupric oxide, which has a very low bioavailability.
Curcumin/Turmeric*	1,500 to 3,000 mg once a day of a formula that includes piperine or bioperine to boost absorption	Do not take curcumin with blood-thinning medications or supplements. Curcumin can also interact with other medications, so speak to your healthcare provider before taking this supplement.
Cysteine	500 to 1,000 mg once a day as n-acetylcysteine, or NAC	When taking NAC supplements, also take extra vitamin C, copper, and zinc.
D-ribose	15,000 mg three times a day	D-ribose can lower blood sugar levels, so check with your healthcare provider before taking this supplement with any diabetes medication, especially insulin.
EPA/DHA (fish oil)*	1,000 to 3,000 mg once a day	Choose a source that contains vitamin E to prevent oxidation.
Gamma-linolenic acid (GLA) as evening primrose oil (EPO)*	240 to 720 mg once a day	It is important to maintain the proper ratio of omega-6 fatty acids to omega-3 fatty acids. (See page 129.) Evening primrose oil may interfere with some medications, such as nonsteroidal anti-inflammatories; can act as a blood thinner; and can lower the seizure threshold. Consult your healthcare provider or pharmacist before taking this supplement.
Glutamine	500 to 1,500 mg three times a day	If you have a sensitivity to monosodium glutamate (MSG), use glutamine with caution. If you are taking medications for seizures, take glutamine only under the direction of your doctor.
Hawthorn*	600 mg dried standardized extract twice a day	Hawthorn can interact with a number of medications. Speak to your healthcare provider or pharmacist to learn if any drugs you're taking might make it unwise to take hawthorn.
Magnesium	50 to 1,000 mg once a day as magnesium citrate	Consult your healthcare provider for dosage if you have kidney disease. Discontinue use and see your doctor if you experience abdominal pain. Take a lower dose if it causes diarrhea.
Malic acid	1,200 to 2,400 mg once a day	Malic acid can reduce blood pressure. If you have low blood pressure, speak to your healthcare provider before using malic acid.

Manganese	2 to 5 mg once a day	Use with caution if you have gallbladder or liver disease.
Methylsulfonylmethane (MSM)	1,000 mg to 3,000 mg three times a day	Use with caution if you are allergic to sulfur. Start by taking 500 mg three times a day, and gradually increase dose. Take with meals to avoid possible heartburn. May cause stomach upset in dosages larger than 6,000 mg.
Phosphatidylserine (PS)	200 to 300 mg twice a day	PS can interact with many drugs. Speak to your healthcare provider before taking it.
Probiotics	20 billion units once a day	If taking an antibiotic, take the probiotics at least two hours before or two hours after using the antibiotics. Do not take them at the same time.
Quercetin*	500 mg three times a day	For best results, take with bromelain and vitamin C. Do not use with blood-thinning medications or supplements.
Selenium	100 to 200 mcg once a day	Do not exceed 200 mcg a day without consulting your healthcare provider.
UltraInflamX	Follow instructions on bottle.	This product, by Metagenics (see Resources), provides macro- and micronutrient support for people with compromised gut function. Do not use if taking a diuretic.
Vitamin A and mixed carotenoids	5,000 IU—half vitamin A and half mixed carotenoids— once a day	Use caution when taking vitamin A supplements because they have the potential to be toxic. Do not take for extended periods of time. Do not take more than 8,000 IU a day if you have liver disease, are a smoker, or have been exposed to asbestos.
Vitamin C	500 to 3,000 mg twice a day	Do not take high doses if you are prone to kidney stones or gout. High doses can also cause diarrhea.
Vitamin D_3	Have your blood levels measured by your healthcare provider, who will determine proper dosage.	
Vitamin E*	400 to 1,000 IU once a day	Take mixed tocopherols, the more active type of vitamin E. Consult your healthcare provider first if you are taking a blood thinner.
Vitamin K*	100 to 1,000 mcg once a day of K_2 or MK-7	If you are on blood-thinning medications, speak to your healthcare provider before using vitamin K.
Zinc	25 to 50 mg once a day as zinc picolinate or zinc citrate	Your copper-to-zinc ratio is very important to your health. (See page 119 for details.) If you are taking zinc and iron supplements, take one in the morning and one in the evening. (Taking them together reduces the efficiency of both.)

*This supplement can have a blood-thinning action. See page 328 for more information.

CHRONIC INFLAMMATION

See Inflammation

CLOSED HEAD INJURY

A closed head injury occurs when there is trauma to the brain without penetration of the skull. The soft tissue of the brain is delicate, and the skull usually serves to protect it. But when a moving head is abruptly stopped—as may occur in a car accident or fall—or when the head is forcibly struck, the brain may hit against the side of the rough, hard skull. The resulting damage, which can include bleeding, swelling, and tearing, can range from mild to serious.

Although doctors used to believe that a closed head injury was less severe than an open head injury (in which the skull has been penetrated), this is not necessarily the case. In fact, an open head injury may actually allow pressure in the brain caused by the accident to be relieved. A closed head injury, on the other hand, allows no outlet for this pressure. Instead, any swelling is constrained, which can cause exacerbated damage to both the brain and the brain stem.

A person who has had a closed head injury may show no immediate signs of being hurt. The three major problems—bleeding, swelling, and tearing—can go undetected after an accident for hours or even days. However, postponing their discovery can allow these problems to become worse, leading to more permanent damage or even death. If you have a head injury, see a doctor, regardless of whether you are aware of any effects. The following supplements should not be started until after any bleeding, swelling, and tearing have been resolved, unless otherwise directed by a healthcare provider.

SUPPLEMENTS TO TREAT CLOSED HEAD INJURY

Supplements	Dosage	Considerations
Calcium	500 mg twice a day as calcium citrate	Although most people are deficient in calcium, there is a danger in taking too much calcium. Do not ingest more than 1,000 to 1,200 mg of calcium a day.
Coenzyme Q_{10}*	100 mg once a day	If you are on blood-thinning medications, speak to your healthcare provider before using CoQ_{10}. Since some medications can cause a deficiency of this nutrient, speak to your healthcare provider to determine if you might need a larger dose.

Copper	2 mg once a day	Your copper-to-zinc ratio is very important for your health. (See page 119 for details.) Also, do not take copper supplement cupric oxide, which has a very low bioavailability.
EPA/DHA (fish oil)*	3,000 mg once a day	Choose a source that contains vitamin E to prevent oxidation.
Magnesium	600 to 800 mg once a day	Consult your healthcare provider for dosage if you have kidney disease. Discontinue use and see your doctor if you experience abdominal pain. Take a lower dose if it causes diarrhea.
Multivitamin	1 tablet once a day or as directed	
Phosphatidylserine (PS)	300 mg once a day	PS can interact with many drugs. Speak to your healthcare provider before taking it.
Vitamin B$_5$ (pantothenic acid)	50 mg twice a day	High doses can deplete your body of other vitamins in the B complex, so take a B-complex vitamin twice a day. Stop taking B$_5$ supplements if you begin having chest pains or breathing problems.
Vitamin B$_6$ (pyridoxine)	50 mg twice a day	Do not take more than 500 mg a day. If you are taking L-dopa for Parkinson's disease, do not take B$_6$ without first consulting your doctor. High doses can deplete your body of other vitamins in the B complex, so take a B-complex vitamin twice a day.
Zinc	25 mg once a day as zinc picolinate or zinc citrate	Your copper-to-zinc ratio is very important to your health. (See page 119 for details.) If you are taking zinc and iron supplements, take one in the morning and one in the evening.

*This supplement can have a blood-thinning action. See page 328 for more information.

COMMON COLD

The common cold is a viral infection of the upper respiratory tract. The most common of all diseases, colds are characterized by congestion, coughing, headache, runny nose, and sneezing. (Although some people exhibit a slight fever, a high temperature is usually indicative of influenza rather than a cold.) Most of these symptoms are the attempts of your immune system to fight the virus. A cold usually clears up in five to ten days, after which there is a several-week period of residual coughing and slight congestion. In older people and individuals with a compromised immune system, the common cold can lead to severe illness and even death.

Colds are extremely contagious, but there are steps you can take to protect yourself. Avoid close contact with infected people. Whenever possible, wash your hands, which can remove viruses before they enter your body. Do not touch your face until you have washed your hands. Also, do not share writing instruments with anyone during the flu season. If you believe you have been exposed to a cold or if your symptoms have already begun, ingest the following supplements. They will help shorten the duration of your cold and lessen its severity.

SUPPLEMENTS TO TREAT THE COMMON COLD

Supplements	Dosage	Considerations
Cysteine	1,000 to 3,000 mg once a day as n-acetylcysteine, or NAC	When taking NAC supplements, also take extra vitamin C, copper, and zinc.
Echinacea	1,000 to 2,000 mg once a day	Do not use long term. Avoid echinacea if you are allergic to plants such as ragweed, chrysanthemums, marigolds, daisies, or dandelions.
Garlic*	10 mg allicin or a total allicin potential of 4,000 mcg (equal to one clove of garlic) once a day	Garlic is a blood thinner. Do not use if you are taking blood-thinning medication or supplements.
Taurine	2,000 mg once a day	Take between meals. Discontinue use if you suddenly have feelings of chest or throat tightness or if you break out in hives. Do not take with aspirin. Have your healthcare provider measure levels before starting taurine therapy.
Vitamin C	1,000 to 2,500 mg twice a day	Do not take high doses if you are prone to kidney stones or gout. High doses can also cause diarrhea.
Zinc	25 to 50 mg once a day as zinc picolinate or zinc citrate	Your copper-to-zinc ratio is very important for your health. (See page 119 for details.) If you are taking zinc and iron supplements, take one in the morning and one in the evening. (Taking them together reduces the efficiency of both.)

*This supplement can have a blood-thinning action. See page 328 for more information.

CONCUSSION

See Closed Head Injury.

CONGESTIVE HEART FAILURE

Congestive heart failure, also called *congestive cardiac failure* or simply *heart failure,* is a condition in which the heart is unable to pump an adequate amount of blood throughout the body. The failing heart keeps working, but not as efficiently as it should.

The symptoms of congestive heart failure can include *edema* (fluid build-up that can result in swollen legs and ankles); shortness of breath; fatigue; and nocturnal cough. Because these can also be signs of other disorders, a physician is needed to confirm the diagnosis.

Congestive heart failure can have many causes, including narrowing of the arteries that supply blood to the heart muscle (coronary artery disease), scar tissue due to past heart attacks, high blood pressure (hypertension), heart valve disease, primary disease of the heart muscle (cardiomyopathy), congenital heart defects, and infection of the heart valves and/or muscles of the heart. If a specific cause can be found, it is generally treated and, if possible, corrected. Other treatments may include rest; dietary modifications, including salt restriction and the avoidance of alcohol; changes in daily activities; and appropriate medications. Supplements that protect and enhance the health of the heart and blood vessels can also be an important part of congestive heart failure management.

SUPPLEMENTS TO TREAT CONGESTIVE HEART FAILURE

Supplements	Dosage	Considerations
Arginine	3,000 to 9,000 mg once a day	Do not take if you have kidney disease, liver disease, or herpes except under a doctor's supervision. Arginine can interact with some medications. Consult with your healthcare provider before beginning this therapy.
Berberine*	300 to 500 mg three times a day of standardized extract	Do not use this supplement during pregnancy. It can cause uterine contractions.
Carnitine*	2,000 mg once a day	Have your healthcare provider measure your TMAO levels before starting long-term supplementation with carnitine.
Carnosine	1,000 mg once a day	Check with your doctor before starting carnosine therapy if you have diabetes, hypertension, kidney disease, or liver damage. Too much carnosine can result in hyperactivity.
Coenzyme Q_{10}*	120 to 400 mg once a day	If you are on blood-thinning medications, speak to your healthcare provider before using CoQ10. Since some medications can cause a deficiency of this nutrient, speak to your healthcare provider to determine if you might need a larger dose.
D-ribose	15,000 mg three times a day	D-ribose can lower blood sugar levels, so check with your healthcare provider before taking this supplement with any diabetes medication, especially insulin.

EPA/DHA (fish oil)*	2,000 to 3,000 mg once a day	For most patients with congestive heart failure, EPA/DHA is very helpful, but for some, it can worsen the condition, so use only under the guidance of your physician. Choose a source that contains vitamin E to prevent oxidation.
Hawthorn*	160 to 900 mg dried standardized extract once a day	Hawthorn can interact with a number of medications. Speak to your healthcare provider or pharmacist to learn if any of the drugs you're taking might make it unwise to take hawthorn.
Iron	Have your doctor measure your iron levels to determine dosage.	Supplement with iron if needed and repeat the laboratory tests every three months.
Magnesium	600 to 800 mg once a day	Consult your healthcare provider for dosage if you have kidney disease. Discontinue use and see your doctor if you experience abdominal pain. Take a lower dose if it causes diarrhea.
Potassium	See your healthcare provider for dosage directions.	
Selenium	100 to 200 mcg once a day	Do not exceed 200 mcg a day without consulting your healthcare provider.
Taurine	2,000 mg twice a day	Take between meals. Discontinue use if you have chest or throat tightness or if you break out in hives. Do not take with aspirin. Have your healthcare provider measure levels before starting taurine therapy.
Vitamin B$_1$ (thiamine)	50 mg twice a day	High doses can deplete your body of other vitamins in the B complex, so take a B-complex vitamin twice a day. Vitamins B$_1$, B$_2$, B$_6$, and B$_9$ have all been shown to benefit heart health.
Vitamin D$_3$	Have your blood levels measured by your healthcare provider, who will determine proper dosage.	
Vitamin E*	400 IU once a day	Take mixed tocopherols, the more active type of vitamin E. Consult your healthcare provider first if you are taking a blood thinner.

*This supplement can have a blood-thinning action. See page 328 for more information.

CROHN'S DISEASE

Crohn's disease is a chronic inflammatory bowel disease. It affects the gastrointestinal tract by causing inflammation and swelling. The cause is unknown, but many doctors believe that the inflammation is due to a misdirected attack by the immune system.

Crohn's disease can attack any part of the gastrointestinal tract, from the mouth to the anus. The name of the exact illness is derived from the location of the problem. *Ileocolitis*, the most prevalent type, affects the large intestine and the part of the small intestine that connects to the large intestine. *Ileitis* is less common, and affects the *ileum*—the part of the small intestine that connects to the colon. Only 20 percent of people with Crohn's disease have *colitis*, which inflames the large intestine.

Crohn's disease is made up of periods of outbreaks followed by periods of remission. Symptoms of outbreaks include abdominal cramps, diarrhea, rectal bleeding, and weight loss. The skin around the anus is often the site of itchiness, fissures, or abscesses. Over the long term, Crohn's disease can damage other organs, such as the eyes and kidneys, and it also increases the risk of cancer of the inflamed areas.

There is no cure for Crohn's disease. Treatment aims to decrease the inflammation and shorten outbreaks, as well as prolonging periods of remission. Doctors usually prescribe anti-inflammatories or antibiotics. Some patients have the most success with *immunosuppressive drugs*—medication that suppresses the immune system. Although these drugs are often effective at restricting the immune system's attack on the body, they also limit the immune system when fighting actual infection or other problems. Therefore, their use can result in a host of additional health issues. The use of supplements to treat Crohn's disease often means that less medication is needed. In some cases, the medication can even be discontinued. Before changing your dosage or stopping your medication, however, please see your healthcare provider.

Be aware that diet also plays a major role in the Crohn's disease process. If you stop eating gluten, dairy, brewer's yeast, and any foods to which you are allergic, you will go a long way toward alleviating the symptoms of Crohn's while decreasing antibody production. Also try to avoid simple sugars, which increase the fermentation of bacteria in the colon and increase transit time.

SUPPLEMENTS TO TREAT CROHN'S DISEASE		
Supplements	Dosage	Considerations
B-complex vitamins	50 mg twice a day	I suggest taking a multivitamin along with your B-complex vitamins. Thiamine, folic acid, B_6, and B_{12} have been shown to be decreased in people with Crohn's disease.
CBD oil (hemp oil)	5 to 500 mg a day in the form of sublingual drops. Start with 5 mg and increase slowly until you find relief.	CBD is generally well tolerated and safe for consumption, even in high doses and with continuous use. However, do not exceed 500 mg a day without consulting your healthcare provider. Make sure to buy a product marked "hemp oil (aerial parts)."

Curcumin/Turmeric*	500 mg three times a day of a formula that includes piperine or bioperine to boost absorption	Do not take curcumin with blood-thinning medications or supplements. Curcumin can also interact with other medications, so speak to your healthcare provider before taking this supplement.
Eleuthero*	50 to 200 mg once a day	Do not use if you have a history of heart disease, hypertension, sleep apnea, narcolepsy, mania, or schizophrenia; if you are pregnant or breastfeeding; or if you have a bleeding disorder.
EPA/DHA (fish oil)*	1,000 to 5,000 mg once a day	Choose a source that contains vitamin E to prevent oxidation. In high doses, fatty acids may cause the blood to thin. If you are taking a blood thinner, do not take EPA/DHA doses above 4,000 mg a day without direct instructions from your doctor. It is important to maintain the proper ratio of omega-6 fatty acids to omega-3 fatty acids. (See page 129.)
Gamma-linolenic acid (GLA) as evening primrose oil (EPO)*	240 to 720 mg once a day	It is important to maintain the proper ratio of omega-6 fatty acids to omega-3 fatty acids. (See page 129.) Evening primrose oil may interfere with some medications, such as nonsteroidal anti-inflammatories; can act as a blood thinner; and can lower the seizure threshold. Consult your healthcare provider or pharmacist before taking this supplement.
Glucosamine sufate	300 to 900 mg once a day	If you are allergic to shellfish, be sure to choose a supplement that is not shellfish based. Consult use with your healthcare provider if you have diabetes, because glucosamine can alter blood sugar levels.
Glutamine	1,000 to 5,000 mg once a day	If you have a sensitivity to monosodium glutamate (MSG), use glutamine with caution. If you are taking medications for seizures, take glutamine only under the direction of your doctor.
Iron	Have your doctor measure your iron levels to determine dosage.	Iron levels are commonly low in patients with Crohn's disease. Supplement with iron if needed, and repeat the laboratory tests every three months.
Kaprex AI	1 softgel capsule twice a day	Made by Metagenics, this multi-nutrient formula supports immune system function. (See Resources.) Do not use if taking an anticoagulant.
Magnesium	400 to 800 mg once a day	Consult your healthcare provider for dosage if you have kidney disease. Discontinue use and see your doctor if you experience abdominal pain. Take a lower dose if it causes diarrhea.
Olive leaf extract*	500 mg to 750 mg a day containing 20 mg of oleuropein per capsule	Olive leaf extracts can interact with many prescription medications, and may increase the effects of blood thinners. Consult your healthcare

		provider before using olive leaf extract if you are taking any medication. Don't use if you are pregnant or breastfeeding.
Phosphatidylcholine (PC)	1,000 to 4,000 mg twice a day	Use with caution if you have malabsorption problems, as this could exacerbate them.
Probiotics	20 billion units once a day	If taking an antibiotic, take the probiotics at least two hours before or after using the antibiotic.
Selenium	200 mcg once a day	Do not exceed 200 mcg a day without consulting your healthcare provider.
Vitamin A and mixed carotenoids	5,000 IU—half vitamin A and half mixed carotenoids —once a day	Use caution when taking vitamin A supplements because they have the potential to be toxic. Do not take for extended periods of time. Do not take more than 8,000 IU a day if you have liver disease, are a smoker, or have been exposed to asbestos.
Vitamin C	500 to 1,500 mg twice a day	Do not take high doses if you are prone to kidney stones or gout. High doses can also cause diarrhea.
Vitamin D$_3$	Have your blood levels measured by your healthcare provider, who will determine proper dosage.	Make sure your healthcare provider monitors you throughout vitamin D therapy. Calcium can be elevated in people with Crohn's disease, and vitamin D can also elevate calcium levels.
Vitamin E*	400 IU once a day	Take mixed tocopherols, the more active type of vitamin E. Consult your healthcare provider first if you are taking a blood thinner.
Vitamin K*	Have your blood levels measured by your healthcare provider, who will determine proper dosage.	If you are on a blood-thinning medication, speak to your healthcare provider before using vitamin K.

*This supplement can have a blood-thinning action. See page 328 for more information.

DEMENTIA

See Alzheimer's Disease.

DEPRESSION

Depression is a state of intense sadness, melancholy, or despair that lasts for a prolonged period of time—sometimes for months. In some cases, it does not seriously affect the individual's ability to function. When it does disrupt function, it is referred to as *clinical depression*. According to the National Institute of Mental Health, one in ten people suffer from a depressive illness of some type each year.

The symptoms of depression can include sadness, fatigue, irritability, apathy, feelings of isolation, loss of interest in favorite activities, hopelessness, insomnia, significant weight changes, aches and pains, and even thoughts of death or suicide. It has been found that symptoms vary according to age, gender, and culture. For instance, a depressed teen-age boy is more likely to experience irritability and grumpiness, while a grown man who is depressed is more likely to experience sleep problems, fatigue, and loss of interest in work and hobbies. Sometimes, there appears to be a cause of the depression, such as loss of a loved one or declining health. In other cases, no obvious cause can be found.

Nutritional deficiencies—deficiencies in the B vitamins, for example—are associated with depression, so a number of supplements can help treat this disorder. But because depression can have a serious impact on your life and even lead to suicide, it is important to consult a physician if you suspect that you or a loved one suffers from this disorder.

A doctor should also be consulted about the nutritional aspect of treatment, as certain medications may contraindicate the use of some supplements. It is important to have tests performed to determine nutrient levels. For instance, your doctor can have your fatty acid and mineral levels analyzed by a laboratory company such as Genova Diagnostics or Doctor's Data. (See Resources for contact information.) A laboratory company such as SpectraCell, on the other hand, can measure your vitamin levels. ZRT Laboratory can measure your neurotransmitter levels. For the best nutritional therapy possible, have your test results reviewed by a personalized medicine practitioner who is fellowship trained. This specialist and your conventional doctor must work together to help treat this disease. Be aware, though, that nutritional therapies are effective only for mild to moderate depression. In addition to using supplements, avoid an excessive intake of caffeine (more than two cups of coffee a day), alcohol, aspartame, monosodium glutamate (MSG), and fructose.

SUPPLEMENTS TO TREAT DEPRESSION

Supplements	Dosage	Considerations
Alpha lipoic acid	100 mg once a day	Alpha lipoic acid can interact with medication taken for diabetes and thyroid problems. Speak to your healthcare provider to see if any of the medications you take make it unwise to use this supplement.
Ashwagandha root	500 to 1,000 mg once a day	High doses can cause gastrointestinal problems.
Asian ginseng*	500 mg once a day	Always take with food. Use with caution if you have high blood pressure. Do not use if you are taking a blood thinner or if you have a hormonally related cancer such as breast, prostate, uterine, or ovarian.

B-complex vitamins	50 mg twice a day	I suggest taking a multivitamin along with your B-complex vitamins.
Calcium	500 mg twice a day	Although most people are deficient in calcium, there is a danger in taking too much calcium. Do not ingest more than 1,000 to 1,200 mg of calcium a day.
Carnitine*	500 to 3,000 mg once a day	Have your healthcare provider measure your TMAO levels before starting long-term supplementation with carnitine.
CBD oil (hemp oil)	5 to 500 mg a day in the form of sublingual drops. Start with 5 mg and increase slowly until you find relief.	CBD is generally well tolerated and safe for consumption, even in high doses and with continuous use. However, do not exceed 500 mg a day without consulting your healthcare provider. Make sure to buy a product marked "hemp oil (aerial parts)."
Chromium	400 mcg once a day as chromium picolinate	Combining with the protein picolinate allows your body to absorb chromium more efficiently. However, some chromium picolinate supplements contain more chromium than necessary. Ask your healthcare provider for a recommendation on chromium consumption.
Cocoa	2.5 g (0.1 ounce) unsweetened cocoa powder (about 0.5 teaspoon)	Cocoa can interact with some medications, so speak to your healthcare provider or pharmacist before starting long-term supplementation. Cocoa also contains caffeine, which can cause side effects in some people.
Coenzyme Q_{10}*	60 to 100 mg once a day	If you are on blood-thinning medications, speak to your healthcare provider before using CoQ_{10}. Since some medications can cause a deficiency of this nutrient, speak to your healthcare provider to determine if you might need a larger dose.
Copper	1 to 3 mg once a day	Your copper-to-zinc ratio is very important for your health. (See page 119 for details.) Also, do not take copper supplement cupric oxide, which has a very low bioavailability.
EPA/DHA (fish oil)*	1,000 to 3,000 mg once a day	Choose a source that contains vitamin E to prevent oxidation.
Gotu kola	9 to 150 mg once a day	Do not take gotu kola if you have liver disease.
Inositol	1,000 to 12,000 mg once a day	May stimulate uterine contractions. Women who wish to become pregnant should consult their doctor regarding its use. Doses larger than 200 mg should be taken only under physician supervision.

Magnesium	600 to 800 mg once a day	Consult your healthcare provider for dosage if you have kidney disease. Discontinue use and see your doctor if you experience abdominal pain. Take a lower dose if it causes diarrhea.
Multivitamin	1 tablet once a day or as directed	
Phosphatidylcholine (PC)	1,000 to 2,000 mg once a day	Use with caution if you have malabsorption problems, as this could exacerbate them.
Phosphatidylserine (PS)	300 mg once a day	PS can interact with many drugs. Speak to your healthcare provider before taking it.
St. John's wort*	900 to 1,800 mg once a day	St. John's wort can interact with many drugs. Speak to your healthcare provider before taking it. If you are exposed to the sun, it may cause a skin rash.
Selenium	200 to 400 mcg once a day	Do not exceed 200 mcg a day without seeing your doctor. If you are considering taking more than 400 mcg, have your selenium levels measured before taking the larger dose.
Tryptophan	1,500 mg twice a day as L-Tryptophan	Check with your doctor before starting an amino acid regimen if you have diabetes, hypertension, kidney disease, or liver disease. Do not take tryptophan if you are pregnant or breastfeeding. Tryptophan can interact with some medications, so consult with your healthcare provider before beginning supplementation.
Tyrosine	1,000 to 4,000 mg once a day	Start at 100 mg a day, and increase the dose gradually. Check with your doctor before starting use if you have diabetes, hypertension, kidney disease, or liver disease.
Valerian	500 mg once a day	Do not take if you have liver disease or if you abuse alcohol. Because valerian can cause sedation, use with caution if you are taking other sedatives, anti-histamine, antidepressants, or anti-anxiety agents.
Vitamin A and mixed carotenoids	5,000 IU—half vitamin A and half mixed carotenoids—once a day	Use caution when taking vitamin A supplements because they have the potential to be toxic. Do not take for extended periods of time. Do not take more than 800 IU a day if you have liver disease, are a smoker, or have been exposed to asbestos.
Vitamin B_1 (thiamine)	50 mg twice a day	High doses can deplete your body of other vitamins in the B complex, so take a B-complex vitamin twice a day.
Vitamin B_6 (pyridoxine)	50 mg twice a day	Do not take more than 500 mg a day. If you are taking L-dopa for Parkinson's disease, do not take B_6 without first consulting your doctor. High doses can deplete your body of other vitamins in the B complex, so take a B-complex vitamin twice a day.

Vitamin B$_9$ (folic acid)	400 mcg twice a day	High doses can deplete your body of other B vitamins, so take a B-complex vitamin twice a day.
Vitamin B$_{12}$ (cobalamin)	500 mcg twice a day	High doses can deplete your body of other B vitamins, so take a B-complex vitamin twice a day.
Vitamin C	500 mg twice a day	Do not take high doses if you are prone to kidney stones or gout. High doses can also cause diarrhea.
Vitamin D$_3$	Have your blood levels measured by your healthcare provider, who will determine proper dosage.	
Zinc	25 to 50 mg once a day as zinc picolinate or zinc citrate	Your copper-to-zinc ratio is very important to your health. (See page 119 for details.) If you are taking zinc and iron supplements, take one in the morning and one in the evening. (Taking them together reduces the efficiency of both.)

*This supplement can have a blood-thinning action. See page 328 for more information.

DERMATITIS

See Eczema.

DIABETES MELLITUS

Diabetes mellitus—better known simply as diabetes—is a chronic disease characterized by abnormally high blood levels of the sugar glucose. There are two main types of diabetes. In *type 1 diabetes* (insulin-dependent diabetes), the pancreas produces little or no insulin, which is the hormone that lowers blood glucose levels. In *type 2 diabetes* (non-insulin-dependent diabetes), the body continues to produce insulin—sometimes at even higher-than-normal levels—but the cells of the body are unable to react properly to the hormone. The majority of people with diabetes have type 2.

More than 80 percent of the United States adult population has blood glucose levels that are not optimal. About 10 million people in the United States have diabetes, and another 500,000 are believed to be undiagnosed. People with hypertension have a two-fold higher prevalence of diabetes and obesity than the general population, and half are insulin resistant. Similarly, people who are obese are twice as likely to have hypertension, hypertriglyceridemia (high triglycerides), or type 2 diabetes than the general population.

The signs and symptoms of diabetes can include frequent urination, excessive thirst, extreme hunger, unusual weight loss or weight gain, increased fatigue, irritability, and blurred vision. When these symptoms occur, it is imperative to seek medical advice, as early detection and treatment of diabetes can improve the chance of avoiding dangerous complications. (See the inset on page 380 for common complications.)

The following are some of the common causes of diabetes.

- Abuse of alcohol
- Decreased estrogen in females
- Decreased testosterone in males
- Eating processed foods
- Elevated DHEA levels
- Excessive caffeine intake
- Excessive dieting
- Excessive progesterone in females (prescribed)
- Genetic susceptibility
- Hypothyroidism (low thyroid function)
- Increased stress
- Increased testosterone in females
- Insomnia
- Lack of exercise
- Nicotine
- Oral contraceptives

It is vital to follow your doctor's recommendations concerning the treatment of diabetes, including the use of medications that lower blood sugar levels. In addition, it is important to choose foods that are low on the glycemic index, and therefore break down slowly during digestion, increasing blood glucose levels very gradually. A careful supplement plan can further improve treatment by resolving common deficiencies and enhancing the body's processing of glucose.

The supplements listed on page 377 can help keep diabetes mellitus under control. They can also help control insulin resistance and hyperinsulinism, conditions in which the body's insulin levels are too high. Both of these conditions can lead to type 2 diabetes. The supplements listed in the table will affect your blood sugar level, so if you already have diabetes, you many need less medication—or you may be able to stop taking your medication altogether. However, this is a decision that must be made with your healthcare provider. Regardless, continue to monitor your blood sugar closely so that it does not fall too low, which can cause hypoglycemia.

You may wish to try a product that contains several of the nutrients listed here. There are several great products that I recommend to my patients. A personalized medicine fellowship physician can help you decide on a product, or you can visit a compounding pharmacist. (See Resource section for information on finding a compounding pharmacist in your area.)

SUPPLEMENTS TO TREAT DIABETES MELLITUS TYPE 2, INSULIN RESISTANCE, AND HYPERINSULINISM

Supplements	Dosage	Considerations
Alpha lipoic acid	100 mg to 400 mg daily	Alpha lipoic acid improves blood sugar levels, so diabetics may be able to take less medication. Alpha lipoic acid also slows the development of diabetic neuropathy. Consult your healthcare provider if you are considering taking more than 500 mg in a day. Larger doses can negatively impact thyroid function.
Arginine	1,000 to 5,000 mg once a day	Do not take if you have kidney disease, liver disease, or herpes except under a doctor's supervision. Arginine can interact with some medications. Consult with your healthcare provider before beginning this therapy.
Asian ginseng*	50 to 200 mg of extract standardized to 4 percent ginsenosides twice a day	Always take with food. Use with caution if you have high blood pressure. Do not use if you are taking a blood thinner or if you have a hormonally related cancer such as breast, prostate, uterine, or ovarian.
B-complex vitamins	50 mg twice a day	I suggest taking a multivitamin along with your B-complex vitamins.
Berberine*	Start with 200 mg twice a day. You may go up to 500 mg three times a day.	Do not use this supplement during pregnancy. It can cause uterine contractions.
Carnitine*	2,000 to 3,000 mg once a day	Have your healthcare provider measure your TMAO levels before starting long-term supplementation with carnitine.
Carnosine	2,000 mg once a day	Check with your doctor before starting carnosine therapy if you have diabetes, hypertension, kidney disease, or liver damage. Too much carnosine can result in hyperactivity.
Chromium	300 to 1,000 mcg once a day as chromium picolinate	Combining with the protein picolinate allows your body to absorb chromium more efficiently. However, some chromium picolinate supplements contain more chromium than necessary. Ask your healthcare provider for a recommendation on chromium consumption.
Coenzyme Q_{10}*	30 to 200 mg daily	If you are on blood-thinning medications, speak to your healthcare provider before using CoQ_{10}. Since some medications can cause a deficiency of this nutrient, speak to your healthcare provider to determine if you might need a larger dose.

Copper	2 to 3 mg once a day	Your copper-to-zinc ratio is very important for your health. (See page 119 for details.) Also, do not take copper supplement cupric oxide, which has a very low bioavailability.
Cysteine	500 mg once a day as n-acetylcysteine, or NAC	When taking NAC supplements, also take extra vitamin C, copper, and zinc.
D-ribose	15,000 mg three times a day	D-ribose can lower blood sugar levels, so check with your healthcare provider before taking this supplement with any diabetes medication, especially insulin.
EPA/DHA (fish oil)*	1,000 to 2,000 mg once a day	Choose a source that contains vitamin E to prevent oxidation.
Fenugreek*	50 mg of seed powder twice a day, or 2 to 4.5 ml of 1:2 liquid extract twice a day	Avoid fenugreek if you are allergic to chickpeas, peanuts, green peas, or soybeans. Fenugreek has mild blood-thinning effects. If you have a bleeding disorder or are taking a medication or supplement that may thin your blood, do not take this herb. Fenugreek may also negatively impact thyroid function.
Fiber, soluble	Suggested daily intake is 25 grams for women and 38 grams for men. Try to get most of your fiber from whole foods.	Choose a fiber supplement with no added sugar, and take with several glasses of water to prevent side effects.
Ginkgo biloba*	120 mg once daily	Do not use with blood-thinning medications or supplements.
Green coffee bean extract	400 mg a day	Because green coffee contains caffeine, you should avoid taking this supplement if you are sensitive to caffeine.
Gymnema sylvestre	400 to 600 mg a day of an extract that contains 24 percent gymnemic acid	Stop taking this supplement two weeks before surgery, as it can interfere with blood sugar control during and after surgical procedures. At high doses, gymnema can cause gastric irritation or liver toxicity.
Inositol	2,000 to 4,000 mg once a day	May stimulate uterine contractions. Women who wish to become pregnant should consult their doctor regarding its use. Doses larger than 200 mg should be taken only under physician supervision.
Magnesium	400 to 800 mg once a day	Consult your healthcare provider for dosage if you have kidney disease. Discontinue use and see your doctor if you experience abdominal pain. Take a lower dose if it causes diarrhea.
Manganese	2 to 5 mg once a day	Use with caution if you have gallbladder or liver disease.
Olive leaf extract*	500 mg to 750 mg a day containing 20 mg of oleuropein per capsule	Olive leaf extracts can interact with many prescription medications, and may increase the effects of blood thinners. Consult your healthcare

		provider before using olive leaf extract if you are taking any medication. Don't use if you are pregnant or breastfeeding.
Quercetin*	300 mg three times a day	For best results, take with bromelain and vitamin C. Do not use with blood-thinning medications or supplements.
Selenium	200 mcg once a day	Do not exceed 200 mcg a day without consulting your healthcare provider.
Taurine	1,000 to 1,500 mg once a day	Take between meals. Discontinue use if you suddenly have feelings of chest or throat tightness or if you break out in hives. Do not take with aspirin. Have your healthcare provider measure levels before starting taurine therapy.
Vanadium*	50 mcg once a day	Do not take more than 50 mcg a day without a doctor's supervision. Do not use if you are taking blood-thinning medications or supplements.
Vitamin B_6 (pyridoxine)	75 mg twice a day	Do not take more than 500 mg a day. If you are taking L-dopa for Parkinson's disease, do not take B_6 without first consulting your doctor. High doses can deplete your body of other vitamins in the B complex, so take a B-complex vitamin twice a day.
Vitamin B_7 (biotin)	8 to 10 mg once a day	Large doses of biotin can deplete your body of other vitamins in the B complex, so take B-complex vitamins twice a day. Biotin can also negatively impact thyroid function.
Vitamin B_{12} (cobalamin)	500 to 1,500 mcg twice a day	High doses can deplete your body of other vitamins in the B complex, so take with a B-complex vitamin twice a day.
Vitamin C	500 to 1,500 mg twice a day	Do not take high doses if you are prone to kidney stones or gout. High doses can also cause diarrhea.
Vitamin D_3	Have your blood levels measured by your healthcare provider, who will determine proper dosage.	
Vitamin E*	400 to 800 IU once a day	Take mixed tocopherols, the more active type of vitamin E. Consult your healthcare provider first if you are taking a blood thinner.
Zinc	20 to 50 mg once a day as zinc picolinate or zinc citrate	Your copper-to-zinc ratio is very important to your health. (See page 119 for details.) If you are taking zinc and iron supplements, take one in the morning and one in the evening. (Taking them together reduces the efficiency of both.)

*This supplement can have a blood-thinning action. See page 328 for more information.

Complications of Diabetes

When you have diabetes, it is vitally important to take good care of yourself. When diabetes is not carefully managed, the resulting complications can be serious, as shown by the following list.

- **Cancer.** People with diabetes have an increased risk of developing any type of cancer—particularly, breast cancer—even if they have no family history of the disorder.

- **Depression.** Depression has been associated with diabetes for almost three hundred years. In one out of every four patients, symptoms are severe enough to warrant treatment.

- **Diabetic neuropathy.** This is one of the most common complications of diabetes. It involves damage to the nerves that run throughout the body, connecting the spinal cord to the skin, muscles, blood vessels, and other organs. (See page 381 for more information on diabetic neuropathy.)

- **Eye problems.** People with diabetes have a higher risk of cataracts than the rest of the population. Early detection and treatment of any eye problem is essential.

- **Foot problems.** Because of poor circulation and/or nerve damage, diabetes can lead to many foot problems.

- **Gastroparesis.** This condition, which involves extremely slow emptying of the stomach, affects people with both type 1 and type 2 diabetes.

- **Heart disease and stroke.** Diabetes involves an increased risk for heart attack, stroke, and complications of the circulatory system.

- **Kidney disease.** Diabetes can damage the kidneys, making them lose their ability to filter out waste products.

- **Memory loss.** Individuals with diabetes commonly experience cognitive decline. The tight control of blood sugar helps to decrease the risk of memory loss.

- **Skin complications.** About a third of those with diabetes have a related skin complication at some time in their lives. Fortunately, when caught early, these problems can usually be resolved.

Diabetic Neuropathy

Diabetic neuropathy is a progressive disorder that affects around 20 percent of diabetics. The body's nerves become damaged, leading to a host of other neuropathic disorders. Symptoms of diabetic neuropathy can include numbness, tingling, paresthesia (feeling of tingling or pricking), weakness, and burning pain. You can help prevent and treat neuropathy by eating a gluten-free diet and controlling your blood sugar. In addition, the following nutrients can slow the progression of diabetic neuropathy.

SUPPLEMENTS TO TREAT DIABETIC NEUROPATHY		
Supplements	**Dosage**	**Considerations**
Alpha lipoic acid	300 to 600 mg once a day	Alpha lipoic acid improves blood sugar levels, so diabetics may be able to take less medication. Alpha lipoic acid also slows the development of diabetic neuropathy. Consult your healthcare provider if you are considering taking more than 500 mg in a day. Larger doses can negatively impact thyroid function.
Carnitine*	2,000 mg once a day	Have your healthcare provider measure your TMAO levels before starting long-term supplementation with carnitine.
Carnosine	1,000 to 2,000 mg once a day	Check with your doctor before starting carnosine therapy if you have diabetes, hypertension, kidney disease, or liver damage. Too much carnosine can result in hyperactivity.
EPA/DHA (fish oil)*	1,000 to 2,000 mg once a day	Choose a source that contains vitamin E to prevent oxidation.
Gamma-linolenic acid (GLA) as evening primrose oil (EPO)*	1,000 mg once a day	It is important to maintain the proper ratio of omega-6 fatty acids to omega-3 fatty acids. (See page 129.) Evening primrose oil may interfere with some medications, such as nonsteroidal anti-inflammatories; can act as a blood thinner; and can lower the seizure threshold. Consult your healthcare provider or pharmacist before taking this supplement.
Vitamin B$_7$ (biotin)	5 mg once a day	Large doses of biotin can deplete your body of other B vitamins, so take B-complex vitamins twice a day. Biotin can also negatively impact thyroid function.
Vitamin B$_{12}$ (cobalamin)	500 to 1,000 mcg twice a day	High doses can deplete your body of other B vitamins, so take B-complex vitamins twice a day.
Vitamin E*	400 to 800 IU once a day	Take mixed tocopherols, the more active type of vitamin E. Consult your healthcare provider first if you are taking a blood thinner.

*This supplement can have a blood-thinning action. See page 328 for more information.

DRY EYES

Dry eyes, also known as *keratoconjunctivitis sicca* (KCS), is an eye disorder that is most often caused by decreased tear production, but may also result from increased evaporation of the tear film due to abnormal tear composition. Symptoms can include dryness, burning, the sensation of having sand or grit in the eye, itching, stinging, tired eyes, redness, a pulling sensation, or a sensation of pressure behind the eye. Generally, both eyes are affected.

Dry eyes are usually age-related. This is especially true when there is an inadequate production of tears. Other causes include the use of contact lenses; eye surgery, including LASIK surgery; health conditions such as diabetes, menopause, rheumatoid arthritis, and lupus; the use of certain medications, such as sedatives, diuretics, tricyclic antidepressants, oral contraceptives, nasal decongestants, and antihistamines; and eye injuries, including thermal and chemical burns.

Most people suffer no long-term effects from dry eyes. But because the condition is uncomfortable, and because it can lead to eye damage if it is left untreated or becomes severe, it is important to identify and eliminate the cause of the condition, and to do what you can to relieve the symptoms. For many people, especially women, appropriate supplementation has been associated with a decreased incidence of dry eyes. *See also* Sjögren's Syndrome.

SUPPLEMENTS TO TREAT DRY EYES

Supplements	Dosage	Considerations
EPA/DHA (fish oil)*	2,000 to 3,000 mg once a day	Choose a source that contains vitamin E to prevent oxidation.
Eye drops that contain carnosine	One to two drops, one to two times a day	
Eye drops that contain vitamin A palmitate	One to two drops, one to two times a day	
Gamma-linolenic acid (GLA) as evening primrose oil (EPO)*	3,000 mg a day	It is important to maintain the proper ratio of omega-6 fatty acids to omega-3 fatty acids. (See page 129.) Evening primrose oil may interfere with some medications, such as nonsteroidal anti-inflammatories; can act as a blood thinner; and can lower the seizure threshold. Consult your healthcare provider or pharmacist before taking this supplement.

*This supplement can have a blood-thinning action. See page 328 for more information.

EATING DISORDER

See Anorexia Nervosa.

ECZEMA

Eczema is a noncontagious, inflammatory skin condition that is characterized by patches of dry, flaking skin that can become cracked and leathery, or blistered and oozing. Severe itching can occur in the affected areas. Eczema most frequently appears on the face and scalp, behind the ears, on the elbows, and in the creases behind the knees. Many cases of this condition begin in infancy, and 20 to 40 percent of those affected as infants continue to have eczema as adults.

The two major types of eczema—*atopic dermatitis* and *contact dermatitis*—are both considered allergic responses. Those with atopic dermatitis often have a family history of eczema or allergic conditions like asthma and hay fever. Contact dermatitis, the more common form of the condition, is often an allergic response to an irritant that has come into contact with the skin. Soaps, wool and synthetic fabrics, dyes, latex, and certain cosmetic products are common culprits. Stressful or emotionally charged situations are also believed to trigger eczema flare-ups, as are extremes in temperature and overly dry air. Cases of eczema can range from very mild to severe and, therefore, will require various treatment protocols. Proper skin care is often sufficient for treating mild cases, while more serious cases may require medication. For this reason, it is important to consult your healthcare provider for the best treatment options for your particular situation.

Often, simple lifestyle changes can help you treat eczema. Helpful strategies include the following:

- Avoidance of allergens such as latex, wool, etc.

- Bleach baths (add a small amount of bleach to water to kill bacteria)

- Controlled temperature and humidity to eliminate excessive heat, cold, and dry air

- Hydration through adequate consumption of water

- Loose-fitting clothes

- Mild soap or gentle soap substitute

- Moisturizing creams

- Wet dressings

SUPPLEMENTS TO TREAT ECZEMA

Supplements	Dosage	Considerations
B-complex vitamins	25 to 50 mg twice a day	I suggest taking a multivitamin along with your B-complex vitamins.
Copper	2 to 3 mg once a day	Your copper-to-zinc ratio is very important for your health. (See page 119 for details.) Also, do not take copper supplement cupric oxide, which has a very low bioavailability.
Dandelion*	100 mg once or twice a day	If you have gallstones or obstructed bile ducts, consult your healthcare practitioner before taking. Do not use dandelion if you are taking a blood-thinning drug or supplement. Avoid if you are allergic to plants such as ragweed, chrysanthemums, marigolds, or daisies.
EPA/DHA (fish oil)*	1,000 to 3,000 once a day	Choose a source that contains vitamin E to prevent oxidation.
Gamma-linolenic acid (GLA) as evening primrose oil (EPO)*	500 to 1,000 mg once a day	It is important to maintain the proper ratio of omega-6 fatty acids to omega-3 fatty acids. (See page 129.) Evening primrose oil may interfere with some medications, such as nonsteroidal anti-inflammatories; can act as a blood thinner; and can lower the seizure threshold. Consult your healthcare provider or pharmacist before taking this supplement.
Glucosamine sulfate	1,000 mg once a day	If you are allergic to shellfish, be sure to choose a supplement that is not shellfish based. Consult use with your healthcare provider if you have diabetes, because glucosamine can alter blood sugar levels.
Methylsulfonylmethane (MSM)	1,000 to 3,000 mg three times a day	Use with caution if you are allergic to sulfur. Start by taking 500 mg three times a day, and gradually increase dose. Take with meals to avoid possible heartburn. May cause stomach upset in dosages larger than 6,000 mg.
Milk thistle	100 to 200 mg twice a day	Do not take if you are allergic to ragweed, chrysanthemums, marigolds, chamomile, or daisies. This supplement reduces the efficiency of certain blood pressure medication and other drugs. Speak to your healthcare provider or pharmacist before taking.
Probiotics	20 billion units once a day	If taking an antibiotic, take the probiotics at least two hours before or two hours after using the antibiotics. Do not take them at the same time.

Taurine	2,000 mg once a day	Take between meals. Discontinue use if you suddenly have feelings of chest or throat tightness or if you break out in hives. Do not take with aspirin. Have your healthcare provider measure levels before starting taurine therapy.
Tea tree oil	Apply the oil directly to the skin once or twice a day	Do not ingest or use in ears.
Vitamin A and mixed carotenoids	25,000 to 50,000 IU—half vitamin A and half mixed carotenoids—once a day for one month	Take these high doses of vitamin A only under the supervision of a healthcare provider. Do not take for extended periods of time. Do not take more than 8,000 IU of vitamin A a day if you have liver disease, are a smoker, or have been exposed to asbestos.
Vitamin C	500 to 1,500 mg twice a day	Do not take high doses if you are prone to kidney stones or gout. High doses can also cause diarrhea.
Vitamin D$_3$	Have your blood levels measured by your healthcare provider, who will determine proper dosage.	
Vitamin E*	400 IU once a day	Take mixed tocopherols, the more active type of vitamin E. Consult your healthcare provider first if you are taking a blood thinner.
Zinc	25 to 75 mg once a day as zinc picolinate or zinc citrate	Your copper-to-zinc ratio is very important to your health. (See page 119.) If you are taking zinc and iron supplements, take one in the morning and one in the evening. (Taking them together reduces the efficiency of both.)

*This supplement can have a blood-thinning action. See page 328 for more information.

ENLARGED PROSTATE

See Benign Prostatic Hyperplasia.

EXHAUSTION

See Adrenal Fatigue and Exhaustion.

EYE HEALTH

See Cataracts; Dry Eyes; Macular Degeneration.

FATIGUE

See Chronic Fatigue Syndrome.

FIBROIDS

Fibroids, which are also known as *leiomyomata,* are benign (non-cancerous) growths on or within the walls of the uterus. By the age of forty, 20 to 40 percent of women develop fibroids. These tumors can be a variety of different sizes and quantities. The resulting symptoms depend upon these factors. If the fibroids are small and do not cause any symptoms, a doctor may recommend that no course of action be taken. However, larger—or multiple—fibroids can cause pain, excessive bleeding, and problems urinating, as well as infertility and premature labor. When fibroids cause serious problems such as these, treatment options include surgery (hysterectomy or myomectomy); medications (such as oral contraceptives or progesterone); and procedures such as high intensity focused ultrasound, which uses ultrasound waves to destroy the fibroid tissue. Women with uterine fibroids have a fourfold increased risk of developing endometrial cancer. Although no substitute for necessary surgery or other medical action, the nutrients in the following table may allow these procedures to be avoided by shrinking the uterine fibroids naturally. You should also avoid drinking caffeine.

Fibroids have estrogen receptors, and are thus responsive to the body's level of estrogen. During periods of pregnancy, when estrogen levels increase, fibroids tend to grow in size. After menopause, on the other hand, when estrogen levels drop significantly, fibroids usually become smaller. For this reason, doctors will often recommend a medication with an estrogen-lowering effect, which will artificially create this situation. Similarly, you may find it effective to take natural progesterone, which directly balances the estrogen in your body. Your doctor will be able to prescribe a specific dosage.

SUPPLEMENTS TO TREAT FIBROIDS		
Supplements	Dosage	Considerations
Alpha lipoic acid	300 mg once a day	Alpha lipoic acid can interact with medication taken for diabetes and thyroid problems. Speak to your healthcare provider to see if any of the medications you take make it unwise to use this supplement.

Carnitine*	1,500 mg once a day	Have your healthcare provider measure your TMAO levels before starting long-term supplementation.
Coenzyme Q_{10}*	100 mg once a day	If you are on blood-thinning medications, speak to your healthcare provider before using CoQ_{10}. Since some medications can cause a deficiency of this nutrient, speak to your healthcare provider to determine if you might need a larger dose.
Digestive enzymes	Follow the manufacturer's instructions. Be sure to take these supplements with or directly before meals.	Do not take digestive enzymes that contain papain if you are allergic to papaya, and avoid enzymes with bromelain if you are allergic to pineapple.
EGCG (green tea extract)*	200 to 400 mg twice a day	Green tea extract can interact with a number of drugs. Check with your healthcare provider before taking this supplement.
Gamma-linolenic acid (GLA) as evening primrose oil (EPO)*	240 to 720 mg once a day	It is important to maintain the proper ratio of omega-6 fatty acids to omega-3 fatty acids. (See page 129.) Evening primrose oil may interfere with some medications, such as nonsteroidal anti-inflammatories; can act as a blood thinner; and can lower the seizure threshold. Consult your healthcare provider or pharmacist before taking this supplement.
Inositol	500 mg twice a day	May stimulate uterine contractions. Women who wish to become pregnant should consult their doctor regarding its use. Doses larger than 200 mg should be taken only under physician supervision.
Magnesium	400 mg once a day	Consult your healthcare provider for dosage if you have kidney disease. Discontinue use and see your doctor if you experience abdominal pain. Take a lower dose if it causes diarrhea.
Milk thistle	100 to 200 mg twice a day	Do not take if you are allergic to ragweed, chrysanthemums, marigolds, chamomile, or daisies. This supplement reduces the efficiency of certain blood pressure medication and other drugs. Speak to your healthcare provider or pharmacist before taking.
Phosphatidylcholine (PC)	2,000 mg once a day	Use with caution if you have malabsorption problems, as this could exacerbate them.

*This supplement can have a blood-thinning action. See page 328 for more information.

FOOD ALLERGIES

Scientists estimate that 60 percent of the US population suffers from food allergies. There are many different foods to which people are allergic, with the eight most common being eggs, fish, milk, peanuts, shellfish, soy, tree nuts, and wheat. Some reactions occur within three hours of eating the offending food, while others may not occur for several days. As you can see on the list below, there are also a large variety of reactions that can occur. They can range from mild to life threatening.

A doctor can help you determine the foods to which you are allergic. Although you may find that you crave these foods, you must eliminate the allergenic (allergy causing) items from your diet. Then, begin supplementation with the nutrients listed in "Supplements to Treat Food Allergies." This will help lessen the severity of your allergy attacks.

■ Symptoms of Food Allergies

- Anal itching
- Anemia
- Anxiety, fear
- Backaches
- Belching
- Cracks at corners of mouth
- Dark circles under eyes
- Depression
- Destructive behavior
- Diarrhea
- Eczema
- Emotional outbursts
- Fluid behind eardrum

- Frequent urination
- Heartburn
- Hearing loss
- Heart palpitations
- Hives
- Hoarseness
- Inability to concentrate
- Indigestion
- Irritable behavior after meals
- Itchy, watery eyes
- Memory loss
- Muscle cramps
- Nervousness

- Panic attacks
- Rapid heartbeat
- Red earlobes
- Red eyeballs
- Red rosy cheeks
- Restlessness
- Ringing in ears (tinnitus)
- Sluggishness
- Spacey feeling
- Spastic colon
- Stomachaches
- Tension headaches
- Tremors
- Wrinkles under eyes

SUPPLEMENTS TO TREAT FOOD ALLERGIES

Supplements	Dosage	Considerations
Alpha lipoic acid	200 to 300 mg once a day	Alpha lipoic acid can interact with medication taken for diabetes and thyroid problems. Speak to your healthcare provider to see if any of the medications you take make it unwise to use this supplement.

B-complex vitamins	25 mg twice a day	I suggest taking a multivitamin along with your B-complex vitamins.
Boswellia*	500 mg capsules or tablets three times a day until symptoms subside. Then take one 500 mg capsule or tablet a day.	Avoid boswellia if you are pregnant, because it can induce miscarriage. Do not take with NSAIDs.
Curcumin/Turmeric*	100 to 1,000 mg once a day of a formula that includes piperine or bioperine to boost absorption	Do not take curcumin with blood-thinning medications or supplements. Curcumin can also interact with other medications, so speak to your healthcare provider before taking this supplement.
Digestive enzymes	Follow the manufacturer's instructions. Be sure to take these supplements with or directly before meals.	Do not take digestive enzymes that contain papain if you are allergic to papaya, and avoid enzymes with bromelain if you are allergic to pineapple.
EPA/DHA (fish oil)*	1,000 to 2,000 once a day	Choose a source that contains vitamin E to prevent oxidation.
Gamma-linolenic acid (GLA) as evening primrose oil (EPO)*	240 mg one to three times a day	It is important to maintain the proper ratio of omega-6 fatty acids to omega-3 fatty acids. (See page 129.) Evening primrose oil may interfere with some medications, such as nonsteroidal anti-inflammatories; can act as a blood thinner; and can lower the seizure threshold. Consult your healthcare provider or pharmacist before taking this supplement.
Ginkgo biloba*	60 mg once or twice a day	Do not use with blood-thinning medications or supplements.
Glutamine	1,000 to 6,000 mg once a day	If you have a sensitivity to monosodium glutamate (MSG), use glutamine with caution. If you are taking medications for seizures, take glutamine only under the direction of your doctor.
Magnesium	400 to 600 mg once a day	Consult your healthcare provider for dosage if you have kidney disease. Discontinue use and see your doctor if you experience abdominal pain. Take a lower dose if it causes diarrhea.
Methylsulfonylmethane (MSM)	1,000 to 3,000 mg three times a day	Use with caution if you are allergic to sulfur. Start by taking 500 mg three times a day, and gradually increase dose. Take with meals to avoid possible heartburn. May cause stomach upset in dosages larger than 6,000 mg.
Perilla seed extract*	5,000 to 10,000 mg once a day	Use with caution if taking aspirin, nonsteroidal anti-inflammatory drugs (NSAIDs), ginkgo, or garlic.
Probiotics	20 billion units once a day	If taking an antibiotic, take the probiotics at least two hours before or two hours after using the antibiotics. Do not take them at the same time.

Quercetin*	500 to 1,000 mg once a day	For best results, take with bromelain and vitamin C. Do not use with blood-thinning medications or supplements.
Selenium	200 to 400 mcg once a day	Do not exceed 200 mcg a day without seeing your doctor. If you are considering taking more than 400 mcg, have your selenium levels measured before taking the larger dose.
Stinging nettle*	300 mg with each meal, up to three times a day	Stinging nettle can interfere with many medications. Speak to your healthcare provider or pharmacist before taking this supplement.
Vitamin C	500 to 1,000 mg twice a day	Do not take high doses if you are prone to kidney stones or gout. High doses can also cause diarrhea.
Vitamin E*	400 to 800 IU once a day	Take mixed tocopherols, the more active type of vitamin E. Consult your healthcare provider first if you are taking a blood thinner.
Zinc	25 mg once a day as zinc picolinate or zinc citrate	Your copper-to-zinc ratio is very important to your health. (See page 119 for details.) If you are taking zinc and iron supplements, take one in the morning and one in the evening. (Taking them together reduces the efficiency of both.)

*This supplement can have a blood-thinning action. See page 328 for more information.

GINGIVITIS

See Periodontal Disease.

GOUT

Uric acid, a byproduct of your metabolism, is usually oxidized by the enzyme uricase so that it can be eliminated by the body. But some people do not produce enough of this digestive enzyme, so the uric acid begins to first collect and then crystallize in their blood and tissues. Once crystallized, the acid becomes sharp and pokes into joints, causing the severe pain and inflammation of gout. Also called *metabolic arthritis,* gout is one of the most miserable forms of arthritis, but it is also one of the most treatable. Although it can occur in any joint in the body, it happens most often in the big toe.

The first stage of gout is symptomless. During this time, the uric acid level in your body rises. The second stage occurs when the uric acid begins to crystallize and causes pain in your joints. The attack may or may not be severe, and usually recedes afterwards for at least a few months and possibly even several years. However, in the third stage of gout, attacks occur with much greater frequency and severity. The disorder can even begin to affect your vital organs.

To test for gout, a doctor extracts fluid from your inflamed joint. If you test positive, talk to your healthcare provider about avoiding niacin (vitamin B$_3$), which competes with uric acid for excretion and may make attacks worse. Vitamin A supplements, too, have been implicated as a possible contributor to gout. Also avoid alcohol, anchovies, baker's and brewer's yeast, game meat, herring, high doses (1,000 micrograms a day or more) of molybdenum, high fructose corn syrup, sugar, mackerel, offal (organ meats), red meat, sardines, and shellfish.

You must see a doctor if you have gout. It is treatable—although not curable—and can be dangerous if not treated before the problem becomes serious. The following supplements will help until you can see a doctor, who will probably prescribe anti-inflammatory medication. It will also be beneficial if during gout attacks, you eat only nuts, raw fruits and vegetables (particularly cherries and strawberries), and seeds. Medical studies have shown that drinking cherry juice or eating cherries can lower uric acid levels in the body. It is recommended that during attacks, you eat a half-pound of cherries a day or drink four to eight ounces of Bing sweet cherry juice or tart cherry juice a day. A medical trial also revealed that acupuncture is an effective therapy for an acute attack of gout.

SUPPLEMENTS TO TREAT GOUT		
Supplements	Dosage	Considerations
Alpha lipoic acid	200 mg once a day	Alpha lipoic acid can interact with medication taken for diabetes and thyroid problems. Speak to your healthcare provider to see if any of the medications you take make it unwise to use this supplement.
Bilberry*	60 mg once a day	Bilberry may interfere with iron absorption and blood clotting. High doses should be used with caution by people with bleeding disorders.
Carnitine*	1,000 mg once a day	Have your doctor measure your TMAO levels before starting long-term supplementation with carnitine.
Chamomile*	400 to 1,000 mg daily in capsule form, or 3 cups of tea daily	Consult your healthcare practitioner before taking if you are on a blood thinner. Do not take if you are allergic to plants such as ragweed, aster, daisies, and, chrysanthemums. Also avoid if you have a hormonally related cancer, such as breast, prostate, uterine, or ovarian.

Chromium	400 to 1,000 mcg once a day as chromium picolinate	Combining with the protein picolinate allows your body to absorb chromium more efficiently. However, some chromium picolinate supplements contain more chromium than necessary. Ask your healthcare provider for a recommendation on chromium consumption.
Coenzyme Q_{10}*	120 mg once a day	If you are on blood-thinning medications, speak to your healthcare provider before using CoQ_{10}. Since some medications can cause a deficiency of this nutrient, speak to your healthcare provider to determine if you might need a larger dose.
EPA/DHA (fish oil)*	2,000 mg once a day	Choose a source that contains vitamin E to prevent oxidation.
Grape seed extract*	300 to 900 mg once a day	Do not use with blood-thinning medications or supplements.
Milk thistle	300 mg once a day	Do not take if you are allergic to ragweed, chrysanthemums, marigolds, chamomile, or daisies. This supplement reduces the efficiency of certain blood pressure medications and other drugs. Speak to your healthcare provider or pharmacist before taking.
Quercetin*	500 mg once a day	For best results, take with bromelain and vitamin C. Do not use with blood-thinning medications or supplements.
Vitamin B_9 (folic acid)	800 mcg twice a day	High doses can deplete your body of other B vitamins, so take a B-complex vitamin twice a day.
Vitamin C	500 to 1,500 mg twice a day	Do not take high doses if you are prone to kidney stones or gout. High doses can also cause diarrhea.
Vitamin E*	400 IU once a day	Take mixed tocopherols, the more active type of vitamin E. Consult your healthcare provider first if you are taking a blood thinner.

*This supplement can have a blood-thinning action. See page 328 for more information.

HAIR LOSS

Hair loss is a common occurrence. Most often, it is the result of aging and genetics, with both men and women tending to lose hair thickness as they grow older. About 25 percent of men begin to bald by their thirties, with 66 percent either having a balding pattern or being completely bald by the age of sixty. Almost 50 percent of all women experience hair loss due to aging. However, there can be other causes of hair loss, including fungal infections of the scalp; high fever; cancer chemotherapy; radiation therapy; hyperthyroidism (an overactive thyroid gland); autoimmune diseases such as lupus;

nutritional deficiencies; emotional stress; gastrointestinal tract imbalances; polycystic ovary disease; some medications; toxic metals; low progesterone levels in women; conversion of testosterone to dihydrotestosterone in men or women; and trichotillomania—a mental disorder that causes an individual to pull out his or her own hair. Even excessive shampooing and blow-drying can cause the hair to break and thin.

Dietary deficiencies have proven to be a major cause of non-age-related hair loss. In one study, extensive hair loss due to shedding (telogen effluvium) occurred in patients after two to five months of following a vigorous weight-loss program. If you are trying to lose weight, make sure to take a multivitamin and to avoid diets that are based on nutrient-poor foods.

People with celiac disease can experience hair loss when antibodies to gliadin (a main protein from gluten) cause cross-reacting antibodies that attack the hair follicles, leading to alopecia areata (spot baldness). If you have positive gluten antibodies, this may be a reason for your hair loss. Make sure you avoid all intake of gluten.

Iron deficiency has also been shown to be a common cause of diffuse hair loss. If your iron levels fall too low, hair growth and regeneration are decreased. If you are experiencing hair loss, be sure to see your healthcare provider and have your iron levels measured.

Clearly, it is important to know the cause of hair thinning and, if possible, to eliminate it. It is also important to eat a well-balanced diet and take in adequate levels of hair-healthy nutrients. The following supplements have been found helpful in maintaining a thick head of hair and slowing hair loss.

SUPPLEMENTS TO TREAT HAIR LOSS		
Supplements	Dosage	Considerations
B-complex vitamins	50 mg twice a day	I suggest taking a multivitamin along with your B-complex vitamins.
Rosemary	1,000 to 2,000 mg once a day in pill form, and/or a few drops of 6- to 10-percent rosemary essential oil massaged into scalp for 2 minutes	Do not use rosemary if you have epilepsy, since this herb can induce seizures.
Saw palmetto*	250 mg twice a day	Speak to your healthcare provider before using this supplement if you have a sex hormone-related disorder or if you are taking birth control pills.
Vitamin B_7 (biotin)	5 to 10 mg once a day	Large doses of biotin can deplete your body of other vitamins in the B complex, so take B-complex vitamins twice a day. Biotin can also negatively impact thyroid function.

| Vitamin D$_3$ | Have your blood levels measured by your healthcare provider, who will determine proper dosage. | |
| Zinc | 25 mg once a day as zinc picolinate or zinc citrate | Your copper-to-zinc ratio is very important for your health. (See page 119 for details.) If you are taking zinc and iron supplements, take one in the morning and one in the evening. |

*This supplement can have a blood-thinning action. See page 328 for more information.

HASHIMOTO'S THYROIDITIS

Hashimoto's thyroiditis, or *chronic lymphocytic thyroiditis*, is the most common type of *thyroiditis*—an inflammation of the thyroid gland. An autoimmune disease, Hashimoto's thyroiditis is genetic and much more prevalent in women than men.

The thyroid gland regulates growth and metabolism. When the immune system attacks the thyroid gland, as it does in Hashimoto's thyroiditis, growth and metabolism slow down. Weight gain is a common symptom, as are constipation, cramps, depression, fatigue, goiters, muscle weakness, and sensitivity to cold. *Hypothyroidism*—low levels of the thyroid hormones—often occurs. However, some people with Hashimoto's thyroiditis exhibit no symptoms.

If you suspect Hashimoto's thyroiditis, see your healthcare provider, who can perform a simple blood test to make this determination and, if necessary, prescribe thyroid hormone replacement to alleviate your condition. Once you begin taking thyroid medication, visit your doctor regularly to make sure that you are taking the proper amount. It may be beneficial to follow a gluten-free diet. You can also take the nutrients listed in the following table to discourage the immune system from attacking the thyroid gland.

SUPPLEMENTS TO TREAT HASHIMOTO'S THYROIDITIS

Supplements	Dosage	Considerations
Eleuthero*	50 to 200 mg once a day	Do not use if you have a history of heart disease, hypertension, sleep apnea, narcolepsy, mania, or schizophrenia; if you are pregnant or breastfeeding; or if you have a bleeding disorder.
EPA/DHA (fish oil)*	1,000 to 5,000 mg once a day	Choose a source that contains vitamin E to prevent oxidation. In high doses, fatty acids may thin the blood. If you are taking a blood thinner, do not take EPA/DHA without direct instructions from your doctor. It is important to maintain the proper ratio of omega-6 to omega-3 fatty acids. (See page 129.)

Glucosamine sulfate	300 to 900 mg once a day	If you are allergic to shellfish, be sure to choose a supplement that is not shellfish based. Consult use with your healthcare provider if you have diabetes because glucosamine can alter blood sugar levels.
Glutamine	1,000 to 5,000 mg	If you have a sensitivity to monosodium glutamate (MSG), use glutamine with caution. If you are taking medications for seizures, take glutamine only under the direction of your doctor.
Magnesium	400 to 800 mg once a day	Consult your healthcare provider for dosage if you have kidney disease. Discontinue use and see your doctor if you experience abdominal pain. Take a lower dose if it causes diarrhea.
Olive leaf extract*	500 to 750 mg a day containing 20 mg of oleuropein per capsule	Olive leaf extracts can interact with many prescription medications, and may increase the effects of blood thinners. Consult your healthcare provider before using olive leaf extract if you are taking any medication. Don't use if you are pregnant or breastfeeding.
Probiotics	20 billion units once a day	If taking an antibiotic, take the probiotics at least two hours before or two hours after using the antibiotics. Do not take them at the same time.
Selenium	200 to 400 mcg once a day	Do not exceed 200 mcg a day without seeing your doctor. If you are considering taking more than 400 mcg, have your selenium levels measured before taking the larger dose.
Vitamin B_3 (niacin)	50 mg twice a day	Do not drink alcohol or hot drinks within one hour of taking niacin. High doses can deplete your body of other vitamins in the B complex, so take a B-complex vitamin twice a day.
Vitamin C	500 to 1,500 mg twice a day	Do not take high doses if you are prone to kidney stones or gout. High doses can also cause diarrhea.
Vitamin D_3	Have your blood levels measured by your healthcare provider, who will determine proper dosage.	
Vitamin E*	400 IU once a day	Take mixed tocopherols, the more active type of vitamin E. Consult your healthcare provider first if you are taking a blood thinner.

*This supplement can have a blood-thinning action. See page 328 for more information.

HEAD INJURY

See Closed Head Injury.

HEADACHES

See Migraine Headaches.

HEART FAILURE

See Congestive Heart Failure.

HEPATITIS C

Hepatitis C is a blood-borne infectious disease of the liver caused by the hepatitis C virus. It is the leading cause of liver transplants in the United States.

In the first six months of infection with the virus—the period referred to as *acute hepatitis C*—60 to 70 percent of the people infected have no symptoms at all, while others experience decreased appetite, fatigue, abdominal pain, jaundice, itching, or flu-like symptoms. When infection with the virus continues for more than six months—a condition called *chronic hepatitis C*—again, there may be no symptoms at all. Some individuals, though, experience weight loss, flu-like symptoms, low-grade fever, muscle pain, joint pain, itching, abdominal pain, nausea, diarrhea, and more. If left untreated, this disorder can progress and cause inflammation of the liver, liver scarring, and cirrhosis. It should be noted, though, that the majority of those infected with hepatitis C experience either no symptoms or such mild symptoms that they do not seek treatment.

Hepatitis C is spread through contact with infected blood, and may be contracted through IV drug use; transfusions with unscreened blood; occupational exposure to blood; and even shared personal items such as razors. The condition has also been known to spread through sex with an infectious person, and from mother to infant during childbirth. Today, transmission usually occurs through sharing needles or other equipment during IV drug use.

Prompt medical treatment of hepatitis C is important to avoid progression of the disease, and nutritional supplements are not meant to replace drugs such as sofosbuvir, which, when used in combination with other medications, has a greater than 90-percent cure rate. However, the supplements recommended below can be useful as an adjunct therapy for this disorder. Avoid high doses of vitamin A, beta-carotene, and niacin if you have hepatitis, and be sure to consult your physician before beginning a supplementation program.

SUPPLEMENTS TO TREAT CHRONIC HEPATITIS C

Supplements	Dosage	Considerations
Alpha lipoic acid	400 to 600 mg once a day	Alpha lipoic acid can interact with medication taken for diabetes and thyroid problems. Speak to your healthcare provider to see if any of the medications you take make it unwise to use this supplement.
Astragalus*	250 to 500 mg standardized extract three to four times a day	Do not use after organ transplant or if you have an allergy to gum tragacanth. Also do not use for an extended period of time. Speak to your healthcare provider to see if any of the medications you take make it unwise to use astragalus.
B-complex vitamins	50 mg twice a day	I suggest taking a multivitamin along with your B-complex vitamins.
Carnitine*	500 to 3,000 mg once a day	Have your healthcare provider measure your TMAO levels before starting long-term supplementation with carnitine.
Coenzyme Q_{10}*	100 to 400 mg once a day	If you are on blood-thinning medications, speak to your healthcare provider before using CoQ_{10}. Since some medications can cause a deficiency of this nutrient, speak to your healthcare provider to determine if you might need a larger dose.
Cysteine	1,000 mg once a day as n-acetylcysteine, or NAC	When taking NAC supplements, also take extra vitamin C, copper, and zinc.
Lysine	1,000 to 3,000 mg once a day	Do not take if you have diabetes or are allergic to eggs, milk, or wheat. Do not take for more than six months because it can cause an imbalance of arginine unless arginine is also supplemented.
Milk thistle	100 to 200 mg twice a day	Do not take if you are allergic to ragweed, chrysanthemums, marigolds, chamomile, or daisies. This supplement reduces the efficiency of certain blood pressure medication and other drugs. Speak to your healthcare provider or pharmacist before taking.
Olive leaf extract*	500 mg to 750 mg a day containing 20 mg of oleuropein per capsule	Olive leaf extracts can interact with many prescription medications, and may increase the effects of blood thinners. Consult your healthcare provider before using olive leaf extract if you are taking any medication. Don't use if you are pregnant or breastfeeding.
Phosphatidylcholine (PC)	2,000 to 10,000 mg once a day	Use with caution if you have malabsorption problems, as this could exacerbate them.
Probiotics	20 billion units once a day	If taking an antibiotic, take the probiotics at least two hours before or two hours after using the antibiotics. Do not take them at the same time.

Selenium	200 mcg once a day	Do not exceed 200 mcg a day without consulting your healthcare provider.
Taurine	1,000 to 3,000 mg	Take between meals. Discontinue use if you suddenly have feelings of chest or throat tightness or if you break out in hives. Do not take with aspirin. Have your healthcare provider measure levels before starting taurine therapy.
Vitamin B9 (folic acid)	500 mcg twice a day	High doses can deplete your body of other B vitamins, so take a B-complex vitamin twice a day.
Vitamin B12 (cobalamin)	5,00 to 1,000 mcg twice a day	High doses can deplete your body of other vitamins in the B complex, so take a B-complex vitamin twice a day.
Vitamin C	500 to 2,500 mg twice a day	Do not take high doses if you are prone to kidney stones or gout. High doses can also cause diarrhea.
Vitamin D3	Have your blood levels measured by your healthcare provider, who will determine proper dosage.	
Vitamin E*	400 IU once a day	Take mixed tocopherols, the more active type of vitamin E. Consult your healthcare provider first if you are taking a blood thinner.
Vitamin K*	45 mg a day of K2	This dose has been shown to help prevent the development of liver carcinoma in women with cirrhosis due to chronic hepatitis. If you are on a blood thinner, do not take vitamin K except under the direction of your doctor.

*This supplement can have a blood-thinning action. See page 328 for more information.

HIGH BLOOD PRESSURE (HYPERTENSION)

Blood pressure is the measurement of the blood's force in the arteries as the heart pushes the blood through the body. High blood pressure, also called *hypertension,* occurs when too much pressure is exerted on the artery walls by the blood.

While researchers don't fully understand the cause of high blood pressure, they have identified several factors that contribute to the disorder. These factors include arteriosclerosis (hardening of the arteries), thickening of the artery walls, and excessive contraction of the small arteries. Researchers have also identified a number of risk factors for high blood pressure. (See the inset on page 399.)

While some people with early-stage hypertension experience dull headaches, dizziness, or nosebleeds, most sufferers have no symptoms whatsoever. Nevertheless, when untreated, high blood pressure increases the risk of serious health problems, including heart attack, stroke, and cognitive decline. This is why it is sometimes referred to as the "silent killer."

Lifestyle changes are very important to decrease your risk of developing hypertension and to treat it if it begins. The Dietary Approaches to Stop Hypertension (DASH) diet, Mediterranean diet, vegetarian diet, and raw foods have all been shown to be beneficial to lower blood pressure. There are also some foods that have been shown to reduce blood pressure, such as bananas, onions, leafy greens, red beets, whole oats, garlic, soy, flaxseed, and pomegranate juice. Using sesame oil as your cooking oil may also lower your blood pressure according to a medical study. In addition, studies reveal that the consumption of 2.5 grams a day of unsweetened cocoa powder, which is rich in flavanols, lowers blood pressure in individuals that already have hypertension. (See page 280 for more information on cocoa.)

Risk Factors for High Blood Pressure

Although scientists don't know exactly why some people have high blood pressure and some do not, they have identified a number of risk factors for this very common disorder. The following are some of the factors associated with hypertension.

- Alcohol abuse.

- Excess weight.

- Genetics.

- Hypothyroidism (low thyroid function).

- Lack of exercise.

- Poor diet—especially one that is high in sodium, saturated fat, trans fatty acids, sugar, refined carbohydrates, and caffeine. Likewise, excessive alcohol intake may lead to high blood pressure

- Smoking.

- Stress.

- Toxic cadmium exposure.

- Toxic lead exposure.

- Use of certain drugs, including amphetamine-like medications; cocaine; steroids; cyclosporine; decongestants; ephedra; erthropoietin; certain antidepressants; nonsteroidal anti-inflammatory drugs (NSAIDs), such as aspirin; COX inhibitors; birth control pills; and synthetic hormone replacement.

Although medications can reduce blood pressure to normal levels, they can also have a range of side effects, including depression; constipation;

dizziness; fatigue; deficiencies of potassium, magnesium, and other nutrients; kidney damage; impaired sexual function; and decreased alertness and memory. Fortunately, certain supplements can help you lower your blood pressure without the use of drugs. (See the table below.) Other supplements can be used *with* drugs to augment their effects. Just keep in mind that hypertension is a serious disorder, so whether you are using these supplements to minimize or eventually discontinue your use of antihypertensive drugs, you must work with a physician to make sure that your blood pressure is being properly controlled. If you are currently taking blood pressure medication, *do not* stop taking it without the approval of your doctor.

It is critical to recognize that a good diet and regular exercise are extremely important in lowering and then maintaining your blood pressure. In addition, stress-reducing techniques such as prayer, medication, tai chi, yoga, exercise, and breathing techniques can further help you lower your blood pressure.

SUPPLEMENTS THAT CAN LOWER BLOOD PRESSURE

Supplements	Dosage	Considerations
Alpha lipoic acid	300 mg once a day	Alpha lipoic acid can interact with medication taken for diabetes and thyroid problems. Speak to your healthcare provider to see if any of the medications you take make it unwise to use this supplement.
Arginine	2,000 mg three times a day	Do not take if you have kidney disease, liver disease, or herpes except under a doctor's supervision. Arginine can interact with some medications. Consult with your healthcare provider before beginning this therapy.
B-complex vitamins	50 mg twice a day	I suggest taking a multivitamin along with your B-complex vitamins.
Calcium	500 mg twice a day	Although most people are deficient in calcium, there is a danger in taking too much. Do not ingest more than 1,000 to 1,200 mg of calcium a day.
Carnitine*	1,000 to 2,000 mg once a day	Have your healthcare provider measure your TMAO levels before starting long-term supplementation.
Cocoa	2.5 g (0.1 ounce) unsweetened cocoa powder (about 0.5 teaspoon)	Cocoa can interact with some medications, so speak to your healthcare provider or pharmacist before starting long-term supplementation. Be aware that cocoa contains caffeine.
Coenzyme Q_{10}*	60 to 120 mg once a day	If you are on blood-thinning medications, speak to your healthcare provider before using CoQ_{10}. Since some medications can cause a deficiency of this nutrient, speak to your healthcare provider to determine if you might need a larger dose.

Cysteine	1,000 mg once a day as n-acetylcysteine, or NAC	When taking NAC supplements, also take extra vitamin C, copper, and zinc.
EPA/DHA (fish oil)*	3,000 to 4,000 mg once a day	Choose a source that contains vitamin E to prevent oxidation. In high doses, fatty acids may cause the blood to thin. If you are taking a blood thinner, do not take EPA/DHA without direct instructions from your doctor. It is important to maintain the proper ratio of omega-6 fatty acids to omega-3 fatty acids. (See page 129.)
Garlic*	10 mg allicin or a total allicin potential of 4,000 mcg (equal to one clove of garlic) once a day	Garlic is a blood thinner. Do not use if you are taking any kind of blood-thinning medication or supplements.
Hawthorn*	160 to 900 mg of dried standardized extract once a day	Hawthorn can interact with a number of medications. Speak to your healthcare provider or pharmacist to learn if any drugs you're taking might make it unwise to take hawthorn.
Lycopene	10 to 20 mg once a day	May cause GI problems such as diarrhea and gas.
Magnesium	600 to 800 mg once a day	Consult your healthcare provider for dosage if you have kidney disease. Discontinue use and see your doctor if you experience abdominal pain. Take a lower dose if it causes diarrhea.
Potassium	See your healthcare provider for dosage directions.	
Quercetin*	50 mg three times a day	For best results, take with bromelain and vitamin C. Do not use with blood-thinning medications or supplements.
Taurine	1,000 to 1,500 mg once a day	Take between meals. Discontinue use if you suddenly have feelings of chest or throat tightness or if you break out in hives. Do not take with aspirin. Have your healthcare provider measure levels before starting taurine therapy.
Vitamin C	500 mg twice a day	Do not take high doses if you are prone to kidney stones or gout. High doses can also cause diarrhea.
Vitamin D$_3$	Have your blood levels measured by your healthcare provider, who will determine proper dosage.	
Vitamin E*	400 to 800 IU once a day	Take mixed tocopherols, the more active type of vitamin E. Consult your healthcare provider first if you are taking a blood thinner.
Zinc	25 mg once a day as zinc picolinate or zinc citrate	Your copper-to-zinc ratio is very important to your health. (See page 119 for details.) If you are taking zinc and iron supplements, take one in the morning and one in the evening. (Taking them together reduces the efficiency of both.)

*This supplement can have a blood-thinning action. See page 328 for more information.

Medications That Can Lower Blood Pressure

Your doctor may feel that it is necessary for you to take one of the following types of medications. Yet, as stated above, many blood pressure medications cause a wide range of side effects. There are often nutrients that can be taken to augment the effects of the medication, so that a lower dosage can be used. This often causes many of the negative effects to subside. You may even find that the nutrient can replace the medication. Before taking any nutrients on the following lists, however, discuss your options with your healthcare provider.

Diuretics

Diuretics can lower your blood pressure quite effectively. Unfortunately, they can also increase your risk of other health problems. The following nutrients may allow you to decrease—and possibly eliminate—your dosage of diuretics while continuing to lower your blood pressure. However, you should never stop taking your blood pressure medication without your doctor's approval.

- Calcium
- Carnitine
- Coenzyme Q_{10}
- Fiber
- Gamma-linolenic acid (GLA)
- Hawthorn berry
- Magnesium
- Potassium
- Protein
- Taurine
- Vitamin B_6 (pyridoxine)
- Vitamin C

Direct Vasodilators

Direct vasodilators are drugs that decrease blood pressure by widening blood vessels. Yet they can cause serious side effects, including headaches, dizziness, upset stomach, and joint pain. Although these side effects may subside when the vasodilator is combined with a beta blocker medication, beta blockers can cause other problems, including worsened asthma and severe depression. Instead of taking a beta blocker with your direct vasodilator medication, try adding any of the following nutrients to your regimen. You may even find that taking the vasodilator is no longer necessary—but do not stop taking it or a beta blocker without the approval of your doctor.

- Alpha lipoic acid
- Arginine
- Calcium
- Coenzyme Q_{10}
- Fiber
- Garlic
- Magnesium
- Omega-3 fatty acids
- Potassium
- Soy
- Taurine
- Vitamin C
- Vitamin E

Angiotensin-Converting Enzyme Inhibitors

Angiotensin-converting enzyme inhibitors—or ACE Inhibitors—are vasodilators that act by restricting the production of the enzyme angiotensin II. This enzyme causes blood vessels to constrict, which results in their becoming more narrow. Restricting this enzyme allows the blood more room to move through the blood vessels, decreasing pressure. However, ACE Inhibitors can also decrease your body's store of important trace minerals such as copper, selenium, and zinc while increasing your potassium levels. The following foods and supplements can limit these side effects and increase the effectiveness of your ACE Inhibitor. You may also find it helpful to take a multivitamin.

- Casein (a phosphoprotein found in milk and cheese)
- Egg yolks
- Garlic
- Gelatin
- Hawthorn berry
- Hydrolyzed wheat germ isolate
- Hydrolyzed whey protein
- Omega-3 fatty acids
- Pycnogenol
- Sake
- Sardines
- Seaweed
- Tuna
- Zinc

Angiotensin II Receptor Blockers

Angiotensin II receptor blockers (ARBs) are vasodilators that can help lower your blood pressure by blocking the effects of the enzyme angiotensin II. ARBs are often effective for people for whom ACE inhibitors have failed. The most common side effect is dizziness, but some people also experience fever, nasal congestion, back pain, and more. The nutrients on the following list can help you avoid these possible side effects while allowing you to continue your medication. You may even find that you are able to decrease your dosage, but don't change your dosage without first consulting your healthcare provider.

- Coenzyme Q_{10}
- Fiber
- Gamma-linolenic acid (GLA)
- Garlic
- Potassium
- Vitamin B_6 (pyridoxine)
- Vitamin C

Central Alpha Agonists

By stimulating alpha-receptors in the brain, central alpha agonists widen the peripheral arteries, releasing the pressure on the blood flow. However, these medications can cause dizziness, dry mouth, sedation, and rebound hypertension, so they are usually reserved as a last resort. The following nutrients can be taken with central alpha agonists to improve their function and reduce side effects. It can also be helpful to restrict dietary sodium.

- Coenzyme Q_{10}
- Docosahexaenoic acid (DHA)
- Fiber
- Garlic
- Gamma-linolenic acid (GLA)
- Potassium

- Protein
- Taurine
- Zinc
- Vitamin B_6 (pyridoxine)
- Vitamin C

Calcium Channel Blockers

Calcium channel blockers decrease blood pressure by limiting the movement of calcium into the blood vessels. The negative effect of these medications is that they can change the strength of the heart muscle's contractions. The following nutrients can help counter this effect as well as lower blood pressure.

- Alpha lipoic acid
- Calcium
- Cysteine (n-acetylcysteine, or NAC)
- Garlic
- Hawthorn berry

- Magnesium
- Omega-3 fatty acids
- Vitamin B_6 (pyridoxine)
- Vitamin C
- Vitamin E

HIGH CHOLESTEROL (HYPERCHOLESTEROLEMIA)

Cholesterol is a wax-like fatty substance—a lipid—found in the cell membranes of all body tissues. About 75 percent of it is synthesized by the body, with the rest being of dietary origin. Despite cholesterol's bad reputation, it is actually necessary for proper body function, and plays a central role in many biochemical processes, including the production of sex hormones. But at the same time, excessively high levels of cholesterol—referred to as *hypercholesterolemia*—pose a threat to good health.

There are two major forms of cholesterol. *High-density lipoproteins (HDLs)*, which are often referred to as "good cholesterol," carry cholesterol from the blood to the liver for elimination from the body. *Low-density lipoproteins (LDLs)*, or "bad cholesterol," carry cholesterol from the liver to the rest of the body. Your *total cholesterol* considers both LDL and HDL levels, because they are both important for good health. When there are high levels of LDLs in the blood—and especially when this is accompanied by low levels of HDLs—cholesterol can be deposited on the walls of the arteries, causing atherosclerosis (hardening of the arteries). This condition, in turn, is an underlying cause of strokes, heart attacks, and most cardiovascular disease in general.

The following are some of the causes of high cholesterol. The second list examines causes of low cholesterol.

■ Causes of High Cholesterol

- Alcoholism
- Amino acid deficiency
- Biotin deficiency
- Carnitine deficiency
- Deficiency of natural antioxidants, such as vitamin E, selenium, and beta-carotene
- Essential fatty acid deficiency
- Excess dietary starch
- Excess dietary sugar
- Fiber deficiency
- Food allergies

- Hormone deficiency (testosterone, DHEA, estrogen, pregnenolone, progesterone)
- Hydrogenated or processed fats (lard, shortening, cottonseed oil, palm oil, margarine, etc.)
- Hypothyroidism (low thyroid activity)
- Increased tissue damage due to infection, radiation, or oxidative activity (free radical production)
- Liver dysfunction
- Some medications
- Vitamin C deficiency

■ Causes of Low Cholesterol

- Adrenal stress
- Cancer
- Cholesterol-lowering drugs
- Chronic hepatitis
- Essential fatty acid deficiency
- Excessive exercise
- Immune decline

- Liver infection or disease
- Low-fat diets
- Manganese deficiency
- Psychological stress
- Recreational drugs such as marijuana or cocaine

Hypercholesterolemia is also linked to high *triglyceride* levels. This refers to the form that fat takes when it is being stored for energy in your body. Triglycerides, like cholesterol, are vital for human life but unhealthy if they reach too high a level. Your doctor will be able to test your HDL, LDL, and triglyceride levels by taking a simple blood test. (You will need to fast the day of the test. Your doctor will provide you with details.)

Dietary changes are key to lowering both cholesterol and triglycerides. Red meat and other foods high in saturated fats should eaten sparingly, while heart-healthy fish, vegetables, fruits, grains, and nuts should be included in greater amounts. Soy foods, which decrease LDL cholesterol and triglycerides, should also be featured in your diet.

Exercise is vital to achieving and maintaining healthy cholesterol levels. Additionally, certain nutrients—such as those listed in the table "Supplements That Decrease Cholesterol Levels"—can help lower bad cholesterol, raise good cholesterol, and restore heart health. To specifically lower your triglycerides, see the nutrients listed in the table "Supplements That Decrease Triglycerides." Causes of high triglyceride levels can be found in the inset on page 409.

SUPPLEMENTS THAT DECREASE CHOLESTEROL LEVELS

Supplements	Dosage	Considerations
Berberine*	200 to 500 mg of standardized extract two to three times a day	Do not use this supplement during pregnancy. It can cause uterine contractions.
Beta-sitosterol	1,000 mg twice a day	Do not use if you have a rare genetic disorder called phytosterolemia.
Carnitine*	1,000 to 2,000 mg once a day	Have your healthcare provider measure your TMAO levels before starting long-term supplementation with carnitine.
Chromium	200 to 300 mcg once a day as chromium picolinate	Combining with the protein picolinate allows your body to absorb chromium more efficiently. However, some chromium picolinate supplements contain more chromium than necessary. Ask your healthcare provider for a recommendation on chromium consumption.
Coenzyme Q_{10}*	60 to 120 mg once a day	If you are on blood-thinning medications, speak to your healthcare provider before using CoQ_{10}. Since some medications can cause a deficiency of this nutrient, speak to your healthcare provider to determine if you might need a larger dose.
EGCG (green tea extract)*	200 to 400 mg twice a day	Green tea extract can interact with a number of drugs. Check with your healthcare provider before taking this supplement.

Fiber, soluble	Suggested daily intake is 25 grams for women and 38 grams for men. Try to get most of your fiber from whole foods.	Choose a fiber supplement with no added sugar, and take with several glasses of water to prevent side effects.
Garlic*	10 mg allicin or a total allicin potential of 4,000 mcg (equal to one clove of garlic) once a day	Garlic is a blood thinner. Do not use if you are taking any kind of blood-thinning medication or supplements.
Gugulipid*	50 mg twice a day	Gugulipid has demonstrated anticoagulant activity. Do not use if you are taking blood-thinning medications or supplements.
Magnesium	600 mg once a day	Consult your healthcare provider for dosage if you have kidney disease. Discontinue use and see your doctor if you experience abdominal pain. Take a lower dose if it causes diarrhea.
Policosanol*	20 mg once a day of a sugar cane-based policosanol supplement	Discuss use with doctor if taking an anticoagulant.
Red yeast rice	600 to 2,400 mg once a day	Be sure to take with 100 mg of pharmaceutical grade CoQ_{10}. Do not take with a statin drug.
Vitamin B_3	(niacin, non-extended release) 50 mg twice a day	Do not drink alcohol or hot drinks within one hour of taking niacin. High doses can deplete your body of other B vitamins, so take a B-complex vitamin twice a day. Do not take more than 50 mg twice a day except under a doctor's direction.
Vitamin E*	400 IU twice a day	Take tocotrienols, which are known to reduce cholesterol. Consult your healthcare provider first if you are taking a blood thinner.

*This supplement can have a blood-thinning action. See page 328 for more information.

SUPPLEMENTS THAT DECREASE TRIGLYCERIDES

Supplements	Dosage	Considerations
Arginine	2,000 to 4,000 mg once a day	Do not take if you have kidney disease, liver disease, or herpes except under a doctor's supervision. Arginine can interact with some medications. Consult with your healthcare provider before beginning this therapy.
Carnitine*	2,000 mg once a day	Have your healthcare provider measure your TMAO levels before starting long-term supplementation with carnitine.
Chromium	300 mcg once a day as chromium picolinate	Combining with the protein picolinate allows your body to absorb chromium more efficiently. However, some chromium picolinate supplements contain more chromium than necessary. Ask your healthcare provider for a recommendation on chromium consumption.

Coenzyme Q_{10}*	60 to 120 mg once a day	If you are on blood-thinning medications, speak to your healthcare provider before using CoQ_{10}. Since some medications can cause a deficiency of this nutrient, speak to your healthcare provider to determine if you might need a larger dose.
EPA/DHA (fish oil)*	2,000 to 4,000 mg once a day	Choose a source that contains vitamin E to prevent oxidation. In high doses, fatty acids may cause the blood to thin. If you are taking a blood thinner, do not take EPA/DHA without direct instructions from your doctor. It is important to maintain the proper ratio of omega-6 fatty acids to omega-3 fatty acids. (See page 129.)
Gugulipid*	50 mg twice a day	Gugulipid has demonstrated anticoagulant activity. Do not use if you are taking blood-thinning medications or supplements.
Lysine	1,000 to 2,000 mg once a day	Do not take if you have diabetes or are allergic to eggs, milk, or wheat. Do not take for more than six months because it can cause an imbalance of arginine unless arginine is also supplemented.
Magnesium	600 mg once a day	Consult your healthcare provider for dosage if you have kidney disease. Discontinue use and see your doctor if you experience abdominal pain. Take a lower dose if it causes diarrhea.
Methionine	250 to 500 mg once a day	Take with folate and vitamins B_6 and B_{12} to prevent a build-up of homocysteine. May counter the effects of levodopa (a drug used to treat Parkinson's disease) as well as other drugs. Speak to your healthcare provider before taking.
Olive leaf extract*	500 mg twice a day containing 20 mg of oleuropein per capsule	Olive leaf extracts can interact with many prescription medications, and may increase the effects of blood thinners. Consult your healthcare provider before using olive leaf extract if you are taking any medication. Don't use if you are pregnant or breastfeeding.
Policosanol*	10 to 20 mg once a day of a sugar cane-based policosanol supplement	Do not use if you are taking any kind of blood-thinning medication or supplement.
Vitamin B_3 (niacin)	50 mg twice a day	Do not drink alcohol or hot drinks within one hour of taking niacin. High doses can deplete your body of other vitamins in the B complex, so take a B-complex vitamin twice a day.
Vitamin B_5 (pantothenic acid)	50 mg twice a day	High doses can deplete your body of other vitamins in the B complex, so take a B-complex vitamin twice a day. Stop taking B_5 if you begin having chest pains or breathing problems.

Vitamin B₉ (folic acid)	400 to 500 mcg twice a day	High doses can deplete your body of other vitamins in the B complex, so take a B-complex vitamin twice a day.
Vitamin E*	400 IU twice a day	Take tocotrienols, which are known to reduce lipids. Consult your healthcare provider before taking if you are using blood thinners.
Zinc*	25 mg once a day as zinc picolinate or zinc citrate	Your copper-to-zinc ratio is very important to your health. (See page 119 for details.) If you are taking zinc and iron supplements, take one in the morning and one in the evening. (Taking them together reduces the efficiency of both.)

*This supplement can have a blood-thinning action. See page 328 for more information.

Causes of High Triglyceride Levels

Triglycerides are fat cells that are stored in your body and later transferred into energy. While these substances are necessary for health, high levels of triglycerides have been strongly linked to coronary heart disease. The supplements in the table beginning on page 407 may help lower triglyceride levels and increase your heart health. The list below, on the other hand, describes factors and foods that can cause your triglyceride levels to rise.

- Alcohol
- Birth control pills or any other progestin-containing drugs
- Caffeine
- Cakes, cookies, and candies
- Diuretics
- Fruit juice

- Genetics
- High-fat diet
- Lack of physical activity
- Nicotine
- Skipping an early meal and compensating in the evening

- Soft drinks
- Stress
- Too much fruit
- White bread
- White flour
- White sugar

HPV INFECTION

See Cervical Cancer.

HYPERCHOLESTEROLEMIA

See High Cholesterol.

HYPERTENSION

See High Blood Pressure.

HYPERTHYROIDISM

The thyroid gland is the body's internal thermostat. It regulates temperature by secreting hormones that control how quickly the body burns calories and uses energy. Hyperthyroidism occurs when there is an excess of thyroid hormones. As a result, body processes, including metabolism, occur more quickly than they should. Dramatic weight loss, fast heart rate, nervousness, fatigue, weakness, depression, sweating, heat or cold intolerance, and a host of other symptoms can result.

There are many different forms of treatment for hyperthyroidism, including hormone-suppressing medication, antithyroid medications, radioactive iodine, and surgery. Based on the cause of the problem and the individual's age and overall health, the healthcare provider determines which treatment route is most appropriate. The following nutrient list can help ease the problem, but *always* see your physician for ongoing care if you have hyperthyroidism.

SUPPLEMENTS TO TREAT HYPERTHYROIDISM

Supplements	Dosage	Considerations
Carnitine*	3,000 to 4,000 mg once a day	Have your healthcare provider measure your TMAO levels before starting long-term supplementation with carnitine.
Coenzyme Q_{10}*	100 mg to 300 mg once a day	Individuals with hyperthyroidism commonly have low coenzyme Q_{10} levels. If you are on blood-thinning medications, speak to your healthcare provider before using CoQ_{10}. Since some medications can cause a deficiency of this nutrient, speak to your healthcare provider to determine if you might need a larger dose.
Ginger*	250 to 1,000 mg three times a day	Ginger can act as a blood thinner. Check with your healthcare provider or pharmacist before taking this supplement.

Magnesium	400 to 600 mg once a day as magnesium glycinate	Consult your healthcare provider for dosage if you have kidney disease. Discontinue use and see your doctor if you experience abdominal pain. Take a lower dose if it causes diarrhea.
Selenium	200 to 400 mcg once a day	Sometimes larger doses are needed. Increase your dose only under the direction of your doctor. Do not exceed 200 mcg a day without consulting your healthcare provider. If you are considering taking more than 400 mcg, have your selenium levels measured before taking the larger dose.
Vitamin A and mixed carotenoids	5,000 to 10,000 IU—half vitamin A and half mixed carotenoids—once a day	Use caution when taking vitamin A supplements because they have the potential to be toxic. Do not take for extended periods of time. Do not take more than 8,000 IU a day if you have liver disease, are a smoker, or have been exposed to asbestos.
Vitamin C	2,000 to 5,000 mg a day	Do not take high doses if you are prone to kidney stones or gout. High doses can also cause diarrhea.
Vitamin E*	400 IU a day	Take mixed tocopherols, the more active type of vitamin E. Consult your healthcare provider first if you are taking a blood thinner.
Zinc	25 to 50 mg a day as zinc picolinate or zinc citrate	Your copper-to-zinc ratio is very important to your health. (See page 119 for details.) If you are taking zinc and iron supplements, take one in the morning and one in the evening. (Taking them together reduces the efficiency of both.)

*This supplement can have a blood-thinning action. See page 328 for more information.

HYPOTHYROIDISM

The thyroid gland is the body's internal thermostat. It regulates temperature by secreting hormones that control how quickly the body burns calories and uses energy. Hypothyroidism develops due to an underactive thyroid gland that does not produce enough hormones. Common signs and symptoms include fatigue, intolerance to cold, slowed heart rate, unexplained weight gain, muscle weakness, hair loss (including the eyebrows), dry skin, cold hands and feet, decreased sexual interest, insomnia, infertility, puffy face, slow speech, tinnitus (ringing in the ears), and heavy menstrual periods. The severity of symptoms depends on the degree of the hormone deficiency. In a large number of cases, this disorder comes on so gradually that the person is unaware that he or she has a problem. If you suspect you may have this condition, check your thyroid function by following the directions in the inset on page 412.

Hypothyroidism affects about 5 million people in the United States, and five to eight times more women than men. Most cases are the result of an autoimmune disorder known as *Hashimoto's thyroiditis* (see page 394), in which the body develops antibodies that attack the thyroid gland. Other common causes of this disorder include surgical removal of the thyroid and radioactive iodine therapy. Less common causes or contributors include infections of the thyroid, too much or too little dietary iodine, an excess of calcium and copper, and deficiencies of iron, selenium, zinc, and vitamins A, B_2, B_3, B_6, and C. Medications, including beta blockers, lithium, certain oral contraceptives, and chemotherapy drugs, are also possible contributors. It's critical to recognize that the cause of hypothyroidism determines which nutritional therapies can be helpful in treating the disorder. In other words, the nutrients recommended for Hashimoto's thyroiditis are different from those presented in the table that follows, which can help treat hypothyroidism that is *not* autoimmune related. (For supplements that treat Hashimoto's disease, see the table on page 394.)

Certain foods—especially seafood, sea vegetables, and other rich sources of iodine—are recommended for those with an underactive thyroid gland. On the other hand, when eaten raw, cabbage, Brussels sprouts, broccoli, turnips, cauliflower, mustard greens, and spinach can contribute to a low-functioning thyroid. These foods should be eaten in moderation and only when cooked. Other foods that should be eaten only in moderate amounts include almonds, walnuts, peanuts, pine nuts, millet, tapioca, and soy products.

Self-Test for an Underactive Thyroid

The following self-test can give you a good indication of whether or not you have an underactive thyroid.

Keep a thermometer next to your bed. As soon as you awake in the morning, before getting out of bed, tuck the thermometer under your armpit and keep it there for fifteen minutes while lying very still. (Any motion can affect the reading.) Write down the temperature. Do this for three days in a row.* Determine your average temperature by adding up the three readings and dividing by three. If it is below 97.5°F, there is a good chance you may have a low-functioning thyroid. Contact your doctor to discuss your findings.

* Because hormonal shifts affect body temperature, women should not take this test while menstruating or during the middle of a menstrual cycle, when ovulation usually occurs.

SUPPLEMENTS TO TREAT HYPOTHYROIDISM

Supplements	Dosage	Considerations
Ashwagandha root	500 to 1,000 mg once a day	High doses can cause gastrointestinal problems.
B-complex vitamins	50 mg twice a day	I suggest taking a multivitamin along with your B-complex vitamins.
Carnitine*	1,000 to 4,000 mg once a day	Have your healthcare provider measure your TMAO levels before starting long-term supplementation with carnitine.
Chromium	200 to 400 mcg once a day as chromium picolinate	Combining with the protein picolinate allows your body to absorb chromium more efficiently. However, some chromium picolinate supplements contain more chromium than necessary. Ask your healthcare provider for a dosage recommendation.
Coenzyme Q_{10}*	30 to 120 mg once a day	If you are on blood-thinning medications, speak to your healthcare provider before using CoQ_{10}. Since some medications can cause a deficiency of this nutrient, speak to your healthcare provider to determine if you might need a larger dose.
Copper	1 to 3 mg once a day	Your copper-to-zinc ratio is very important for your health. (See page 119 for details.) Also, do not take copper supplement cupric oxide, which has a very low bioavailability.
EPA/DHA (fish oil)*	5,000 to 2,000 mg once a day	Choose a source that contains vitamin E to prevent oxidation.
Gamma-linolenic acid (GLA) as evening primrose oil (EPO)*	240 mg once a day	It is important to maintain the proper ratio of omega-6 fatty acids to omega-3 fatty acids. (See page 129.) Evening primrose oil may interfere with some medications, such as nonsteroidal anti-inflammatories; can act as a blood thinner; and can lower the seizure threshold. Consult your healthcare provider or pharmacist before taking this supplement.
Iodine	100 to 300 mcg once a day	Most table salts contain iodine, but sea salts do not. Before starting iodine supplementation, have your healthcare provider measure your iodine level.
Magnesium	400 to 600 mg once a day	Consult your healthcare provider for dosage if you have kidney disease. Discontinue use and see your doctor if you experience abdominal pain. Take a lower dose if it causes diarrhea.
Milk thistle	200 mg twice a day	Do not take if you are allergic to ragweed, chrysanthemums, marigolds, chamomile, or daisies. This supplement reduces the efficiency of certain blood pressure medication and other drugs. Speak to your healthcare provider or pharmacist before taking.

Sage	300 mg once a day	Do not use if you have a hormonally related cancer, such as breast, prostate, uterine, or ovarian. Use with caution if you have fibroids.
Selenium	200 mcg once a day	Do not exceed 200 mcg a day without seeing your doctor. If you are considering taking more than 400 mcg, have your selenium levels measured before taking the larger dose.
Tyrosine	1,000 mg once a day	Start at 100 mg a day, and increase the dose gradually. Check with your doctor before starting use if you have diabetes, hypertension, kidney disease, or liver disease.
Vitamin A and mixed carotenoids	5,000 to 10,000 IU—half vitamin A and half mixed carotenoids—once a day	Use caution when taking vitamin A supplements because they have the potential to be toxic. Do not take for extended periods of time. Do not take more than 8,000 IU a day if you have liver disease, are a smoker, or have been exposed to asbestos.
Vitamin B_3 (niacin)	50 mg twice a day	Do not drink alcohol or hot drinks within one hour of taking niacin. High doses can deplete your body of other vitamins in the B complex, so take a B-complex vitamin twice a day.
Vitamin B_6 (pyridoxine)	50 mg twice a day	Do not take more than 500 mg a day. If you are taking L-dopa for Parkinson's disease, do not take B_6 without first consulting your doctor. High doses can deplete your body of other vitamins in the B complex, so take a B-complex vitamin twice a day.
Vitamin B_{12} (cobalamin)	500 mcg twice a day	High doses can deplete your body of other vitamins in the B complex, so take B-complex vitamins twice a day.
Vitamin C	500 to 1,500 mg twice a day	Do not take high doses if you are prone to kidney stones or gout. High doses can also cause diarrhea.
Vitamin D_3	Have your blood levels measured by your healthcare provider, who will determine proper dosage.	
Vitamin E*	400 IU once a day	Take mixed tocopherols, the more active type of vitamin E. Consult your healthcare provider first if you are taking a blood thinner.
Zinc	25 to 50 mg once a day as zinc picolinate or zinc citrate	Your copper-to-zinc ratio is very important to your health. (See page 119 for details.) If you are taking zinc and iron supplements, take one in the morning and one in the evening. (Taking them together reduces the efficiency of both.)

*This supplement can have a blood-thinning action. See page 328 for more information.

IBS

See Irritable Bowel Syndrome.

INFLAMMATION

Acute inflammation, characterized by redness, swelling, pain, and heat, is a localized reaction to an injury, infection, or other irritation. It can occur to any organ or tissue, and protects the body from the affected area by allowing the stimuli to be removed and the healing to begin. Sometimes, unfortunately, the immune system may not perform this process properly. Chronic inflammation—the subject of this discussion—occurs when the body's reaction does not lead to healing within a reasonable amount of time. It can last indefinitely and lead to disease and discomfort.

There are many different causes of inflammation, as well as many different diseases to which it can lead. The following all-too-common disorders are associated with chronic inflammation:

- Alzheimer's disease and other forms of dementia
- Arthritis
- Asthma
- Cancer
- Cardiovascular disease
- COPD (chronic obstructive pulmonary disease)
- Depression
- Diabetes
- Hypertension (high blood pressure)
- Inflammatory bowel disease, such as Crohn's disease and ulcerative colitis
- Nonalcoholic fatty liver disease
- Obesity
- Peripheral artery disease
- Psoriasis

Diet is an important part of the battle against chronic inflammation. Avoid consuming soda, sugar, and white flour products, all of which can contribute to this problem. Also consider following the Mediterranean Diet, which emphasizes vegetables, fruits, whole grains, and legumes, which are all anti-inflammatory. The following nutrients will further help reduce both acute and chronic forms of inflammation. *See also* Asthma; Atherosclerosis; Crohn's Disease; Gout; Hashimoto's Thyroiditis; Lupus; Myasthenia Gravis; Rheumatoid Arthritis; Ulcerative Colitis; Wound Healing.

SUPPLEMENTS TO TREAT CHRONIC INFLAMMATION

Supplements	Dosage	Considerations
Bromelain	250 to 750 mg three times a day as part of a digestive enzyme product	Do not take bromelain if you are allergic to pineapple, latex, wheat, celery, carrot, fennel, cypress pollen, or grass pollen.
Curcumin/Turmeric*	100 to 500 mg a day of a formula that includes piperine or bioperine to boost absorption	Do not take curcumin with blood-thinning medications or supplements. Curcumin can also interact with other medications, so speak to a healthcare provider before taking this supplement.
EPA/DHA (fish oil)*	2,000 to 10,000 mg once a day	Choose a source that contains vitamin E to prevent oxidation. In high doses, fatty acids may cause the blood to thin. If you are taking a blood thinner, do not take EPA/DHA without direct instructions from your doctor. It is important to maintain the proper ratio of omega-6 fatty acids to omega-3 fatty acids. (See page 129.)
Glucosamine sulfate	500 to 1,000 mg three times a day	If you are allergic to shellfish, be sure to choose a supplement that is not shellfish based. Consult use with your healthcare provider if you have diabetes, because glucosamine can alter blood sugar levels.
Magnesium	400 to 600 mg once a day as magnesium glycinate	Consult your healthcare provider for dosage if you have kidney disease. Discontinue use and see your doctor if you experience abdominal pain. Take a lower dose if it causes diarrhea.
Methylsulfonylmethane (MSM)	1,000 to 3,000 mg three times a day	Use with caution if you are allergic to sulfur. Start by taking 500 mg three times a day, and gradually increase dose. Take with meals to avoid possible heartburn. May cause stomach upset in dosages larger than 6,000 mg.
Resveratrol	40 mg a day	Do not use resveratrol if you have or have had a hormonally related cancer until more is known about the estrogenic activity of resveratrol.
Vitamin D$_3$	Have your blood levels measured by your healthcare provider, who will determine proper dosage.	
Vitamin E*	1,000 IU once a day of gamma-tocopherol	Consult your healthcare provider first if you are taking a blood thinner.

*This supplement can have a blood-thinning action. See page 328 for more information.

INFLAMMATORY BOWEL DISEASE

See Crohn's Disease; Ulcerative Colitis.

INSOMNIA

Insomnia is a sleep disorder characterized by an inability to sleep and/or an inability to remain asleep for a reasonable period of time. People with this problem have difficulty falling asleep, staying asleep, or sleeping soundly. As a result, they often suffer from daytime fatigue, lack of energy, poor concentration, and irritability. Insomnia is estimated to affect at least half of the adults in the United States.

Factors That Can Contribute to Insomnia

As explained in the text that follows this inset, insomnia can exist on its own, without outside causes, or can be brought about by a variety of activities, lifestyle choices, disorders, and substances. Some people may find that the following factors can cause or contribute to insomnia.

- **Chemical exposure:** Over a hundred chemicals are known to interfere with sleep.
- **Diet:** Caffeinated beverages, food additives, and allergen-containing foods. Eating sugary foods right before bed.
- **Hormonal problems:** Thyroid dysfunction, growth hormone loss, progesterone loss, testosterone loss, estrogen loss, and elevated cortisol.
- **Illnesses:** Urinary disorders, nasal and sinus problems, reflux esophagitis, asthma, gall bladder disease, chronic pain, and emotional disorders such as anxiety and depression.
- **Lack of exercise.**
- **Light.**
- **Medications:** Asthma medications, blood pressure medications, and synthetic progestins.
- **Night work.**
- **Nutritional deficiencies:** Deficiencies of niacin, magnesium, copper, iron, tryptophan, and vitamin B_6.
- **Sleep apnea.**

Insomnia is often categorized in terms of its duration. *Transient insomnia* lasts less than a week; *short-term insomnia* lasts a week to a month; and *chronic insomnia* lasts more than a month. Moreover, insomnia may be considered *primary*, meaning that it exists on its own; or *secondary*, meaning that it has other causes. Secondary insomnias include sleep problems caused by stress; lack of an enforced bedtime during childhood; an underlying psychiatric disorder, such as anxiety or depression; a medical condition, such as restless legs syndrome; or consumption of or withdrawal from alcohol, caffeine, or another substance. (See the inset on page 417 for more factors that can contribute to insomnia.)

When a specific cause for insomnia can be found, the elimination of the causative factor can often end the sleep problem. Healthy habits, such as limited caffeine consumption, a consistent bedtime routine, and exercising in the morning, can also end or minimize insomnia. Moreover, a sound supplement program can relieve sleep problems by eliminating nutritional deficiencies, inducing relaxation, and helping to restore the body's normal rhythms.

SUPPLEMENTS TO TREAT INSOMNIA		
Supplements	Dosage	Considerations
Astragalus*	250 to 500 mg standardized extract three or four times a day	Do not use after organ transplant or if you have an allergy to gum tragacanth. Also do not use for an extended period of time. Speak to your healthcare provider to see if any of the medications you take make it unwise to use astragalus.
CBD oil (hemp oil)	5 to 500 mg a day in the form of sublingual drops. Start with 5 mg and increase slowly until you find relief.	CBD is generally well tolerated and safe for consumption, even in high doses and with continuous use. However, do not exceed 500 mg a day without consulting your healthcare provider. Make sure to buy a product marked "hemp oil (aerial parts)."
Chamomile*	200 to 500 mg twice a day in capsule form, or 1 to 2 cups of tea daily	Consult your healthcare practitioner before taking if you are on a blood thinner. Do not take if you are allergic to plants such as ragweed, aster, daisies, and, chrysanthemums. Also avoid if you have a hormonally related cancer, such as breast, prostate, uterine, or ovarian.
Gamma-aminobutyric acid (GABA)	300 to 900 mg once a day, about thirty minutes before bedtime	Always take with a multivitamin to supply the nutrients that are needed to metabolize GABA.
Inositol	1,000 mg once a day, one hour before bedtime	May stimulate uterine contractions. Women who wish to become pregnant should consult their doctor regarding its use. Doses larger than 200 mg should be taken only under physician supervision.

Magnesium	600 mg once a day, one hour before bedtime	Consult your healthcare provider for dosage if you have kidney disease. Discontinue use and see your doctor if you experience abdominal pain. Take a lower dose if it causes diarrhea.
Melatonin	1 to 3 mg taken thirty to sixty minutes before bedtime	It is best to have your melatonin levels measured to determine the best dose for you. This is especially important if you are taking a dose larger than 3 mg. Too much melatonin can lower serotonin.
Passion flower*	45 drops liquid extract once a day, or 90 mg tablet once a day	Avoid this supplement if you are taking an MAO inhibitor or a sedative medication. Also avoid if you have a bleeding disorder or are taking a blood-thinning drug or supplement. Consult your healthcare provider or pharmacist before using this supplement.
Theanine	100 to 200 mg twice a day as L-theanine	Because theanine lowers blood pressure, you should use with caution if you have low blood pressure.
Tryptophan	1,000 mg at bedtime as L-Tryptophan	Check with your doctor before starting an amino acid regimen if you have diabetes, hypertension, kidney disease, or liver disease. Do not take tryptophan if you are pregnant or breastfeeding. Tryptophan can interact with some medications, so consult with your healthcare provider before beginning supplementation.

*This supplement can have a blood-thinning action. See page 328 for more information.

INSULIN-DEPENDENT DIABETES

See Diabetes Mellitus.

IRRITABLE BOWEL SYNDROME (IBS)

Irritable bowel syndrome, or IBS, is a "functional" disorder of the lower intestinal tract. This means that although no structural abnormalities can be found, the body's function in terms of the movement of the intestines is impaired. IBS is believed to affect up to 20 percent of the US population—about one person in every five. It occurs more often in women than in men.

Bloating and abdominal pain and cramping are the major symptoms of IBS. Other symptoms vary from person to person, and may include constipation, diarrhea, or alternating constipation and diarrhea; nausea; and vomiting. Emotional stress and the consumption of certain foods tend to worsen symptoms. No one knows what causes IBS, and it is usually a lifelong problem.

In many cases, IBS can be controlled through medication and a diet that avoids problem foods. These foods vary from person to person, but often include grains, breads, crackers, cakes, cookies, potatoes, beans, and other carbohydrates that increase the formation of gas. A diet that's low in FOD-MAPs—hard-to-digest carbohydrates that are present in many foods— is recommended for all individuals with IBS. Foods restricted on a low-FODMAP diet include the following:

- Milk and other lactose-containing foods

- Foods with added fructose

- Foods that naturally contain fructose in excess of glucose, such as apples and pears

- Fructan-containing foods, such as wheat, artichokes, onions, garlic, and leeks

- Sorbitol-containing foods, such as stone fruits (peaches, plums, etc.)

- Raffinose-containing foods, such as lentils, cabbage, Brussels sprouts, and legumes

In addition to changing your diet, taking supplements listed in the following table can help relieve the symptoms of IBS.

SUPPLEMENTS TO TREAT IRRITABLE BOWEL SYNDROME

Supplements	Dosage	Considerations
Boswellia extract*	500 mg capsules or tablets three times a day until symptoms subside. Then take one 500 mg capsule or tablet a day.	Take with a meal. Avoid boswellia if you are pregnant, because it can induce miscarriage. Do not take with NSAIDs.
CBD oil (hemp oil)	5 to 500 mg a day in the form of sublingual drops. Start with 5 mg and increase slowly until you find relief.	CBD is generally well tolerated and safe for consumption, even in high doses and with continuous use. However, do not exceed 500 mg a day without consulting your healthcare provider. Make sure to buy a product marked "hemp oil (aerial parts)."
Digestive enzymes	Follow the manufacturer's instructions. Be sure to take these supplements with or directly before meals.	Do not take digestive enzymes that contain papain if you are allergic to papaya, and avoid enzymes with bromelain if you are allergic to pineapple.
EPA/DHA (fish oil)*	1,000 to 2,000 mg once a day	Choose a source that contains vitamin E to prevent oxidation.

Fiber, soluble and insoluble	Suggested daily intake is 25 grams for women and 38 grams for men. Try to get most of your fiber from whole foods.	Choose a fiber supplement with no added sugar, and take with several glasses of water to prevent side effects.
Gamma-linolenic acid (GLA) as evening primrose oil (EPO)*	240 to 720 mg once a day	It is important to maintain the proper ratio of omega-6 fatty acids to omega-3 fatty acids. (See page 129.) Evening primrose oil may interfere with some medications, such as nonsteroidal anti-inflammatories; can act as a blood thinner; and can lower the seizure threshold. Consult your healthcare provider or pharmacist before taking this supplement.
Glutamine	6,000 mg once a day	If you have a sensitivity to monosodium glutamate (MSG), use glutamine with caution. If you are taking medications for seizures, take glutamine only under the direction of your doctor.
Licorice (glycyrrhiza)	200 mg twice a day as deglycyrrizinated licorice (DGL)	Do not use if you have high blood pressure, and discontinue use if you develop high blood pressure while taking supplements.
Magnesium	400 to 800 mg once a day	Consult your healthcare provider for dosage if you have kidney disease. Discontinue use and see your doctor if you experience abdominal pain. Take a lower dose if it causes diarrhea.
Melatonin	1 to 3 mg taken thirty to sixty minutes before bedtime	Melatonin can interact with other drugs, so speak to your doctor before taking this supplement. It is best to have your melatonin levels measured.
Olive leaf extract*	500 mg twice a day containing 20 mg of oleuropein per capsule	Olive leaf extracts can interact with many prescription medications, and may increase the effects of blood thinners. Consult your healthcare provider before using olive leaf extract if you are taking any medication. Don't use if you are pregnant or breastfeeding
Probiotics	20 billion units once a day	If taking an antibiotic, take the probiotics at least two hours before or two hours after using the antibiotics. Do not take them at the same time.
Querectin*	500 to 2,000 mg once a day	For best results, take with bromelain and vitamin C. Do not use with blood-thinning medications or supplements.
UltraInflamX	Follow instructions on bottle.	This is a metagenics product. (See Resources.) Do not use if taking a diuretic.
Vitamin A and mixed carotenoids	5,000 to 10,000 IU—half vitamin A and half mixed carotenoids—once a day	Use caution when taking vitamin A supplements because they have the potential to be toxic. Do not take for extended periods of time. Do not take more than 8,000 IU a day if you have liver disease, are a smoker, or have been exposed to asbestos.

Vitamin B₉ (folic acid)	400 mcg twice a day	High doses can deplete your body of other vitamins in the B complex, so take a B-complex vitamin twice a day.
Vitamin C	500 to 1,500 mg twice a day	Do not take high doses if you are prone to kidney stones or gout. High doses can also cause diarrhea.
Vitamin E*	200 to 400 IU once a day	Take mixed tocopherols, the more active type of vitamin E. Consult your healthcare provider first if you are taking a blood thinner.
Zinc	25 to 75 mg once a day as zinc picolinate or zinc citrate	Your copper-to-zinc ratio is very important to your health. (See page 119 for details.) If you are taking zinc and iron supplements, take one in the morning and one in the evening. (Taking them together reduces the efficiency of both.)

*This supplement can have a blood-thinning action. See page 328 for more information.

LEAKY GUT SYNDROME

A common but poorly recognized problem, leaky gut syndrome occurs when spaces develop between the cells of the gut (the intestines), allowing bacteria, toxins, medications, and partially digested particles of food to leak into the body. This can lead to a host of problems, including poor absorption of nutrients, infection, food allergies, chemical sensitivities, and autoimmune disease.

The symptoms of leaky gut syndrome are wide in range, and include gastrointestinal complaints, such as abdominal pain, constipation, bloating, gas, and diarrhea; neurological problems, such as anxiety, confusion, mood swings, and poor memory; breathing problems, such as shortness of breath and asthma; and various other difficulties, including poor immunity, recurrent bladder infections, chronic joint pain, and fatigue.

Leaky gut syndrome may be due to a number of causes. These include heavy metal toxicity; environmental toxins; nutritional deficiencies; the use of certain medications, such as broad-spectrum antibiotics, birth control pills, prednisone, and non-steroidal anti-inflammatory drugs (NSAIDs); fungal infection; food allergies; excess consumption of refined sugar, caffeine, and alcohol; a deficiency of digestive enzymes or hydrochloric acid in the stomach; and even stress.

A healthy diet can help avoid leaky gut syndrome and can aid in repairing the gut when problems occur. A number of nutritional supplements can also improve gut health.

SUPPLEMENTS TO TREAT LEAKY GUT SYNDROME

Supplements	Dosage	Considerations
Cysteine	500 mg once a day as n-acetylcysteine, or NAC	When taking NAC supplements, also take extra vitamin C, copper, and zinc.
Digestive enzymes	Follow the manufacturer's instructions. Be sure to take these supplements with or directly before meals.	Do not take digestive enzymes that contain papain if you are allergic to papaya, and avoid enzymes with bromelain if you are allergic to pineapple.
EPA/DHA (fish oil)*	500 mg to 1,000 mg three times a day	Choose a source that contains vitamin E to prevent oxidation.
Fiber, soluble and insoluble	Suggested daily intake is 25 grams for women and 38 grams for men. Try to get most of your fiber from whole foods.	Choose a fiber supplement with no added sugar, and take with several glasses of water to prevent side effects.
Gamma-linolenic acid (GLA) as evening primrose oil (EPO)*	500 mg three times a day	It is important to maintain the proper ratio of omega-6 fatty acids to omega-3 fatty acids. (See page 129.) Evening primrose oil may interfere with some medications, such as nonsteroidal anti-inflammatories; can act as a blood thinner; and can lower the seizure threshold. Consult your healthcare provider or pharmacist before taking this supplement.
Glutamine	2,000 to 6,000 mg once a day	If you have a sensitivity to monosodium glutamate (MSG), use glutamine with caution. If you are taking medications for seizures, take glutamine only under the direction of your doctor.
Methylsulfonylmethane (MSM)	1,000 mg three times a day	Use with caution if you are allergic to sulfur. Start by taking 500 mg three times a day, and gradually increase dose. Take with meals to avoid possible heartburn. May cause stomach upset in dosages larger than 6,000 mg.
Probiotics	20 billion units once a day as *Lactobacillus rhamnosus* and *Saccharomyces boulardii*	If taking an antibiotic, take the probiotics at least two hours before or two hours after using the antibiotics. Do not take them at the same time.
Quercetin*	500 mg three times a day	For best results, take with bromelain and vitamin C. Do not use with blood-thinning medications or supplements.
UltraInflamX	Follow instructions on bottle.	This product, by Metagenics (see Resources), provides macro- and micronutrient support for people with compromised gut function. Do not use if taking a diuretic.

Vitamin A and mixed carotenoids	5,000 to 15,000 IU—half vitamin A and half mixed carotenoids—once a day	Use caution when taking vitamin A supplements because they have the potential to be toxic. Do not take for extended periods of time. Do not take more than 8,000 IU a day if you have liver disease, are a smoker, or have been exposed to asbestos.
Vitamin B$_5$ (pantothenic acid)	50 to 100 mg twice a day	High doses can deplete your body of other vitamins in the B complex, so take a B-complex vitamin twice a day. Stop taking B$_5$ supplements if you begin having chest pains or breathing problems.
Vitamin C	500 mg twice a day	Do not take high doses if you are prone to kidney stones or gout. High doses can also cause diarrhea.
Vitamin E*	400 IU once a day	Take mixed tocopherols, the more active type of vitamin E. Consult your healthcare provider first if you are taking a blood thinner.
Zinc	10 to 20 mg a day as zinc picolinate or zinc citrate	Your copper-to-zinc ratio is very important to your health. (See page 119 for details.) If you are taking zinc and iron supplements, take one in the morning and one in the evening. (Taking them together reduces the efficiency of both.)

*This supplement can have a blood-thinning action. See page 328 for more information.

LEG CRAMPS

A leg cramp is a painful, involuntary contraction of a single muscle or group of muscles in the leg. Most commonly, leg cramps occur in the calf muscles, but the thigh muscles can also be affected. Typically, these cramps take place at night, sometimes awakening the individual from sleep, and last anywhere from less than a minute to several minutes before subsiding. They are most often experienced by adolescents and the elderly.

The exact cause of leg cramps is not understood. However, the occurrence of these cramps has been linked to a number of risk factors, including muscle fatigue, heavy exercising, dehydration, excess weight, electrolyte imbalance, and the use of certain medications. Reactive hypoglycemia, an exaggerated fall in blood sugar concentrations due to an excessive secretion of insulin, usually in response to eating, can also cause leg cramps, as can neurological disorders such as Parkinson's disease.

Gentle stretching of the muscles, a well-balanced diet, adequate rest, and warm baths or showers taken before retiring at night can all reduce the occurrence of leg cramps. By helping to ensure electrolyte balance, nutritional supplements can also normalize muscle function and prevent painful contractions.

SUPPLEMENTS TO TREAT LEG CRAMPS

Supplements	Dosage	Considerations
Calcium	500 mg once or twice a day	Although most people are deficient in calcium, there is a danger in taking too much calcium. Do not ingest more than 1,000 to 1,200 mg of calcium each day.
Carnitine*	300 mg three to four times a day	Have your healthcare provider measure your TMAO levels before starting long-term supplementation with carnitine.
EPA/DHA (fish oil)*	1,000 mg once a day	Choose a source that contains vitamin E to prevent oxidation.
Magnesium	600 to 800 mg once a day	Consult your healthcare provider for dosage if you have kidney disease. Discontinue use and see your doctor if you experience abdominal pain. Take a lower dose if it causes diarrhea.
Potassium	See your healthcare provider for dosage directions.	
Vitamin B$_{12}$ (cobalamin)	500 mcg twice a day	High doses can deplete your body of other vitamins in the B complex, so take a B-complex vitamin twice a day.
Vitamin C	200 mg four times a day	Do not take high doses if you are prone to kidney stones or gout. High doses can also cause diarrhea.
Vitamin E*	400 to 800 IU once a day	Take mixed tocopherols, the more active type of vitamin E. Consult your healthcare provider first if you are taking a blood thinner.

LUPUS

The immune system of people who have lupus, also known as *systemic lupus erythematosus,* or SLE, is unable to distinguish between foreign antigens and the person's own body. As a result, the immune system creates antibodies that attack otherwise healthy tissues and organs. The resulting inflammation can cause permanent damage to almost any body part, including the blood, brain, heart, joints, kidneys, liver, lungs, and skin.

About 1.5 million Americans have lupus—approximately 1 in 200 people. It appears most often in people between the ages of fifteen and forty-four, and it affects African Americans and Asians more often than people from other races. It also affects more women than men. In fact, 90 percent of people with SLE are women ages fifteen to forty-five.

The following are common signs and symptoms of lupus:

- Chest pain
- Cold hands and feet (20 percent have Raynaud's syndrome)
- Depression
- Dry eyes and mouth
- Easy bruising
- Edema (tissue swelling)
- Fatigue
- Fever
- Hair loss
- Pain
- Premenstrual flare-ups
- Rashes
- Sun sensitivity

There is also no simple, definitive test to diagnose lupus, and unfortunately, the disease can often be mistaken for other illnesses for months or even years. The course of the disease varies from person to person. Although there is no cure for this chronic autoimmune disease, treatment can make life much more comfortable. Anti-inflammatory or immunosuppressive drugs may be prescribed to shorten or even prevent flare-ups. Steroids may be prescribed, but are usually avoided because of their extensive side effects. Doctors also focus on treating the disease's symptoms. The following supplements may be helpful in managing lupus.

SUPPLEMENTS TO TREAT LUPUS

Supplements	Dosage	Considerations
Alpha-linolenic acid (ALA) as flaxseed oil*	1,000 mg once a day	It is important to maintain the proper ratio of omega-6 fatty acids to omega-3 fatty acids. (See page 129.) Flaxseed oil may interfere with anticoagulants, work as a laxative, or affect blood sugar levels. Consult your healthcare provider or pharmacist before taking this supplement.
Astragalus*	200 to 500 mg standardized extract three times a day	Do not use after organ transplant or if you have an allergy to gum tragacanth. Also do not use for an extended period of time. Speak to your healthcare provider to see if any of the medications you take make it unwise to use astragalus.
D-ribose	15,000 mg three times a day	D-ribose can lower blood sugar levels, so check with your healthcare provider before taking this supplement with any diabetes medication, especially insulin.
Eleuthero*	50 to 200 mg once a day	Do not use if you have a history of heart disease, hypertension, sleep apnea, narcolepsy, mania, or schizophrenia; if you are pregnant or breastfeeding; or if you are taking blood thinners.

EPA/DHA (fish oil)*	1,000 to 5,000 mg once a day	Choose a source that contains vitamin E to prevent oxidation. In high doses, fatty acids may cause the blood to thin. If you are taking a blood thinner, do not take EPA/DHA without direct instructions from your doctor. It is important to maintain the proper ratio of omega-6 fatty acids to omega-3 fatty acids. (See page 129.)
Gamma-linolenic acid (GLA) as evening primrose oil (EPO)*	240 to 720 mg once a day	It is important to maintain the proper ratio of omega-6 fatty acids to omega-3 fatty acids. (See page 129.) Evening primrose oil may interfere with some medications, such as nonsteroidal anti-inflammatories; can act as a blood thinner; and can lower the seizure threshold. Consult your healthcare provider or pharmacist before taking this supplement.
Glucosamine sulfate	300 to 900 mg once a day	If you are allergic to shellfish, be sure to choose a supplement that is not shellfish based. Consult use with your healthcare provider if you have diabetes, because glucosamine can alter blood sugar levels.
Glutamine	1,000 to 5,000 mg once a day	If you have a sensitivity to monosodium glutamate (MSG), use glutamine with caution. If you are taking medications for seizures, take glutamine only under the direction of your doctor.
Gotu kola	60 to 120 mg once a day	Do not take gotu kola if you have liver disease.
Indole-3-carbinol (1-3-C)	300 mg once a day	Low-dose supplementation may cause a mild elevation of liver enzymes and a skin rash.
Magnesium	400 to 800 mg once a day	Consult your healthcare provider for dosage if you have kidney disease. Discontinue use and see your doctor if you experience abdominal pain. Take a lower dose if it causes diarrhea.
Olive leaf extract*	500 mg twice a day containing 20 mg of oleuropein per capsule	Olive leaf extracts can interact with many prescription medications, and may increase the effects of blood thinners. Consult your healthcare provider before using olive leaf extract if you are taking any medication. Don't use if you are pregnant or breastfeeding.
Probiotics	20 billion units once a day	If taking an antibiotic, take the probiotics at least two hours before or two hours after using the antibiotics. Do not take them at the same time.
Selenium	100 to 200 mcg once a day	Do not exceed 200 mcg a day without consulting your healthcare provider.
Vitamin C	500 to 1,500 mg twice a day	Do not take high doses if you are prone to kidney stones or gout. High doses can also cause diarrhea.

| Vitamin E* | 400 IU once a day | Take mixed tocopherols, the more active type of vitamin E. Consult your healthcare provider first if you are taking a blood thinner. |

*This supplement can have a blood-thinning action. See page 328 for more information.

MACULAR DEGENERATION

Macular degeneration is the progressive destruction of the *macula,* an oval spot in the eye that is responsible for central vision and is specialized for fine detail. Because this condition usually affects the elderly, it is also referred to as *age-related macular degeneration,* or AMD. In the United States, macular degeneration is the leading cause of vision loss and blindness in those over sixty-five years of age.

There are two types of macular degeneration. *Dry (non-neovascular) macular degeneration* is an early stage of the disease, and is diagnosed when deteriorating tissue begins to accumulate as yellowish spots known as drusen. *Wet (neovascular) macular degeneration* occurs when new blood vessels grow beneath the retina, leaking blood and fluid, and permanently damaging retinal cells.

Macular degeneration usually results in a slow and painless loss of vision, although more rapid vision loss sometimes occurs. Early signs of AMD-related vision loss include shadowy areas in central vision, or unusually fuzzy or distorted vision. Even before symptoms appear, your healthcare provider may detect AMD through a retinal examination.

As already mentioned, macular degeneration is usually associated with aging. Specific variants of one or more genes have also been linked to AMD. Other risk factors include smoking, high blood pressure, light eye color, not wearing sunglasses when exposed to sunlight, obesity, the use of certain drugs, and a poor diet—especially one that is high in fat. Many researchers believe that certain nutrients can help lower the risk for AMD.

SUPPLEMENTS TO PREVENT AND TREAT MACULAR DEGENERATION

Supplements	Dosage	Considerations
Alpha lipoic acid	300 to 400 mg once a day	Alpha lipoic acid can interact with medication taken for diabetes and thyroid problems. Speak to your healthcare provider to see if any of the medications you take make it unwise to use this supplement.
Bilberry*	120 mg once a day	Bilberry may interfere with iron absorption and blood clotting. High doses should be used with caution by people with bleeding disorders.

Carnitine*	200 mg once a day	Have your healthcare provider measure your TMAO levels before starting long-term supplementation with carnitine.
Coenzyme Q_{10}*	100 mg once a day	If you are on blood-thinning medications, speak to your healthcare provider before using CoQ_{10}. Since some medications can cause a deficiency of this nutrient, speak to your healthcare provider to determine if you might need a larger dose.
Copper	2 mg once a day	Your copper-to-zinc ratio is very important for your health. (See page 119 for details.) Also, do not take copper supplement cupric oxide, which has a very low bioavailability.
Cysteine	1,000 to 3,000 mg once a day as n-acetylcysteine, or NAC	When taking NAC supplements, also take extra vitamin C, copper, and zinc.
EPA/DHA (fish oil)*	1,000 to 2,000 mg once a day	Choose a source that contains vitamin E to prevent oxidation.
Ginkgo biloba*	120 mg once a day	Do not use with blood-thinning medications or supplements.
Grape seed extract*	100 to 200 mg once a day	Caution is advised when taking supplements containing grape seed polyphenols with vitamin C if you have hypertension. The combination may increase your blood pressure. Do not use with blood-thinning medications or supplements.
Lutein	6 to 12 mg once a day	
Melatonin	1 to 3 mg taken thirty to sixty minutes before bedtime	Melatonin can interact with other drugs, so speak to your healthcare provider before taking this supplement.
Selenium	200 to 300 mcg once a day	Do not exceed 200 mcg a day without consulting your healthcare provider.
Taurine	3,000 mg once a day	Take between meals. Discontinue use if you suddenly have feelings of chest or throat tightness or if you break out in hives. Do not take with aspirin. Have your healthcare provider measure levels before starting taurine therapy.
Vitamin A and mixed carotenoids	5,000 to 10,000 IU—half vitamin A and half mixed carotenoids—once a day	Use caution when taking vitamin A supplements because they have the potential to be toxic. Do not take for extended periods of time. Do not take more than 8,000 IU a day if you have liver disease, are a smoker, or have been exposed to asbestos.
Vitamin B_6 (pyridoxine)	50 mg twice a day	A study showed a relationship between high serum homocysteine levels and age-related macular degeneration. Taking vitamins B_6, B_9, and B_{12} together can lower homocysteine levels. Do not take more than 500 mg a day. If you are taking L-dopa for Parkinson's disease, do not take

		B6 without first consulting your doctor. High doses can deplete your body of other vitamins in the B complex, so take a B-complex vitamin twice a day. If you know you have the MTHFR genotype, take in the form of pyridoxal 5-phosphate.
Vitamin B9 (folate)	200 to 400 mcg twice a day	High doses can deplete your body of other vitamins in the B complex, so take a B-complex vitamin twice a day. If you know you have the MTHFR genotype, take the active form of L-5-methyltetrahydrofolate.
Vitamin B12 (cobalamin)	500 mcg twice a day	High doses can deplete your body of other vitamins in the B complex, so take a B-complex vitamin twice a day. If you know you have the MTHFR genotype, take in the form of methylcobalamin.
Vitamin C	1,000 to 1,500 mg twice a day	Do not take high doses if you are prone to kidney stones or gout. High doses can also cause diarrhea.
Vitamin E*	400 to 800 IU once a day	Take mixed tocopherols, the more active type of vitamin E. Consult healthcare provider first if you are taking a blood thinner.
Zeaxanthin	4 mg once a day	
Zinc	25 to 80 mg once a day as zinc picolinate or zinc citrate	Your copper-to-zinc ratio is very important to your health. (See page 119 for details.) If you are taking zinc and iron supplements, take one in the morning and one in the evening. (Taking them together reduces the efficiency of both.)

*This supplement can have a blood-thinning action. See page 328 for more information.

MEMORY PROBLEMS

See Alzheimer's Disease.

MENSTRUAL CRAMPS

Menstrual cramps are dull or throbbing pains felt throughout the lower abdomen. They affect almost 50 percent of menstruating women just before and during their periods. The medical term for menstrual cramps is *dysmenorrhea*. The pain tends to be intermittent, and while it's strongest in the abdomen, it can radiate to the back and inner thighs. The severity of the symptoms varies among women. Common additional problems include backache, headache, dizziness, nausea, vomiting, and diarrhea. These symptoms may resolve after two or three hours, but they can last up to three days.

A study showed that people who eat breakfast every day have less severe dysmenorrhea than those who eat breakfast infrequently. You can also reduce the severity of this problem by taking the supplements recommended in the table below.

SUPPLEMENTS TO TREAT MENSTRUAL CRAMPS		
Supplements	Dosage	Considerations
B-complex vitamins	50 mg twice a day	I suggest taking a multivitamin along with your B-complex vitamins.
Calcium	500 mg once or twice a day	Although most people are deficient in calcium, there is a danger in taking too much calcium. Do not ingest more than 1,000 to 1,200 mg of calcium a day.
EPA/DHA (fish oil)*	2,000 to 3,000 mg once a day. Begin taking this supplement seven to ten days before your period begins.	Choose a source that contains vitamin E to prevent oxidation.
Gamma-linolenic acid (GLA) as evening primrose oil (EPO)*	500 to 1,000 mg once a day	It is important to maintain the proper ratio of omega-6 fatty acids to omega-3 fatty acids. (See page 129.) Evening primrose oil may interfere with some medications, such as nonsteroidal anti-inflammatories; can act as a blood thinner; and can lower the seizure threshold. Consult your healthcare provider or pharmacist before taking this supplement.
Ginger*	100 mg once a day	Ginger can act as a blood thinner. Check with your healthcare provider or pharmacist before taking this supplement.
Magnesium	300 to 500 mg once a day as magnesium glycinate	Consult your healthcare provider for dosage if you have kidney disease. Discontinue use and see your doctor if you experience abdominal pain. Take a lower dose if it causes diarrhea.
Pycnogenol (OPCs)*	30 mg once a day	Pycnogenol may affect blood sugar levels.
Valerian	Take as a combination herbal remedy that also includes black cohosh, blackhaw, cramp bark, and rose tea.	Valerian can cause sedation, so use with caution if you are taking other sedatives, antihistamines, antidepressants, or anti-anxiety agents.
Vitamin B_{12} (cobalamin)	500 mcg twice a day	High doses can deplete your body of other vitamins in the B complex, so take a B-complex vitamin twice a day.
Vitamin E*	200 to 400 IU once a day	Take mixed tocopherols, the more active type of vitamin E. Consult your healthcare provider first if you are taking a blood thinner.

*This supplement can have a blood-thinning action. See page 328 for more information.

MIGRAINE HEADACHES

A migraine headache is a moderate to severe headache, usually occurring on one side of the head only. It can last from several hours to three days, and is often accompanied by gastrointestinal problems such as nausea and vomiting. Other symptoms characteristic of migraines include pain that has a pulsating or throbbing quality, pain that worsens with physical activity, and sensitivity to light and sound.

Fifteen to thirty minutes before the migraine begins, some people experience an *aura*—a "warning" that comes in the form of sparkling flashes of light, dazzling zigzag lines, slowly spreading blind spots, tingling sensations in an arm or leg, or even speech problems. Although auras typically occur before the onset of a migraine, they sometimes continue after the headache starts or even occur after it begins.

Headaches are one of the most common reasons patients see a healthcare provider, and about 30 million Americans suffer from migraine headaches. The prevalence is highest in woman and in people that live in North America.

Experts are still debating the causes and mechanisms of migraine headaches. We do know that migraines can have various triggers, including hormonal changes; the consumption of certain foods, such as aged cheese, wine, chocolate, fermented and marinated foods, and monosodium glutamate; stress; sensory stimuli such as bright lights and sun glare; changes in the sleep-wake cycle; poor sleep practices; changes in the weather; the use of certain medications; aspartame; MSG; low melatonin levels; and neurotransmitter imbalances.

If you suffer from migraine headaches, it makes sense to avoid potential triggers. Some people have found that consuming caffeine can stop some attacks. In addition, certain nutrients are known to help prevent the occurrence of migraines.

SUPPLEMENTS TO TREAT MIGRAINE HEADACHES

Supplements	Dosage	Considerations
Alpha lipoic acid	300 mg once a day	Alpha lipoic acid can interact with medication taken for diabetes and thyroid problems. Speak to your healthcare provider to see if any of the medications you take make it unwise to use this supplement.
B-complex vitamins	50 mg twice a day	I suggest taking a multivitamin along with your B-complex vitamins.

Calcium	500 mg twice a day	Although most people are deficient in calcium, you can take too much calcium. Do not ingest more than 1,000 to 1,200 mg of calcium a day.
Carnitine*	1,000 to 3,000 once a day	Have your healthcare provider measure your TMAO levels before starting long-term supplementation with carnitine.
CBD oil (hemp oil)	5 to 500 mg a day in the form of sublingual drops. Start with 5 mg and increase slowly until you find relief.	CBD is generally well tolerated and safe for consumption, even in high doses and with continuous use. However, do not exceed 500 mg a day without consulting your healthcare provider. Make sure to buy a product marked "hemp oil (aerial parts)."
Coenzyme Q_{10}*	100 mg three times a day	If you are on blood-thinning medications, speak to your healthcare provider before using CoQ_{10}. Since some medications can cause a deficiency of this nutrient, speak to your healthcare provider to determine if you might need a larger dose.
Curcumin/Turmeric*	100 to 1,000 mg once a day of a formula that includes piperine or bioperine to boost absorption	Do not take curcumin with blood-thinning medications or supplements. Curcumin can also interact with other medications, so speak to your healthcare provider before taking this supplement.
EPA/DHA (fish oil)*	1,000 to 2,000 mg once a day	Choose a source that contains vitamin E to prevent oxidation.
Feverfew*	100 mg once a day standardized to 0.2 to 0.4 percent parthenolide	If you are allergic to plants in the daisy family (such as chamomile or ragweed), do not take feverfew. This supplement also has the potential to interact with anticoagulant drugs such as coumadin. To stop use, taper doses if you've been taking the supplement for a long time. Abrupt cessation may lead to nervousness, headache, insomnia, or joint pain.
Ginger*	500 mg twice a day	Ginger can act as a blood thinner. Check with your healthcare provider or pharmacist before taking this supplement.
Ginkgo biloba*	60 to 120 mg once or twice a day	Do not use with blood-thinning medications or supplements.
Magnesium	600 to 800 mg once a day	Consult your healthcare provider for dosage if you have kidney disease. Discontinue use and see your doctor if you experience abdominal pain. Take a lower dose if it causes diarrhea.
Melatonin	1 to 3 mg taken thirty to sixty minutes before bedtime	Melatonin can interact with other drugs, so speak to your healthcare provider before taking this supplement.
Probiotics	20 billion units once a day	If taking an antibiotic, take the probiotics at least two hours before or two hours after using the antibiotics. Do not take them at the same time.

Selenium	200 mcg once a day	Do not exceed 200 mcg a day without consulting your healthcare provider.
Vitamin B₂ (riboflavin)	50 to 100 mg twice a day	High doses can deplete your body of other B vitamins, so take a B-complex vitamin twice a day.
Vitamin B₉ (folic acid)	200 to 400 mcg twice a day	High doses can deplete your body of other B vitamins, so take a B-complex vitamin twice a day.
Vitamin C	500 to 1,500 mg twice a day	Do not take high doses if you are prone to kidney stones or gout. High doses can also cause diarrhea.
Vitamin D₃	Have your blood levels measured by your healthcare provider, who will determine proper dosage.	
Vitamin E*	400 to 800 IU once a day	Take mixed tocopherols, the more active type of vitamin E. Consult your healthcare provider first if you are taking a blood thinner.
Zinc	25 mg twice a day as zinc picolinate or zinc citrate	Your copper-to-zinc ratio is very important to your health. (See page 119 for details.) If you are taking zinc and iron supplements, take one in the morning and one in the evening. (Taking them together reduces the efficiency of both.)

*This supplement can have a blood-thinning action. See page 328 for more information.

MULTIPLE SCLEROSIS

Multiple sclerosis (MS) is a degenerative disease of the nervous system that affects the brain, spinal cord, and optic nerves. In this disorder, the myelin sheaths that protect the nerve fibers degenerate, leaving the nerves vulnerable to damage. Areas of the body that are controlled by the damaged nerves become impaired. Symptoms vary, depending on which nerves are involved, and commonly include visual disturbances, muscle fatigue, slurred speech, numbness, dizziness, thinking and memory problems, and impaired balance and coordination. Women are more commonly affected than men, with 60 percent of people with MS being female. The disorder is usually diagnosed in young adults between the ages of twenty and forty.

Although the exact cause of MS is not known, most researchers believe that an unknown virus triggers the autoimmune process responsible for damaging the myelin sheaths. Heredity seems to play a role: 15 percent of those with this disease have a close relative who is also affected. It is estimated that ten to fifteen genes may affect the risk of an individual developing MS.

Multiple sclerosis is much more prevalent in colder climates. This may be due to the lower levels of vitamin D generally found in people in northern areas because of decreased exposure to the sun. Furthermore, a meta-analysis showed that exposure to organic solvents was associated with an increased risk. Allergies to mold, tobacco, and house dust may also be triggering factors for MS, and exacerbations of this disorder may be related to allergic reactions to foods.

Currently, there is no cure for MS, although a number of promising treatments are being investigated. Nutritional supplements, moderate exercise, and the avoidance of stress have all been shown to be helpful, especially during the early stages of the disease. Proper diet is also important. Several studies have shown that a low-fat, high-fiber diet can help decrease the number of new MS lesions. Saturated fats, especially those found in meat (red meat in particular) and dairy products, should be avoided, as well as hydrogenated and partially hydrogenated fats. The diet should include lots of fresh fruits and vegetables, especially leafy greens, as well as foods that contain beneficial omega-3 fatty acids. It can also be helpful to avoid gluten.

SUPPLEMENTS TO TREAT MULTIPLE SCLEROSIS

Supplements	Dosage	Considerations
Alpha lipoic acid	300 to 400 mg once a day	Alpha lipoic acid can interact with medication taken for diabetes and thyroid problems. Speak to your healthcare provider to see if any of the medications you take make it unwise to use this supplement.
Carnitine*	2,000 mg to 3,000 mg twice a day	Have your healthcare provider measure your TMAO levels before starting long-term supplementation with carnitine.
CBD oil (hemp oil)	5 to 500 mg a day in the form of sublingual drops. Start with 5 mg and increase slowly until you find relief.	CBD is generally well tolerated and safe for consumption, even in high doses and with continuous use. However, do not exceed 500 mg a day without consulting your healthcare provider. Make sure to buy a product marked "hemp oil (aerial parts)."
Cocoa	2.5 g (0.1 ounce) unsweetened cocoa powder (about 0.5 teaspoon)	Cocoa can interact with some medications, so speak to your healthcare provider or pharmacist before starting long-term supplementation. Cocoa also contains caffeine, which can cause side effects in some people.
Coenzyme Q_{10}*	300 to 500 mg once a day	If you are on blood-thinning medications, speak to your healthcare provider before using CoQ_{10}. Since some medications can cause a deficiency of this nutrient, speak to your healthcare provider to determine if you might need a larger dose.

Copper	1 to 2 mg once a day	Your copper-to-zinc ratio is very important for your health. (See page 119 for details.) Also, do not take copper supplement cupric oxide, which has a very low bioavailability.
Cysteine	200 mg once a day as N-acetylcysteine, or NAC	When taking NAC supplements, also take extra vitamin C, copper, and zinc.
D-ribose	15,000 mg three times a day	D-ribose can lower blood sugar levels, so check with your healthcare provider before taking this supplement with any diabetes medication, especially insulin.
EPA/DHA (fish oil)*	1,000 to 3,000 mg once a day	Choose a source that contains vitamin E to prevent oxidation.
Gamma-linolenic acid (GLA) as evening primrose oil (EPO)*	300 to 720 mg once a day	It is important to maintain the proper ratio of omega-6 fatty acids to omega-3 fatty acids. (See page 129.) Evening primrose oil may interfere with some medications, such as nonsteroidal anti-inflammatories; can act as a blood thinner; and can lower the seizure threshold. Consult your healthcare provider or pharmacist before taking this supplement.
Ginkgo biloba*	120 mg twice a day	Do not use with blood-thinning medications or supplements.
Glutathione	250 to 500 mg as liposomal glutathione in the form of a liquid or lozenge.	Check with your doctor before starting glutathione therapy if you have diabetes, hypertension, kidney disease, or liver disease. Do not use if you have a sulfite sensitivity.
Magnesium	400 to 600 mg once a day	Consult your healthcare provider for dosage if you have kidney disease. Discontinue use and see your doctor if you experience abdominal pain. Take a lower dose if it causes diarrhea.
Phosphatidylcholine (PC)	500 to 1,000 mg once a day	Use with caution if you have malabsorption problems, as this could exacerbate them.
Phosphatidylserine (PS)	200 to 300 mg once a day	PS can interact with many drugs. Speak to your healthcare provider before taking it.
Selenium	200 mcg once a day	Do not exceed 200 mcg a day without consulting your healthcare provider.
Threonine	3 to 7.5 g a day as L-Threonine	To determine the exact dose that you need, have your healthcare provider measure your amino acid levels.
Vitamin B_3 (niacin)	50 mg twice a day	High doses can deplete your body of other vitamins in the B complex, so take a B-complex vitamin twice a day.
Vitamin B_6 (pyridoxine)	50 mg twice a day	Do not take more than 500 mg a day. If you are taking L-dopa for Parkinson's disease, do not take B_6 without first consulting your doctor.

		High doses can deplete your body of other vitamins in the B complex, so take a B-complex vitamin twice a day.
Vitamin B$_9$ (folic acid)	200 to 400 mcg twice a day	High doses can deplete your body of other vitamins in the B complex, so take a B-complex vitamin twice a day.
Vitamin B$_{12}$ (cobalamin)	500 mcg twice a day	Check with your physician to see if intramuscular (IM) injection may be more beneficial for you. High doses can deplete your body of other B vitamins, so take a B-complex vitamin twice a day.
Vitamin C	500 mg twice a day	Do not take high doses if you are prone to kidney stones or gout. High doses can also cause diarrhea.
Vitamin D$_3$	Have your blood levels measured by your healthcare provider, who will determine proper dosage.	
Vitamin E*	400 IU once a day	Take mixed tocopherols, the more active type of vitamin E. Consult your healthcare provider first if you are taking a blood thinner.
Zinc	10 to 15 mg once a day as zinc picolinate or zinc citrate	Your copper-to-zinc ratio is very important to your health. (See page 119 for details.) If you are taking zinc and iron supplements, take one in the morning and one in the evening. (Taking them together reduces the efficiency of both.)

*This supplement can have a blood-thinning action. See page 328 for more information.

MUSCLE CRAMPS

See Leg Cramps.

MYASTHENIA GRAVIS

Myasthenia gravis is a chronic autoimmune disease in which the immune system attacks the body's own proteins as foreign antigens. Specifically, the immune system targets and interferes with acetylcholine, a neurotransmitter that transmits messages between the nerves and muscles. In myasthenia gravis, the body produces antibodies against its own acetylcholine receptors and blocks them from binding acetylcholine. This results in moderate to severe muscle weakness that can occur throughout the body. Symptoms tend to be exacerbated by activity and improved with rest.

The muscle weakness is usually first seen in the eye. The following are common symptoms of this disease process.

- Blurred or double vision
- Chronic muscle fatigue
- Drooping eyelid
- Hoarse voice
- Impaired speech
- Shortness of breath or difficulty breathing
- Trouble chewing and swallowing
- Unstable or waddling gait
- Weakness and tingling sensation in the arms and legs

Myasthenia gravis affects an estimated 20 individuals per 100,000 people in the United States. Women typically develop the disease more frequently than men and at a younger age. Although initial signs of myasthenia gravis may emerge at any age, women most commonly develop symptoms under the age of forty, while symptoms among men usually develop later in life, after the age of sixty.

Myasthenia gravis can be treated by either addressing the symptoms or trying to suppress the autoimmune disease. The symptoms can be treated by increasing muscle strength through medication. To suppress the disease, doctors can prescribe immunosuppressant drugs, which discourage the immune system from attacking acetylcholine. However, because immunosuppressant drugs can have side effects, they are usually recommended for only a short period of time and when found to be necessary. Anticholinesterase agents, on the other hand, both treat the weakened muscles and suppress the immune system. Newer and more costly therapies include plasma exchange and intravenous immunoglobulin therapy. A patient could also decide to have the thymus gland removed, a procedure that is often effective—but it can sometimes take years for the effects to be felt. Newer therapies being considered for treatment of myasthenia gravis include rituximab (Rituxan) and eculizumab (Soliris). Speak to your doctor about these promising therapies.

Because myasthenia gravis can restrict vitally important muscles, such as the lungs, patients can have life-threatening episodes. In these situations, immediate professional medical help is critical.

SUPPLEMENTS TO TREAT MYASTHENIA GRAVIS

Supplements	Dosage	Considerations
Alpha-linolenic acid (ALA) as flaxseed oil*	1,000 mg once a day	It is important to maintain the proper ratio of omega-6 fatty acids to omega-3 fatty acids. (See page 129.) Flaxseed oil may interfere with anticoagulants, work as a laxative, or affect blood sugar levels. Consult your healthcare provider or pharmacist before taking this supplement.

Astragalus*	200 to 500 mg standardized extract three times a day	Do not use after organ transplant or if you have an allergy to gum tragacanth. Also do not use for an extended period of time. Speak to your healthcare provider to see if any of the medications you take make it unwise to use astragalus.
Cat's claw*	50 mg twice a day	Do not take if you have leukemia or if you are pregnant or breastfeeding. Do not take if you have a bleeding disorder or are taking a blood-thinning drug or supplement. Cat's claw can lower blood pressure, so use with caution if you are taking a drug that lowers blood pressure. Discontinue use two weeks before surgery.
Coenzyme Q_{10}*	300 to 400 mg a day	If you are on blood-thinning medications, speak to your healthcare provider before using CoQ_{10}. Since some medications can cause a deficiency of this nutrient, speak to your healthcare provider to determine if you might need a larger dose.
Curcumin/Turmeric*	100 to 500 mg once a day of a formula that includes piperine or bioperine to boost absorption	Do not take curcumin with blood-thinning medications or supplements. Curcumin can also interact with other medications, so speak to your healthcare provider before taking this supplement.
EGCG (green tea extract)*	800 mg a day EGCG	Green tea extract can interact with a number of drugs. Check with your healthcare provider before taking this supplement.
Eleuthero*	50 to 200 mg once a day	Do not use if you have a history of heart disease, hypertension, sleep apnea, narcolepsy, mania, or schizophrenia, or if you are pregnant or breastfeeding.
EPA/DHA (fish oil)*	1,000 to 5,000 mg once a day	Choose a source that contains vitamin E to prevent oxidation. In high doses, fatty acids may cause the blood to thin. If you are taking a blood thinner, do not take EPA/DHA without direct instructions from your doctor. It is important to maintain the proper ratio of omega-6 fatty acids to omega-3 fatty acids. (See page 129.)
Gamma-linolenic acid (GLA) as evening primrose oil (EPO)*	240 to 720 mg once a day	It is important to maintain the proper ratio of omega-6 fatty acids to omega-3 fatty acids. (See page 129.) Evening primrose oil may interfere with some medications, such as nonsteroidal anti-inflammatories; can act as a blood thinner; and can lower the seizure threshold. Consult your healthcare provider or pharmacist before taking this supplement.

Glucosamine sulfate	300 to 900 mg once a day	If you are allergic to shellfish, be sure to choose a supplement that is not shellfish based. Consult use with your healthcare provider if you have diabetes, because glucosamine can alter blood sugar levels.
Glutamine	1 to 5 g once a day	If you have a sensitivity to monosodium glutamate (MSG), use glutamine with caution. If you are taking medications for seizures, take glutamine only under the direction of your doctor.
Magnesium	400 to 800 mg once a day	Consult your healthcare provider for dosage if you have kidney disease. Discontinue use and see your doctor if you experience abdominal pain. Take a lower dose if it causes diarrhea.
Olive leaf extract*	500 mg twice a day containing 20 mg of oleuropein per capsule	Olive leaf extracts can interact with prescription medications, and may increase the effects of blood thinners. Consult your healthcare provider before using olive leaf extract if you are taking any medication. Don't use if you are pregnant or breast-feeding.
Probiotics	20 billion units once a day	If taking an antibiotic, take the probiotics at least two hours before or two hours after using the antibiotics. Do not take them at the same time.
Selenium	200 to 300 mcg once a day	Do not exceed 200 mcg a day without consulting your healthcare provider.
Vitamin C	500 to 1,500 mg twice a day	Do not take high doses if you are prone to kidney stones or gout. High doses can also cause diarrhea.
Vitamin D$_3$	Have your blood levels measured by your healthcare provider, who will determine proper dosage.	
Vitamin E*	400 IU once a day	Take mixed tocopherols, the more active type of vitamin E. Consult your healthcare provider first if you are taking a blood thinner.

*This supplement can have a blood-thinning action. See page 328 for more information.

NON-INSULIN-DEPENDENT DIABETES

See Diabetes Mellitus.

OBESITY

See Weight Gain and Obesity.

OSTEOARTHRITIS

There are over 100 different types of arthritis. More than 66 million Americans (almost one in three adults) have some type of arthritis. *Osteoarthritis* is the most common form and is the leading cause of joint pain and disability in middle-aged and older individuals.

Also known as *osteoarthrosis, degenerative arthritis,* and *degenerative joint disease,* osteoarthritis is a gradual wearing down of *cartilage*—the firm, elastic tissue that connects bones with muscles and protects the joints. This can cause swelling and inflammation of the joints, reduced mobility, and muscle spasms. Simple movement often causes pain, which is usually characterized by either a sharp ache or burning sensation. Painful *bone spurs*—abnormal growths of bone—can form as well. It is most likely to occur in the hips, knees, spine, feet, and hands. Osteoarthritis occurs equally in men and women. However, symptoms appear to be worse and occur earlier in women than in men.

There are two forms of osteoarthritis: primary and secondary. *Primary osteoarthritis* is due to the wear and tear of the body as part of the aging process, which is why it usually starts after the age of forty-five. When the cartilage becomes damaged, enzymes are released that destroy collagen, the major component of connective tissue. As an individual ages, the ability to restore and make normal collagen decreases.

Secondary osteoarthritis has a specific cause, such as an injury or illness. Any of the following can lead to secondary osteoarthritis:

- Congenital abnormalities
- Formation of calcium deposits in joints and surrounding tissues
- Infection
- Long-term use of medications
- Obesity
- Surgery
- Trauma
- Toxic metals

People with osteoarthritis tend to feel best in the morning, with symptoms becoming progressively worse as the day continues. Osteoarthritis is irreversible, so treatment aims to reduce pain and improve mobility.

Diet has been shown to play a role in osteoarthritis. Eating the wrong foods can make this condition worse, while eating wisely can help you better manage symptoms. Decrease your intake of acid-producing foods—such as sugar and meat—and increase your consumption of foods that are anti-inflammatory, such as fruits, vegetables, and olive oil. The following are the foods most commonly linked to arthritis. If these foods make your symptoms worse, try to avoid them.

- Beef
- Chocolate
- Corn
- Dairy products
- Eggs
- Green beans
- Nuts (especially peanuts)
- Oranges
- Soy
- Sugar
- Wheat (avoiding all gluten can be helpful)
- Yeast (both baker's and brewer's)
- Foods in the nightshade family: eggplant, paprika, peppers, potatoes, and tomatoes

Losing weight—and therefore placing less pressure on joints—has been shown to be one of the most beneficial therapies for osteoarthritis. Nutritional therapies can also be effective.

SUPPLEMENTS TO TREAT OSTEOARTHRITIS		
Supplements	Dosage	Considerations
Bitter melon	500 to 1,000 mg capsule daily, or 50 to 100 ml juice daily	Do not use if you are pregnant or breastfeeding, if you are male and trying to initiate a pregnancy, or if you are female and trying to get pregnant. If you have blood sugar problems, monitor your blood sugar on a regular basis during treatment.
Boron	1,000 mcg once a day	
Boswellia*	400 mg once a day	Avoid boswellia if you are pregnant, because it can induce miscarriage. Do not take with NSAIDs.
Cat's claw*	50 mg twice a day	Do not take if you have leukemia or if you are pregnant or breastfeeding. Do not take if you have a blooding disorder or are taking a blood-thinning drug or supplement. Cat's claw can lower blood pressure, so use with caution if you are taking a drug that lowers blood pressure. Discontinue use two weeks before surgery.
Chondroitin sulfate	500 to 2,000 mg once a day	Do not take if you have asthma or prostate cancer, or if you are pregnant or breastfeeding. Also avoid if you are taking a blood-thinning drug or supplement.
Copper	1 to 2 mg once a day	Your copper-to-zinc ratio is very important for your health. (See page 119 for details.) Also, do not take copper supplement cupric oxide, which has a very low bioavailability.

Curcumin/Turmeric*	100 to 500 mg once a day of a formula that includes piperine or bioperine to boost absorption	Do not take curcumin with blood-thinning medications or supplements. Curcumin can also interact with other medications, so speak to your healthcare provider before taking this supplement.
EPA/DHA (fish oil)*	1,000 to 2,000 mg once a day	Choose a source that contains vitamin E to prevent oxidation.
Gamma-linolenic acid (GLA) as evening primrose oil (EPO)*	240 to 720 mg once a day	It is important to maintain the proper ratio of omega-6 fatty acids to omega-3 fatty acids. (See page 129.) Evening primrose oil may interfere with some medications, such as nonsteroidal anti-inflammatories; can act as a blood thinner; and can lower the seizure threshold. Consult your healthcare provider or pharmacist before taking this supplement.
Ginger*	100 mg once a day	Ginger can act as a blood thinner. Check with your healthcare provider or pharmacist before taking this supplement.
Glucosamine sulfate	1,000 mg three times a day	If you are allergic to shellfish, be sure to choose a supplement that is not shellfish based. Consult use with your healthcare provider if you have diabetes, because glucosamine can alter blood sugar levels.
Manganese	5 to 10 mg once a day	Use with caution if you have gallbladder or liver disease.
Methylsulfonylmethane (MSM)	1,000 to 3,000 mg three times a day	Use with caution if you are allergic to sulfur. Start by taking 500 mg three times a day, and gradually increase dose. Take with meals to avoid possible heartburn. May cause stomach upset in dosages larger than 6,000 mg.
Quercetin*	500 to 1,000 mg once a day	For best results, take with bromelain and vitamin C. Do not use with blood-thinning medications or supplements.
UltraInflamX	Follow instructions on bottle.	This product, by Metagenics (see Resources), provides macro- and micronutrient support for people with compromised gut function. Do not use if taking a diuretic.
Vitamin C	1,000 to 2,000 mg a day	Do not take high doses if you are prone to kidney stones or gout. High doses can also cause diarrhea.
Vitamin D_3	Have your blood levels measured by your healthcare provider, who will determine proper dosage.	
Zinc	35 to 50 mg a day as zinc picolinate or zinc citrate	Your copper-to-zinc ratio is very important to your health. (See page 119 for details.) If you are taking zinc and iron supplements, take one in the morning and one in the evening.

*This supplement can have a blood-thinning action. See page 328 for more information.

OSTEOPOROSIS

Osteoporosis is a progressive disease in which the bones become porous and brittle, making them susceptible to fracture. In North America, Europe, Australia, and Asia, it is estimated that one in every three women age fifty-five years old and older will have a fracture from osteoporosis in her lifetime. Globally, about 1.7 billion hip fractures occur each year. Although one-third of the cases of osteoporosis involve men, osteoporosis occurs primarily in postmenopausal women. In most cases, the bone loss does not cause any symptoms, so the condition usually goes unnoticed until a break occurs.

Osteoporosis tends to occur more often in small, fine-boned individuals, rather than those with larger, denser bones. It is particularly threatening to women after menopause because that is when the ovaries stop producing estrogen and progesterone, which help maintain and build bone mass.

Diet is believed to play an important part in the risk for osteoporosis. Nutrient deficiencies that can contribute to osteoporosis include calcium, which is essential for healthy bones, and vitamin D, which helps the body absorb calcium. If the body does not get a sufficient amount of calcium through foods and/or supplements, it will rob this essential mineral from the bones. Other dietary factors that increase the risk of osteoporosis include an excessive consumption of protein, salt, sugar, caffeine, and carbonated soft drinks. Foods containing oxalic acid—such as spinach, Swiss chard, beet and dandelion greens, rhubarb, asparagus, and chocolate—should also be avoided, because oxalic acid binds with calcium and decreases its absorption.

Smoking and alcohol consumption are additional risk factors for osteoporosis, as are a number of medications. Certain blood thinners, steroids, seizure medications, chemotherapy drugs, lithium, and tetracycline can all lead to bone loss.

An important but little-recognized risk factor for osteoporosis is chronic stress. Chronic stress creates abnormal levels of the stress hormone cortisol, which inhibits bone-building activity, leading to low bone density.

A genetic variant regulating a gene responsible for bone density also can play a role. Speak to your doctor about gene testing that can determine if you have a genetic predisposition for osteoporosis.

Some surgeries, too, can increase the risk of osteoporosis. Intestinal bypass surgery for weight control, removal of part or all of the intestine, and total thyroidectomy (removal of the thyroid gland) can all adversely affect bone density.

Finally, the following disorders are associated with an increased risk of developing osteoporosis.

- Anorexia nervosa
- Celiac disease
- COPD (chronic obstructive pulmonary disease)
- Crohn's disease
- Cushing's disease
- Diabetes mellitus
- Fat malabsorption
- Gallbladder disease
- History of chronic low back pain for more than ten years
- History of stress fractures
- Hypercalciuria (excessive loss of calcium in the urine)
- Hyperhomocysteinemia (high homocysteine level)
- Hypochlorhydria (inadequate production of hydrochloric acid)
- Kidney disease
- Lactose intolerance
- Multiple myeloma
- Primary biliary cirrhosis
- Rheumatoid arthritis
- Scoliosis

Although some risk factors, like age and gender, cannot be changed, there is much you can do to reduce the risk of osteoporosis. Improving your diet, decreasing your alcohol intake, and starting a bone-building exercise program—one that includes weight-bearing exercises like the use of elliptical training machines and walking—can improve your bone health. The supplements recommended in the table below can also be helpful.

SUPPLEMENTS TO TREAT OSTEOPOROSIS		
Supplements	Dosage	Considerations
Boron	5 to 10 mg once a day	
Calcium	500 mg twice a day	Although most people are deficient in calcium, there is a danger in taking too much calcium. Do not ingest more than 1,000 to 1,200 mg of calcium a day.
Copper	1 to 2 mg once a day	Your copper-to-zinc ratio is very important for your health. (See page 119 for details.) Also, do not take copper supplement cupric oxide, which has a very low bioavailability.
EPA/DHA (fish oil)*	500 to 1,000 mg once a day	Choose a source that contains vitamin E to prevent oxidation.
Gamma-linolenic acid (GLA) as evening primrose oil (EPO)*	240 mg once a day	It is important to maintain the proper ratio of omega-6 fatty acids to omega-3 fatty acids. (See page 129.) Evening primrose oil may interfere with some medications, such as nonsteroidal anti-inflammatories; can act as a blood thinner;

		and can lower the seizure threshold. Consult your healthcare provider or pharmacist before taking this supplement.
Magnesium	400 to 800 mg once a day	Consult your healthcare provider for dosage if you have kidney disease. Discontinue use and see your doctor if you experience abdominal pain. Take a lower dose if it causes diarrhea.
Manganese	5 to 10 mg once a day	Use with caution if you have gallbladder or liver disease.
Potassium	See your healthcare provider for dosage directions.	Consume foods high in potassium, such as those listed on page 85.
Vitamin B_6 (pyridoxine)	50 mg twice a day	Taking vitamins B_6, B_9, and B_{12} together can lower levels of homocysteine, which is a risk factor for osteoporosis. Do not take more than 500 mg a day. If you are taking L-dopa for Parkinson's disease, do not take B_6 without first consulting your doctor. High doses can deplete your body of other vitamins in the B complex, so take a B-complex vitamin twice a day. If you have high homocysteine levels, take in the form of pyridoxal 5-phosphate.
Vitamin B_9 (folate)	200 to 400 mcg twice a day	High doses can deplete your body of other vitamins in the B complex, so take a B-complex vitamin twice a day. If you have high homocysteine levels, take the active form L-5-methyltetrahydrofolate.
Vitamin B_{12} (cobalamin)	500 mcg twice a day	High doses can deplete your body of other vitamins in the B complex, so take a B-complex vitamin twice a day. If you have high homocysteine levels, take in the form of methylcobalamin.
Vitamin C	500 mg twice a day	Vitamin C increases calcium absorption by 100 percent, making it important in lowering the risk of osteoporosis. Do not take high does if you are prone to kidney stones or gout.
Vitamin D_3	Have your blood levels measured by your healthcare provider, who will determine proper dosage.	
Vitamin K*	150 mcg once a day of K_2 or MK-7. K_2 is particularly effective at maintaining bone structure.	If you are on blood-thinning medications, speak to your healthcare provider before using vitamin K.
Zinc	25 mg once a day as zinc picolinate or zinc citrate	Your copper-to-zinc ratio is very important to your health. (See page 119 for details.) If you are taking zinc and iron supplements, take one in the morning and one in the evening.

*This supplement can have a blood-thinning action. See page 328 for more information.

OVARIAN CYSTS

See Polycystic Ovary Syndrome.

PARKINSON'S DISEASE

Also known as *palsy* or *paralysis agitans,* Parkinson's disease is a degenerative condition that affects the nervous system. In people who do not have Parkinson's, the neurotransmitter *dopamine* and the neurotransmitter *acetylcholine* act together to transmit messages between nerve cells that control muscle function. Acetylcholine sends the signal that causes muscles to contract, while dopamine keeps the contractions at manageable levels. In people with Parkinson's, the amount of dopamine becomes inadequate as dopamine-producing neurons die, and the imbalance between these two chemicals causes involuntary tremors and muscle stiffness.

In the United States, this disorder affects at least 1 million people, and worldwide, more than 7 million are affected. Annually, about 50,000 new cases are reported in the US alone. Parkinson's disease is slightly more common in men than women, and white individuals are 1.5 percent more likely to get Parkinson's than individuals from other races. The incidence increases with age, with the average age of onset being about sixty.

Parkinson's disease usually starts with mild tremors in a hand or leg that worsen when the individual is resting. As the disease progresses, so does the trembling, which eventually affects both sides of the body. Later symptoms typically include stiffness, muscle weakness, a shaking head, and a shuffling gait. A "pill-rolling" movement in which the thumb and forefinger rub together is another characteristic of the disease. Speech becomes impaired, and everyday activities require assistance. The condition also involves cognitive disturbances, which lead to dementia in 80 percent of patients by the tenth year. Neuropsychiatric symptoms such as depression are also quite common.

The cause of Parkinson's disease is not known. One popular theory suggests that an accumulation of environmental toxins in the body may be a factor. Likewise, some of the biochemical changes that occur in Parkinson's disease are related to oxidative stress. For that reason, the disorder may be associated with a dysfunction of the mitochondria, one of the main sources of oxidative stress.

SUPPLEMENTS TO TREAT PARKINSON'S DISEASE

Supplements	Dosage	Considerations
Alpha lipoic acid	100 to 600 mg once a day	Alpha lipoic acid can interact with medication taken for diabetes and thyroid problems. Speak to your healthcare provider to see if any of the medications you take make it unwise to use this supplement.
Carnitine*	1,500 to 3,000 mg once a day	Have your healthcare provider measure your TMAO levels before starting long-term supplementation with carnitine.
CBD oil (hemp oil)	5 to 500 mg a day in the form of sublingual drops. Start with 5 mg and increase slowly until you find relief.	CBD is generally well tolerated and safe for consumption, even in high doses and with continuous use. However, do not exceed 500 mg a day without consulting your healthcare provider. Make sure to buy a product marked "hemp oil (aerial parts)."
Choline	2,600 mg a day	Choline supplementation can allow a 50-percent reduction of levodopa dose. Because choline can worsen levodopa side effects and lead to increased dyskinesia, you should work with your doctor to regulate the dose.
Cocoa	2.5 g (0.1 ounce) unsweetened cocoa powder (about 0.5 teaspoon)	Cocoa can interact with some medications, so speak to your healthcare provider or pharmacist before starting long-term supplementation. Cocoa also contains caffeine, which can cause side effects in some people.
Coenzyme Q_{10}*	400 to 1,600 mg once a day	If you are on blood-thinning medications, speak to your healthcare provider before using CoQ_{10}. Since some medications can cause a deficiency of this nutrient, speak to your healthcare provider to determine if you might need a larger dose.
Cysteine	500 to 2,000 mg once a day as n-acetylcysteine, or NAC	When taking NAC supplements, also take extra vitamin C, copper, and zinc. N-acetyl-cysteine directly encourages production of glutathione, which is present in lower levels in people with Parkinson's.
D-ribose	15,000 mg three times a day	D-ribose can lower blood sugar levels, so check with your healthcare provider before taking this supplement with any diabetes medication, especially insulin.
EPA/DHA (fish oil)*	2,000 mg once a day	Choose a source that contains vitamin E to prevent oxidation. Be aware that in large doses—above 3,000 mg a day—fish oil can act like a blood thinner.

Ginkgo biloba*	240 to 360 mg once a day	Do not use with blood-thinning medications or supplements. Ginkgo biloba can interact with a wide range of medications, so speak to your healthcare provider or pharmacist to learn if you can safely use this supplement.
Glutathione	250 to 500 mg of liposomal glutathione in liquid or pill form	Check with your doctor before starting glutathione therapy if you have diabetes, hypertension, kidney disease, or liver disease. Do not use if you have a sulfite sensitivity. If you opt to take NAC, there is no need to take glutathione.
Grape seed extract*	50 to 200 mg once a day	Do not use with blood-thinning medications or supplements.
Milk thistle	200 mg twice a day	Do not take if you are allergic to ragweed, chrysanthemums, marigolds, chamomile, or daisies. This supplement reduces the efficiency of certain blood pressure medication and other drugs. Speak to your healthcare provider or pharmacist before taking it.
Phosphatidylserine (PS)	300 to 500 mg once a day	PS can interact with many drugs, such as anticholinergic medications, and drugs given for Alzheimer's disease. Speak to your healthcare provider or pharmacist before taking it.
Probiotics	20 billion units once a day	If taking an antibiotic, take the probiotics at least two hours before or two hours after using the antibiotics. Do not take them at the same time.
Selenium	200 mcg once a day	Do not exceed 200 mcg a day without consulting your healthcare provider. Larger doses of selenium can lead to toxicity.
Vitamin C	500 to 2,500 mg twice a day	Vitamin C helps preserve the energy producing capacity of the mitochondria, which is affected by the administration of L-dopa. Do not take high doses of vitamin C if you are prone to kidney stones or gout. High doses can also cause diarrhea.
Vitamin D_3	Have your blood levels measured by your healthcare provider, who will determine proper dosage.	
Vitamin E*	800 to 1,200 IU once a day	Take mixed tocopherols, the more active type of vitamin E. Consult your healthcare provider first if you are taking a blood thinner. If you experience diarrhea, flatulence, nausea, and/or heart palpitations, reduce your dose.

*This supplement can have a blood-thinning action. See page 328 for more information.

PCOS

See Polycystic Ovary Syndrome.

PERIODONTAL DISEASE

Periodontal disease refers to any infection of the tissues that support the teeth. This infection begins just below the gumline, where it causes the tooth attachment and the gums to break down. This type of disease is classified according to its severity, of which there are two major stages—gingivitis and periodontitis. *Gingivitis*, which affects only the gums, is a milder and reversible form of the disease. Left untreated, it can lead to *periodontitis* (also called *pyorrhea*), a more serious, destructive condition that erodes the underlying bone and leads to tooth loss. Periodontal disease is also a major risk factor for heart disease. In the United States, more than 75 percent of adults over age thirty-five have some degree of periodontal disease.

Poor nutrition and inadequate oral hygiene are key factors in the development of periodontal disease. Other factors that can increase the risk of developing periodontal disease include excessive alcohol and sugar consumption, tobacco chewing or smoking, and a number of medications, including certain cancer therapy drugs, steroids, and oral contraceptives. Individuals with systemic diseases such as diabetes are also at greater risk.

Although there are several signs that can signal a possible periodontal problem—gums that are red, swollen, and tender; persistent bad breath; gums that bleed easily; permanent teeth that begin to separate or loosen; and gums that have receded from the teeth—it is possible to experience no warning signs at all! This is one reason that regular dental checkups are so important. Of course, good daily hygiene, which includes brushing and flossing, is essential as well.

SUPPLEMENTS TO TREAT PERIODONTAL DISEASE

Supplements	Dosage	Considerations
Calcium	500 mg once a day	Although most people are deficient in calcium, there is a danger in taking too much calcium. Do not ingest more than 1,000 to 1,200 mg of calcium each day.
Carnitine*	1,000 to 2,000 mg once a day	Have your healthcare provider measure your TMAO levels before starting long-term supplementation with carnitine.
Coenzyme Q_{10}*	100 to 300 mg once a day	If you are on blood-thinning medications, speak to your healthcare provider before using CoQ10. Since some medications can cause a deficiency of this nutrient, speak to your healthcare provider to determine if you might need a larger dose.

Copper	2 mg once a day	Your copper-to-zinc ratio is very important for your health. (See page 119 for details.) Also, do not take copper supplement cupric oxide, which has a very low bioavailability.
EPA/DHA (fish oil)*	2,000 mg once a day	Choose a source that contains vitamin E to prevent oxidation. Be aware that in large doses—above 3,000 mg a day—fish oil can act like a blood thinner.
Probiotics	20 billion units once a day	If taking an antibiotic, take the probiotics at least two hours before or two hours after using the antibiotics. Do not take them at the same time.
Vitamin A and mixed carotenoids	25,000 IU—half vitamin A and half mixed carotenoids— once a day, short term only (one to two months)	Use caution when taking vitamin A supplements because they have the potential to be toxic. Do not take for extended periods of time. Do not take more than 8,000 IU a day if you have liver disease, are a smoker, or have been exposed to asbestos. Do not take amounts of 25,000 IU or higher without a doctor's supervision.
Vitamin B_6 (pyridoxine)	50 mg twice a day	Do not take more than 500 mg a day. If you are taking L-dopa for Parkinson's disease, do not take B_6 without first consulting your doctor. High doses can deplete your body of other vitamins in the B complex, so also take a B-complex vitamin twice a day.
Vitamin B_9 (folic acid)	400 mcg twice a day	High doses can deplete your body of other vitamins in the B complex, so also take a B-complex vitamin twice a day.
Vitamin C	1,000 mg twice a day	Do not take high doses if you are prone to kidney stones or gout. High doses can also cause diarrhea.
Vitamin E*	400 IU once a day	Take mixed tocopherols, the more active type of vitamin E. Consult your healthcare provider first if you are taking a blood thinner. If you experience diarrhea, flatulence, nausea, and/or heart palpitations, reduce your dose.
Zinc	25 mg once a day as zinc picolinate or zinc citrate	Your copper-to-zinc ratio is very important to your health. (See page 119 for details.) If you are taking zinc and iron supplements, take one in the morning and one in the evening. (Taking them together reduces the efficiency of both.)

*This supplement can have a blood-thinning action. See page 328 for more information.

PERIODONTITIS

See Periodontal Disease.

PIMPLES

See Acne.

PMS

See Premenstrual Syndrome.

POLYCYSTIC OVARY SYNDROME (PCOS)

Polycystic Ovary Syndrome (PCOS), also known as *Stein-Leventhal syndrome,* is an endocrine disorder in which multiple cysts develop in the ovaries. Worldwide, PCOS is the most common endocrine disorder in women of reproductive age, and it affects nearly 10 percent of the women in the United States.

PCOS can have very serious health consequences, including insulin resistance; type 2 diabetes; an increased risk of uterine cancer; and an increased risk of heart disease due to high cholesterol, high blood pressure, and elevated c-reactive protein and homocysteine. In addition, individuals with PCOS have a higher rate of metabolic syndrome, which dramatically increases the risk of heart disease. They also have a greater risk of infertility. Depression and anxiety are common among women with PCOS.

Many scientists believe that PCOS has a hereditary component—that women with PCOS have a gene that triggers conditions associated with PCOS. This belief seems to be borne out by the fact that if a woman is diagnosed with the disorder, her sister has a 40-percent chance of developing PCOS, as well.

A woman with PCOS may have any number of the following symptoms and signs: irregular menstruation and/or menstruation cycles; lack of ovulation; and elevated levels of male hormones, such as testosterone. Obesity, often concentrated at the torso; pain during sexual intercourse; larger than normal ovaries; excess hair on face or body; acne; and sleep apnea are also common signs and symptoms of PCOS.

A variety of medications—such as hormonal birth control and anti-androgen drugs—are used to treat women with PCOS. Doctors also recommend regular exercise and a diet that is either low in carbohydrates or low on the glycemic index. Stress reduction is important, as well, as stress may be a contributing factor to PCOS. Finally, the addition of the nutrients recommended in the following table can make treatment of PCOS more successful.

SUPPLEMENTS TO TREAT PCOS

Supplements	Dosage	Considerations
Alpha lipoic acid	100 to 400 mg once a day	Alpha lipoic acid can interact with medication taken for diabetes and thyroid problems. Speak to your healthcare provider to see if any of the medications you take make it unwise to use this supplement.
B-complex vitamins	50 mg twice a day	I suggest taking a multivitamin along with your B-complex vitamins.
Carnitine*	1,000 to 3,000 mg once a day	Have your healthcare provider measure your TMAO levels before starting long-term supplementation with carnitine.
Chromium	600 to 1,000 mcg once a day as chromium picolinate	Combining with the protein picolinate allows your body to absorb chromium more efficiently. However, some chromium picolinate supplements contain more chromium than necessary. Ask your healthcare provider for a product recommendation.
Copper	1 to 3 mg once a day	Your copper-to-zinc ratio is very important for your health. (See page 119 for details.) Also, do not take copper supplement cupric oxide, which has a very low bioavailability
EGCG (green tea extract)*	270 mg EGCG a day	Green tea extract can interact with a number of drugs. Check with your healthcare provider before taking this supplement.
EPA/DHA (fish oil)*	1,000 to 2,000 mg once a day	Choose a source that contains vitamin E to prevent oxidation.
Gamma-linolenic acid (GLA) as evening primrose oil (EPO)*	240 to 480 mg once a day	It is important to maintain the proper ratio of omega-6 fatty acids to omega-3 fatty acids. (See page 129.) Evening primrose oil may interfere with some medications, such as nonsteroidal anti-inflammatories; can act as a blood thinner; and can lower the seizure threshold. Consult your healthcare provider or pharmacist before taking this supplement.
Inositol	6,000 mg twice a day	May stimulate uterine contractions. Women who wish to become pregnant should consult their doctor regarding its use. Doses larger than 200 mg should be taken only under physician supervision.
Licorice (glycyrrhiza)	300 mg twice a day	Do not use if you have high blood pressure, and discontinue use if you develop high blood pressure while taking licorice. Because licorice can interact poorly with other medication, consult your healthcare provider before starting supplementation.

Magnesium	400 to 800 mg once a day	Consult your healthcare provider for dosage if you have kidney disease. Discontinue use and see your doctor if you experience abdominal pain. Take a lower dose if it causes diarrhea.
Saw palmetto*	250 mg twice a day	Speak to your healthcare provider before using this supplement if you have a sex hormone-related disorder or if you are taking birth control pills.
Stinging nettle*	300 mg twice a day with meals	Stinging nettle can interfere with many medications. Speak to your healthcare provider or pharmacist before taking this supplement.
Taurine	500 to 2,000 mg once a day	Take between meals. Discontinue use if you suddenly have feelings of chest or throat tightness or if you break out in hives. Do not take with aspirin. Have your healthcare provider measure levels before starting taurine therapy.
Vitamin C	1,000 to 3,000 mg once a day	Do not take high doses if you are prone to kidney stones or gout. High doses can also cause diarrhea.
Vitamin D_3	Have your blood levels measured by your healthcare provider, who will determine proper dosage.	Vitamin D deficiency is common in women with PCOS.
Vitamin E*	400 to 800 IU once a day	Take mixed tocopherols, the more active type of vitamin E. Consult your healthcare provider first if you are taking a blood thinner.
Zinc	25 to 50 mg once a day as zinc picolinate or zinc citrate	Your copper-to-zinc ratio is very important to your health. (See page 119 for details.) If you are taking zinc and iron supplements, take one in the morning and one in the evening.

*This supplement can have a blood-thinning action. See page 328 for more information.

PREMENSTRUAL SYNDROME (PMS)

Premenstrual syndrome (PMS) is experienced by some women one to two weeks before they begin menstruating each month and continues until menstruation starts. It may even last one or two days after the period begins. Some of the emotional symptoms include tension, anxiety, irritability, mood swings, confusion, and depression. Physical symptoms include weight gain from water retention, cravings for salty foods or sweets, backache, sensitivity of breasts, swelling of feet or ankles, acne, bladder irritation, hives or rashes, headache, palpitations, and joint or muscle pain, to name just a few. Many women experience some of these symptoms during menstruation, but for women with PMS, the severity of these symptoms is disabling and interferes with their regular lives. PMS affects between 60 and 75 percent of women in the United States. Generally, the problems and symptoms recur in predictable patterns, but some months may bring more severe symptoms than others.

The cause of PMS is unknown and debated, although many people believe hormones to be at the root of the problem. Treatment—such as anti-inflammatories, diuretics, anti-anxiety medication, antidepressants, and medications that influence hormone production—tend to deal with different causes and different symptoms. Every woman is unique and may find success with a different method. However, before beginning one of the aforementioned treatments, some people find that a simple change to a more healthy, well-balanced diet with less sugar, salt, and candy in the one to two weeks before menstruation can help immensely. Other women find that their symptoms are improved after implementing a healthier diet with the addition of the nutrients recommended in the table below.

Some women experience symptoms that are even more severe. These women have *premenstrual dysphoric disorder (PMDD)*. Sufferers of PMDD should see their healthcare provider.

SUPPLEMENTS TO TREAT PREMENSTRUAL SYNDROME

Supplements	Dosage	Considerations
B-complex vitamins	50 mg mg once a day	I suggest taking a multivitamin along with your B-complex vitamins.
Calcium	500 mg twice a day	Although most people are deficient in calcium, there is a danger in taking too much calcium. Do not ingest more than 1,000 to 1,200 mg of calcium a day.
Carnitine*	500 mg once a day	Have your healthcare provider measure your TMAO level before starting long-term supplementation with carnitine.
Chromium	400 mcg once a day as chromium picolinate	Combining with the protein picolinate allows your body to absorb chromium more efficiently. However, some chromium picolinate supplements contain more chromium than necessary. Ask your healthcare provider for a recommendation.
Copper	1 to 2 mg once a day	Your copper-to-zinc ratio is very important for your health. (See page 119 for details.) Also, do not take copper supplement cupric oxide, which has a very low bioavailability.
EPA/DHA (fish oil)*	1,000 to 2,000 mg a day	Choose a source that contains vitamin E to prevent oxidation.
Gamma-linolenic acid (GLA) as evening primrose oil*	1,000 to 2,000 mg a day	It is important to maintain the proper ratio of omega-6 fatty acids to omega-3 fatty acids. (See page 129.) Evening primrose oil may interfere with some medications, such as nonsteroidal

		anti-inflammatories; can act as a blood thinner; and can lower the seizure threshold. Consult your healthcare provider or pharmacist before taking this supplement.
Ginkgo biloba*	120 to 180 mg once a day	Do not use with blood-thinning medications or supplements.
Magnesium	400 to 800 mg once a day	Consult your healthcare provider for dosage if you have kidney disease. Discontinue use and see your doctor if you experience abdominal pain. Take a lower dose if it causes diarrhea.
Manganese	2 to 5 mg once a day	Use with caution if you have gallbladder or liver disease.
St. John's Wort*	500 mg twice a day	St. John's wort can interact with many drugs. Speak to your healthcare provider before taking it. If you are exposed to the sun, it may cause a skin rash.
Taurine	500 mg once a day	Take between meals. Discontinue use if you suddenly have feelings of chest or throat tightness or if you break out in hives. Do not take with aspirin. Have your healthcare provider measure levels before starting taurine therapy.
Vitamin A and mixed carotenoids	5,000 to 8,000 IU—half vitamin A and half mixed carotenoids—once a day	Use caution when taking vitamin A supplements because they have the potential to be toxic. Do not take for extended periods of time. Do not take more than 5,000 IU a day if you have liver disease, are a smoker, or have been exposed to asbestos.
Vitamin B_6 (pyridoxine)	50 mg twice a day	Do not take more than 500 mg a day. If you are taking L-dopa for Parkinson's disease, do not take B_6 without first consulting your doctor. High doses can deplete your body of other vitamins in the B complex, so take a B-complex vitamin twice a day.
Vitamin B_{12} (cobalamin)	500 mcg twice a day	High doses can deplete your body of other vitamins in the B complex, so take a B-complex vitamin twice a day.
Vitamin C	1,000 mg once a day	Do not take high doses if you are prone to kidney stones or gout. High doses can also cause diarrhea.
Vitamin E*	400 to 800 IU once a day	Take mixed tocopherols, the more active type of vitamin E. Consult your healthcare provider first if you are taking a blood thinner.
Zinc	25 to 50 mg once a day as zinc picolinate or zinc citrate	Your copper-to-zinc ratio is very important to your health. (See page 119 for details.) If you are taking zinc and iron supplements, take one in the morning and one in the evening. (Taking them together reduces the efficiency of both.)

*This supplement can have a blood-thinning action. See page 328 for more information.

PROSTATE DISORDER

See Benign Prostatic Hyperplasia.

PSORIASIS

A common skin disorder that affects 2 percent of the population, psoriasis is characterized by thick patches of raised, reddish skin that is covered by what looks like silvery-white scales. In this condition, the body produces new skin cells at a much faster rate than normal; however, the old skin cells on the surface are shed at a slower, more normal rate. Because of this, the cells beneath the surface of the skin accumulate and form thick patches, while the "scales" on top are actually unshed dead skin cells. These patches, which typically appear on the scalp, elbows, knees, and lower back, often itch and may crack and bleed.

Although psoriasis is not contagious, it generally occurs in members of the same family. Flare-ups are followed by periods of healing, although the condition never disappears. The duration and severity of the cases range from some being so mild that people don't even realize they have the condition, while others are so severe that the patches may cover large areas of the body. The cause of psoriasis is not known, although breakouts can be triggered by stress, infection, overexposure to the sun, and alcohol abuse. Medications, including beta blockers and nonsteroidal anti-inflammatory drugs (NSAIDS), are other possible triggers.

Psoriasis is not curable, but it is treatable. Keeping this condition under control requires lifelong therapy. Treatments, which can be recommended by a healthcare professional, will vary depending on the severity of the condition. Dietary changes can be helpful. Avoid gluten and foods from the nightshade family, such as tomatoes, eggplant, white potatoes, peppers, and paprika. Also avoid high-sugar foods, alcohol, and foods to which you are allergic. Studies have also shown that it can be beneficial to eat oily fish, which is rich in omega-3 fatty acids.

SUPPLEMENTS TO TREAT PSORIASIS

Supplements	Dosage	Considerations
B-complex vitamins	50 mg twice a day	I suggest taking a multivitamin along with your B-complex vitamins.

Copper	2 to 3 mg once a day	Your copper-to-zinc ratio is very important for your health. (See page 119 for details.) Also, do not take copper supplement cupric oxide, which has a very low bioavailability.
Curcumin/Turmeric*	100 to 1,000 mg once a day of a formula that includes piperine or bioperine to boost absorption	Do not take curcumin with blood-thinning medications or supplements. Curcumin can also interact with other medications, so speak to your healthcare provider before taking this supplement.
Dandelion*	100 mg once or twice a day	If you have gallstones or obstructed bile ducts, consult your healthcare practitioner before taking. Do not use dandelion if you are taking a blood-thinning drug or supplement. Avoid if you are allergic to plants such as ragweed, chrysanthemums, marigolds, or daisies.
EPA/DHA (fish oil)*	1,000 to 3,000 mg once a day	Choose a source that contains vitamin E to prevent oxidation.
Gamma-linolenic acid (GLA) as evening primrose oil (EPO)*	500 to 1,000 mg once a day	It is important to maintain the proper ratio of omega-6 fatty acids to omega-3 fatty acids. (See page 129.) Evening primrose oil may interfere with some medications, such as nonsteroidal anti-inflammatories; can act as a blood thinner; and can lower the seizure threshold. Consult your healthcare provider or pharmacist before taking this supplement.
Glucosamine sulfate	1,000 mg once a day	If you are allergic to shellfish, be sure to choose a supplement that is not shellfish based. Consult use with your healthcare provider if you have diabetes, because glucosamine can alter blood sugar levels.
Methylsulfonylmethane (MSM)	1,000 to 3,000 mg three times a day	Use with caution if you are allergic to sulfur. Start by taking 500 mg three times a day, and gradually increase dose. Take with meals to avoid possible heartburn. May cause stomach upset in dosages larger than 6,000 mg.
Milk thistle	100 mg twice a day	Do not take if you are allergic to ragweed, chrysanthemums, marigolds, chamomile, or daisies. This supplement reduces the efficiency of certain blood pressure medication and other drugs. Speak to your healthcare provider or pharmacist before taking.
Probiotics	20 billion units once a day	If taking an antibiotic, take the probiotics at least two hours before or two hours after using the antibiotics. Do not take them at the same time.
Taurine	2,000 mg once a day	Take between meals. Discontinue use if you suddenly have feelings of chest or throat tightness or if you break out in hives. Do not take with aspirin. Have your healthcare provider measure levels before starting taurine therapy.

Tea tree oil gel	Apply directly to skin once or twice a day.	Do not ingest or use in ears.
Vitamin A and mixed carotenoids	50,000 IU—half vitamin A and half mixed carotenoids—once a day for one month, only under the supervision of your healthcare provider	Use caution when taking vitamin A supplements because they have the potential to be toxic. Do not take for extended periods of time. Do not take more than 8,000 IU a day if you have liver disease, are a smoker, or have been exposed to asbestos. Do not take amounts of 25,000 IU or higher without a doctor's supervision.
Vitamin C	500 to 1,500 mg twice a day	Do not take high doses if you are prone to kidney stones or gout. High doses can also cause diarrhea.
Vitamin D$_3$	Have your blood levels measured by your healthcare provider, who will determine proper dosage.	
Vitamin E*	400 IU once a day	Take mixed tocopherols, the more active type of vitamin E. Consult your healthcare provider first if you are taking a blood thinner.
Zinc	25 to 75 mg once a day as zinc picolinate or zinc citrate	Your copper-to-zinc ratio is very important to your health. (See page 119 for details.) If you are taking zinc and iron supplements, take one in the morning and one in the evening. (Taking them together reduces the efficiency of both.)

*This supplement can have a blood-thinning action. See page 328 for more information.

PYORRHEA

See Periodontal Disease.

RHEUMATOID ARTHRITIS

Rheumatoid arthritis (RA) is an autoimmune disease in which the body's immune system mistakenly attacks healthy tissue and joints, resulting in chronic inflammation. It is a debilitating disease because it can create a severe lack of mobility. Rheumatoid arthritis causes pain, stiffness, swelling, and even destruction of the joints during periods of inflammation, which are followed by periods of remission. This chronic illness can affect any joint in the body. It usually starts with small joints, such as those in the hands, and progresses to other joints. Its effect is symmetrical, meaning that it affects both sides of the body equally. For most people, the effects are worst upon wakening and gradually subside as the day progresses.

Rheumatoid arthritis is usually diagnosed between the ages of forty and fifty, and it is more common in women than men. Patients with RA have a higher risk of cardiovascular disease, pulmonary hypertension, and myocardial infarction (heart attack).

Although there is no known cause, many people believe that rheumatoid arthritis is related to a prior infection from a bacteria, fungus, or virus. Others believe that the disease is genetic, and still others think it is the result of lifestyle choices, such as smoking and gluten intake. Scientists are currently studying rheumatoid arthritis in an effort to pinpoint its cause.

Treatment for rheumatoid arthritis addresses the inflammatory component of the disease while also attempting to stabilize the immune system. Your healthcare provider may prescribe medications that can slow the progress of RA. Diet, too, can be helpful. A study has shown that people who follow a Mediterranean eating plan have less symptoms of RA and improved joint function. Eating organic foods and avoiding any foods to which you are allergic can also be beneficial. In addition, try to avoid the following foods, which may worsen the disorder:

- Beef
- Cheese and other dairy products
- Coffee
- Corn
- Eggs
- Foods from the nightshade family, such as eggplant, peppers, potatoes, and tomatoes
- Gluten
- Grapefruit
- Lemons
- Malt
- Oats
- Oranges
- Peanuts
- Pork
- Rye
- Soy
- Sugar

SUPPLEMENTS TO TREAT RHEUMATOID ARTHRITIS

Supplements	Dosage	Considerations
Alpha lipoic acid	300 to 400 mg once a day	Alpha lipoic acid can interact with medication taken for diabetes and thyroid problems. Speak to your healthcare provider to see if any of the medications you take make it unwise to use this supplement.
Arginine	2,000 mg once a day	Do not take if you have kidney disease, liver disease, or herpes except under a doctor's supervision. Arginine can interact with some medications. Consult with your healthcare provider before beginning this therapy.
B-complex vitamins	50 mg twice a day	I suggest taking a multivitamin along with your B-complex vitamins.

Boswellia*	400 to 800 mg three times a day	Avoid boswellia if you are pregnant, because it can induce miscarriage. Do not take with NSAIDs.
Bromelain	Use as part of a digestive enzyme product	Do not take bromelain if you are allergic to pineapple, latex, wheat, celery, carrot, fennel, cypress pollen, or grass pollen.
Carnitine*	500 to 1,000 mg once a day	Have your healthcare provider measure your TMAO levels before starting long-term supplementation with carnitine.
Coenzyme Q$_{10}$*	100 to 200 mg once a day	If you are on blood-thinning medications, speak to your healthcare provider before using CoQ$_{10}$. Since some medications can cause a deficiency of this nutrient, speak to your healthcare provider to determine if you might need a larger dose.
Copper	2 mg once a day	Your copper-to-zinc ratio is very important for your health. (See page 119 for details.) Also, do not take copper supplement cupric oxide, which has a very low bioavailability.
Curcumin/Turmeric*	100 to 1,000 mg once a day of a formula that includes piperine or bioperine to boost absorption	Do not take curcumin with blood-thinning medications or supplements. Curcumin can also interact with other medications, so speak to your healthcare provider before taking this supplement.
Cysteine	500 to 1,000 mg once a day as n-acetylcysteine, or NAC	When taking NAC supplements, also take extra vitamin C, copper, and zinc.
EGCG (green tea extract)*	500 to 1,000 mg once or twice a day	Green tea extract can interact with a number of drugs. Check with your healthcare provider before taking this supplement.
EPA/DHA (fish oil)*	3,000 to 9,000 mg a day	Choose a source that contains vitamin E to prevent oxidation. In high doses, fatty acids may cause the blood to thin. If you are taking a blood thinner, do not take EPA/DHA without direct instructions from your doctor. It is important to maintain the proper ratio of omega-6 fatty acids to omega-3 fatty acids. (See page 129.)
Gamma-linolenic acid (GLA) as evening primrose oil (EPO)*	1,000 mg once a day	It is important to maintain the proper ratio of omega-6 fatty acids to omega-3 fatty acids. (See page 129.) Evening primrose oil may interfere with some medications, such as nonsteroidal anti-inflammatories; can act as a blood thinner; and can lower the seizure threshold. Consult your healthcare provider or pharmacist before taking this supplement.
Ginger*	100 mg once a day	Ginger can act as a blood thinner. Check with your healthcare provider or pharmacist before taking this supplement.

Glutamine	1,500 mg once a day	If you have a sensitivity to monosodium glutamate (MSG), use glutamine with caution. If you are taking medications for seizures, take glutamine only under the direction of your doctor.
Grape seed extract*	300 to 600 mg once a day	Do not use with blood-thinning medications or supplements.
Magnesium	600 mg once a day	Consult your healthcare provider for dosage if you have kidney disease. Discontinue use and see your doctor if you experience abdominal pain. Take a lower dose if it causes diarrhea.
Methylsulfonylmethane (MSM)	1,000 to 3,000 mg three times a day	Use with caution if you are allergic to sulfur. Start by taking 500 mg three times a day, and gradually increase dose. Take with meals to avoid possible heartburn. May cause stomach upset in doses larger than 6,000 mg.
Probiotics	20 billion units a day	If taking an antibiotic, take the probiotics at least two hours before or two hours after using the antibiotics. Do not take them at the same time.
Quercetin*	500 mg once a day	For best results, take with bromelain and vitamin C. Do not use with blood-thinning medications or supplements.
Selenium	100 to 200 mcg once a day	Do not exceed 200 mcg a day without consulting your healthcare provider.
Vitamin C	500 to 1,000 mg twice a day	Do not take high doses if you are prone to kidney stones or gout. High doses can also cause diarrhea.
Vitamin D$_3$	Have your blood levels measured by your healthcare provider, who will determine proper dosage.	
Zinc	25 mg once a day as zinc picolinate or zinc citrate	Your copper-to-zinc ratio is very important to your health. (See page 119 for details.) If you are taking zinc and iron supplements, take one in the morning and one in the evening. (Taking them together reduces the efficiency of both.)

*This supplement can have a blood-thinning action. See page 328 for more information.

SCLERODERMA (SYSTEMIC SCLEROSIS)

Scleroderma is a chronic, degenerative disease that causes excess buildup of *collagen*—a protein chemical that strengthens connective tissue. It is then deposited throughout the skin or other organs. The collagen build-up usually appears as small white lumps under the skin that burst and become white fluid.

There are three types of scleroderma. *Limited scleroderma* is a localized disorder. The skin, particularly of the extremities, becomes hard and thick, and may also appear red and scaly. Although it can affect the muscles as well as the skin, the disease travels slowly and does not usually spread to the organs. *Diffuse scleroderma*, also called *systemic sclerosis* and *CREST syndrome*, is a generalized disorder that spreads quickly through the body and can affect many of the body's organs. It is the most serious and potentially fatal type of scleroderma. *Morphea scleroderma*, or *linear scleroderma*, can affect different parts of the skin but does not interfere with the body's other structures.

People with scleroderma may experience a wide array of symptoms. Their skin may appear shiny, discolored, or hard, and may be itchy. They may feel fatigued or short of breath, or experience pain in their joints or numbness in their toes or fingers. They may also lose weight or experience damage to the affected system. There is no cure for scleroderma, but there is much that can be done to alleviate many of the symptoms. Your doctor can suggest therapy for your specific ailments. You should also moisturize your skin, refrain from smoking, practice good sleep habits, avoid strong detergents, and reduce stress as much as possible. These safeguards, as well as the nutrients listed in the table below, will help reduce the effects of scleroderma.

SUPPLEMENTS TO TREAT SCLERODERMA		
Supplements	Dosage	Considerations
Alpha-linolenic acid (ALA) as flaxseed oil*	1,000 mg once a day	It is important to maintain the proper ratio of omega-6 fatty acids to omega-3 fatty acids. (See page 129.) Flaxseed oil may interfere with anticoagulants, work as a laxative, or affect blood sugar levels. Consult your healthcare provider or pharmacist before taking this supplement.
Carnitine*	1,000 to 2,000 mg once a day	Have your healthcare provider measure your TMAO levels before starting long-term supplementation with carnitine.
Cysteine	1,000 mg once a day as n-acetylcysteine, or NAC	When taking NAC supplements, also take extra vitamin C, copper, and zinc.
EPA/DHA (fish oil)*	1,000 to 4,000 mg once a day	Choose a source that contains vitamin E to prevent oxidation. In high doses, fatty acids may cause the blood to thin. If you are taking a blood thinner, do not take EPA/DHA without direct instructions from your doctor. It is important to maintain the proper ratio of omega-6 fatty acids to omega-3 fatty acids. (See page 129.)
Gamma-linolenic acid (GLA) as evening primrose oil (EPO)*	240 to 720 mg once a day	It is important to maintain the proper ratio of omega-6 fatty acids to omega-3 fatty acids. (See page 129.) Evening primrose oil may interfere with

		some medications, such as nonsteroidal anti-inflammatories; can act as a blood thinner; and can lower the seizure threshold. Consult your healthcare provider before taking this supplement.
Glucosamine sulfate	300 to 900 mg once a day	If you are allergic to shellfish, be sure to choose a supplement that is not shellfish based. Consult your healthcare provider if you have diabetes, because glucosamine can alter blood sugar levels.
Glutamine	1,000 to 6,000 mg once a day	If you have a sensitivity to monosodium glutamate (MSG), use glutamine with caution. If you are taking medications for seizures, take glutamine only under the direction of your doctor.
Gotu kola	60 to 120 mg a day	Do not take gotu kola if you have liver disease.
Probiotics	20 billion units once a day	If taking an antibiotic, take the probiotics at least two hours before or two hours after using the antibiotics. Do not take them at the same time.
Selenium	200 mcg once a day	Do not consume more than 200 mcg a day without consulting your healthcare provider.
Vitamin C	500 to 2,500 mg twice a day	Do not take high doses if you are prone to kidney stones or gout. High doses can also cause diarrhea.
Vitamin D$_3$	Have your blood levels measured by your healthcare provider, who will determine proper dosage.	
Vitamin E*	400 to 800 IU once a day	Take mixed tocopherols, the more active type of vitamin E. Consult your healthcare provider first if you are taking a blood thinner.

*This supplement can have a blood-thinning action. See page 328 for more information.

SJÖGREN'S SYNDROME

Sjögren's syndrome is a common autoimmune disease that affects several million people in the United States. It occurs when the body's white blood cells attack the exocrine glands that produce moisture. The eyes, mouth, nose, skin, and vagina can become dry; the voice can become hoarse; and major organs can be damaged. Some people experience mild symptoms, while others become severely ill from the disease. Like many other autoimmune diseases, Sjögren's syndrome can be difficult to diagnose because of the wide range of symptoms as well as the similarity of these symptoms to those of other disorders.

A large majority of people with this illness are women. In 50 percent of cases, Sjögren's syndrome occurs alone. The other 50 percent of cases affect people who also have one of the following autoimmune diseases: rheumatoid arthritis, lupus, diffuse scleroderma, or dermatomyositis.

There is no cure for Sjögren's syndrome; therefore, care focuses on treating the symptoms. There are various moisture replacement therapies that are quite effective. Your doctor will be able to recommend the appropriate course of action for you. There are also immunosuppressive medications that hinder the immune system's function. In addition, you can help control this disorder through diet. Studies have shown that many people with Sjogren's do better if they avoid all gluten and dairy products. The supplements recommended in the table below can also be beneficial.

SUPPLEMENTS TO TREAT SJÖGREN'S SYNDROME

Supplements	Dosage	Considerations
Alpha-linolenic acid (ALA) as flaxseed oil*	1,000 mg once a day	It is important to maintain the proper ratio of omega-6 fatty acids to omega-3 fatty acids. (See page 129.) Flaxseed oil may interfere with anticoagulants, work as a laxative, or affect blood sugar levels. Consult your healthcare provider or pharmacist before taking this supplement.
Coenzyme Q_{10}*	100 mg a day	If you are on blood-thinning medications, speak to your healthcare provider before using CoQ_{10}. Since some medications can cause a deficiency of this nutrient, speak to your healthcare provider to determine if you might need a larger dose.
Cysteine	200 mg three times a day as n-acetylcysteine, or NAC	When taking NAC supplements, also take extra vitamin C, copper, and zinc.
Eleuthero*	50 to 200 mg once a day	Do not use if you have a history of heart disease, hypertension, sleep apnea, narcolepsy, mania, or schizophrenia, or if you are pregnant or breastfeeding.
EPA/DHA (fish oil)*	1,000 to 5,000 mg once a day	Choose a source that contains vitamin E to prevent oxidation. In high doses, fatty acids may cause the blood to thin. If you are taking a blood thinner, do not take EPA/DHA without direct instructions from your doctor. It is important to maintain the proper ratio of omega-6 fatty acids to omega-3 fatty acids. (See page 129.)
Gamma-linolenic acid (GLA) as evening primrose oil (EPO)*	240 to 720 mg once a day	It is important to maintain the proper ratio of omega-6 fatty acids to omega-3 fatty acids. (See page 129.) Evening primrose oil may interfere with some medications, such as nonsteroidal anti-inflammatories; can act as a blood thinner; and can lower the seizure threshold. Consult your healthcare provider or pharmacist before taking this supplement.

Glucosamine sulfate	300 to 900 mg once a day	If you are allergic to shellfish, be sure to choose a supplement that is not shellfish based. Consult your healthcare provider if you have diabetes, because glucosamine can alter blood sugar levels.
Glutamine	1 to 5 g once a day	If you have a sensitivity to monosodium glutamate (MSG), use glutamine with caution. If you are taking medications for seizures, take glutamine only under the direction of your doctor.
Iron	Have your doctor measure your iron levels to determine dosage.	Supplement with iron if needed and repeat the laboratory tests every three months. Studies show that people with Sjögren's syndrome are frequently deficient in iron, B_9, and B_{12}.
Magnesium	400 to 800 mg once a day	Consult your healthcare provider for dosage if you have kidney disease. Discontinue use and see your doctor if you experience abdominal pain. Take a lower dose if it causes diarrhea.
Olive leaf extract*	500 mg twice a day containing 20 mg of oleuropein per capsule	Olive leaf extract can interact with prescription medications, and may increase the effects of blood thinners. Consult your doctor before using olive leaf extract if you are taking any medication. Don't use if you are pregnant or breastfeeding.
Probiotics	20 billion units once a day	If taking an antibiotic, take the probiotics at least two hours before or two hours after using the antibiotics. Do not take them at the same time.
Selenium	200 mcg once a day	Do not exceed 200 mcg a day without consulting your healthcare provider.
Vitamin B_9 (folate)	Have your doctor measure your B_9 levels to determine dosage.	Supplement with B_9 if needed and repeat the laboratory tests every three months. Studies show that people with Sjögren's syndrome are frequently deficient in iron, B_9, and B_{12}. High doses of this supplement can deplete your body of other vitamins in the B complex, so take a B-complex vitamin twice a day.
Vitamin B_{12} (folate)	Have your doctor measure your B_{12} levels to determine dosage.	Supplement with B_{12} if needed and repeat the laboratory tests every three months. Studies show that people with Sjögren's syndrome are frequently deficient in iron, B_9, and B_{12}. High doses of this supplement can deplete your body of other vitamins in the B complex, so take a B-complex vitamin twice a day.
Vitamin C	500 to 1,500 mg twice a day	Do not take high doses if you are prone to kidney stones or gout. High doses can also cause diarrhea.
Vitamin E*	400 IU once a day	Take mixed tocopherols, the more active type of vitamin E. Consult your healthcare provider first if you are taking a blood thinner.

*This supplement can have a blood-thinning action. See page 328 for more information.

SKIN DISORDERS

See Acne; Eczema; Psoriasis.

SLEEP DISORDERS

See Insomnia.

STRESS

See Adrenal Fatigue and Exhaustion; Anxiety.

STROKE

Also called a *cerebrovascular accident,* a stroke occurs when the blood supply to the brain is interrupted, and the brain is deprived of the oxygen it needs to function. An *ischemic* stroke, the most common type, is caused by a blocked blood vessel in the brain. A *hemorrhagic* stroke develops when an artery in the brain leaks or bursts. Brain damage can begin within minutes, so it is important to recognize stroke symptoms and act fast. Quick treatment can help limit damage to the brain and increase the chance of a full recovery.

Symptoms of a stroke, which happen quickly, typically include numbness or paralysis on one side of the body (usually the face, arm, or leg); dim, blurry, or double vision; difficulty speaking and understanding; dizziness; unsteadiness when walking; and severe headache. (See the "Warning" on page 468.) About 80 percent of strokes are caused by atherosclerosis, which results from a gradual build-up of plaque on artery walls, eventually causing them to close. High blood pressure is another major risk factor.

After experiencing a stroke, following your doctor's orders is crucial for stabilizing your condition and reducing the risk of having another one. In addition to any prescribed medications and therapies, eating a well-balanced diet that includes lots of fresh vegetables, whole grains, and lean protein is recommended. This type of diet will help protect blood vessels, oxygenate tissues, and fight damaging free radicals. The following nutritional supplement program is designed to further support stroke recovery. However, if your stroke was hemorrhagic, do not take these nutrients until your physician confirms that there is no further risk of bleeding.

WARNING

If you experience any symptoms of a stroke, immediately call 911 or another emergency service. If the symptoms occur, but go away quickly, be sure to contact your doctor immediately. You may have had a *transient ischemic attack (TIA)*. Also known as a *mini-stroke,* a TIA is often a warning that a stroke may occur soon. Seeking immediate treatment can help prevent it.

SUPPLEMENTS FOR STROKE RECOVERY

Supplements	Dosage	Considerations
Carnitine*	400 mg once a day	Have your healthcare provider measure your TMAO levels before starting long-term supplementation.
Coenzyme Q_{10}*	150 to 200 mg once a day	If you are on blood-thinning medications, speak to your healthcare provider before using CoQ_{10}. Since some medications can cause a deficiency of this nutrient, speak to your healthcare provider to determine if you might need a larger dose.
EPA/DHA (fish oil)*	1,000 to 2,000 mg once a day	Choose a source that contains vitamin E to prevent oxidation.
Magnesium	400 to 600 mg a day as magnesium glycinate	Consult your healthcare provider for dosage if you have kidney disease. Discontinue use and see your doctor if you experience abdominal pain. Take a lower dose if it causes diarrhea.
Phosphatidylserine (PS)	100 to 300 mg once a day	PS can interact with many drugs. Speak to your healthcare provider before taking it.
Potassium	See your healthcare provider for dosage directions.	Consume foods high in potassium such as those listed on page 85.
Quercetin*	500 mg twice a day	For best results, take with bromelain and vitamin C. Do not use with blood-thinning medications or supplements.
Vitamin B_3 (niacin)	50 mg twice a day	Do not drink alcohol or hot drinks within one hour of taking niacin. High doses can deplete your body of other vitamins in the B complex, so take a B-complex vitamin twice a day.
Vitamin B_6 (pyridoxine)	50 mg twice a day	Do not take more than 500 mg a day. If you are taking L-dopa for Parkinson's disease, do not take B_6 without first consulting your doctor. High doses can deplete your body of other vitamins in the B complex, so take a B-complex vitamin twice a day. If you have high homocysteine levels, take in the form of pyridoxal 5-phosphate.

Vitamin B9 (folate)	400 mcg twice a day	High doses can deplete your body of other vitamins in the B complex, so take a B-complex vitamin twice a day. If you have high homocysteine levels, take the active form L-5-methyltetrahydrofolate.
Vitamin B12 (cobalamin)	500 mcg twice a day	High doses can deplete your body of other vitamins in the B complex, so take a B-complex vitamin twice a day. If you have high homocysteine levels, take in the form of methylcobalamin.
Vitamin C	1,000 to 2,000 a day	Do not take high doses if you are prone to kidney stones or gout. High doses can also cause diarrhea.

*This supplement can have a blood-thinning action. See page 328 for more information.

SYSTEMIC SCLEROSIS

See Scleroderma.

THYROID DISORDERS

See Hashimoto's Thyroiditis; Hyperthyroidism; Hypothyroidism.

TRAUMATIC HEAD INJURY

See Closed Head Injury.

TYPE 1 DIABETES

See Diabetes Mellitus.

TYPE 2 DIABETES

See Diabetes Mellitus.

ULCERATIVE COLITIS

Ulcerative colitis (UC) is a disorder that causes inflammation of the inner lining of the digestive tract, along with sores (*ulcers*). This disorder is referred to as an inflammatory bowel disease (IBD), which is a general term for conditions that cause inflammation of the small intestine and colon. More than 500,000 Americans have ulcerative colitis.

There are several types of this disorder, with each form occurring in a specific location. The different forms include *ulcerative proctitis,* in which inflammation is confined to the rectum, causing rectal bleeding and/or pain; *left-sided colitis,* which extends from the rectum to the left side of the colon, resulting in bloody diarrhea, abdominal cramping and pain, and weight loss; *pan colitis,* which affects the entire colon, causing bloody diarrhea, abdominal cramping, weight loss, fatigue, and night sweats; and *fulminant colitis,* a rare form that affects the entire colon and causes severe pain, diarrhea, and sometimes dehydration. Other areas of the body can also be affected by UC, including the skin, eyes, hepatobiliary system (the liver, gallbladder, and bile ducts), and the musculoskeletal system. Individuals with ulcerative colitis also have an increased risk of developing colon cancer.

No one knows exactly what causes ulcerative colitis, but researchers are exploring possible connections to viral or bacterial infection, poor diet, heredity, and use of antibiotics. Until the cause is found, treatments aim at reducing inflammation. Medications, including anti-inflammatory drugs, are often prescribed, and surgery is sometimes needed.

Diet has been found to have a significant effect on ulcerative colitis, and each person may find that certain foods exacerbate symptoms. Keep a diary of your food intake and flare-ups to determine if some foods worsen your symptoms. For instance, numerous studies have shown that food allergies may be the cause of and/or exacerbate ulcerative colitis. Have your doctor test you for both IgE and IgG types of food allergies, and strictly avoid foods to which you are allergic.

People with ulcerative colitis often do better without gluten. Therefore, you should avoid all gluten intake. In a number of cases, lactose intolerance may be a factor, so also avoid dairy products except those that are lactose-free. In addition, the following foods and liquids have been shown to aggravate symptoms in some individuals:

- Alcohol
- Carbonated beverages
- High-fiber foods
- Nuts
- Seeds
- Spicy foods

The supplements recommended in the following table can play an important role in relieving inflammation and helping the digestive tract to heal.

SUPPLEMENTS TO TREAT ULCERATIVE COLITIS

Supplements	Dosage	Considerations
Aloe vera juice	25 ml (about 1 ounce) up to four times a day	Taking aloe vera before a meal may help prevent indigestion. If your stools get loose, cut down on your dosage. Do not exceed the manufacturer's recommendations.
CBD oil (hemp oil)	5 to 500 mg a day in the form of sublingual drops. Start with 5 mg and increase slowly until you find relief.	CBD is generally well tolerated and safe for consumption, even in high doses and with continuous use. However, do not exceed 500 mg a day without consulting your healthcare provider. Make sure to buy a product marked "hemp oil (aerial parts)."
Curcumin/Turmeric*	100 to 500 mg once a day of a formula that includes piperine or bioperine to boost absorption	Do not take curcumin with blood-thinning medications or supplements. Curcumin can also interact with other medications, so speak to your healthcare provider before taking this supplement.
Cysteine	500 mg once a day as n-acetylcysteine, or NAC	When taking NAC supplements, also take extra vitamin C, copper, and zinc.
Digestive enzymes	Follow the manufacturer's instructions. Be sure to take these supplements with or directly before meals.	Do not take digestive enzymes that contain papain if you are allergic to papaya, and avoid enzymes with bromelain if you are allergic to pineapple. Use with caution if you have a severe ulcer.
EGCG (green tea extract)*	800 mg a day	Green tea extract can interact with a number of drugs. Check with your healthcare provider before taking this supplement.
EPA/DHA (fish oil)*	1,000 mg three times a day, or up to 5,000 mg three times a day	Choose a source that contains vitamin E to prevent oxidation. In high doses, fatty acids may cause the blood to thin. If you are taking a blood thinner, do not take EPA/DHA without direct instructions from your doctor. It is important to maintain the proper ratio of omega-6 fatty acids to omega-3 fatty acids. (See page 129.)
Fiber, soluble, as psyllium	20 g ground psyllium seeds twice daily with water	Choose a fiber supplement with no added sugar. Supplement with several glasses of water.
Gamma-linolenic acid (GLA) as evening primrose oil (EPO)*	500 mg three times a day	It is important to maintain the proper ratio of omega-6 fatty acids to omega-3 fatty acids. (See page 129.) Evening primrose oil may interfere with some medications, such as nonsteroidal anti-inflammatories; can act as a blood thinner; and can lower the seizure threshold. Consult your healthcare provider or pharmacist before taking this supplement.

Glutamine	2,000 to 6,000 mg daily	If you have a sensitivity to monosodium glutamate (MSG), use glutamine with caution. If you are taking medication for seizures, take glutamine only under the direction of your doctor.
Licorice, deglycyrrhizinated (DGL)	500 mg three times a day taken approximately 20 minutes before a meal and at bedtime.	Do not use if you have high blood pressure, and discontinue use if you develop high blood pressure while taking licorice. Because licorice can interact poorly with some medication, consult your healthcare provider before starting supplementation.
Magnesium	400 to 600 mg a day as magnesium glycinate	Consult your healthcare provider for dosage if you have kidney disease. Discontinue use and see your doctor if you experience abdominal pain. Take a lower dose if it causes diarrhea. Most people with UC have low magnesium levels.
Methylsulfonylmethane (MSM)	1,000 mg three times a day up to 3,000 mg three times a day	Use with caution if you are allergic to sulfur. Start by taking 500 mg three times a day, and gradually increase dose. Take with meals to avoid possible heartburn. May cause stomach upset in dosages larger than 6,000 mg.
Phosphatidylcholine (PC)	1,000 to 2,000 mg twice a day of enteric-coated tablets	Use with caution if you have malabsorption problems, as this could exacerbate them. Studies have shown that in patients with UC, the PC content of the mucus layer is decreased by about 70 percent.
Probiotics	20 billion units once a day	If taking an antibiotic, take the probiotics at least two hours before or two hours after using the antibiotics. Do not take them at the same time. In several studies, VSL #3 (which contains a combination of different good bacteria) was shown to be effective for UC. Supplementing with probiotics increases the efficacy of conventional treatment and also prevents pouchitis flare-ups.
Quercetin*	500 mg three times a day	For best results, take with bromelain and vitamin C. Do not use with blood-thinning medications or supplements.
UltraInflamX	Follow instructions on bottle.	This is a Metagenics product. (See Resources.) Do not use if taking a diuretic.
Vitamin A and mixed carotenoids	5,000 to 20,000 IU—half vitamin A and half mixed carotenoids—once a day	Use caution when taking vitamin A supplements because they have the potential to be toxic. Do not take for extended periods of time. Do not take more than 8,000 IU a day if you have liver disease, are a smoker, or have been exposed to asbestos.
Vitamin B$_5$ (pantothenic acid)	50 to 100 mg twice a day	High doses can deplete your body of other vitamins in the B complex, so take a B-complex vitamin twice a day. Stop taking B$_5$ supplements if you begin having chest pains or breathing problems.

Vitamin B$_6$ (pyridoxine)	50 mg twice a day	Do not take more than 500 mg a day. If you are taking L-dopa for Parkinson's disease, do not take B$_6$ without first consulting your doctor. High doses can deplete your body of other vitamins in the B complex, so take a B-complex vitamin twice a day.
Vitamin B$_9$ (folic acid)	400 to 800 mcg twice a day	High doses can deplete your body of other vitamins in the B complex, so take a B-complex vitamin twice a day. Many people with UC have decreased folic acid levels.
Vitamin C	500 mg twice a day	Do not take high doses if you are prone to kidney stones or gout. High doses can also cause diarrhea.
Vitamin D$_3$	Have your blood levels measured by your healthcare provider, who will determine proper dosage.	Studies have shown that patients with UC and other inflammatory bowel disease have low vitamin D levels.
Vitamin E*	400 IU once a day	Take mixed tocopherols, the more active type of vitamin E. Consult your healthcare provider first if you are taking a blood thinner.
Vitamin K*	500 mcg a day of K$_2$ or MK-7	If you are on blood-thinning medications, speak to your healthcare provider before using vitamin K. Some people with UC have low vitamin K levels.
Zinc	10 to 20 mg three times a day as zinc picolinate or zinc citrate	Your copper-to-zinc ratio is very important to your health. (See page 119 for details.) If you are taking zinc and iron supplements, take one in the morning and one in the evening. (Taking them together reduces the efficiency of both.)

*This supplement can have a blood-thinning action. See page 328 for more information.

UTERINE FIBROIDS

See Fibroids.

VARICOSE VEINS

Dark blue or purple in color, varicose veins are veins that are swollen, bulging, and often appear twisted—like cords. They are unsightly and can form anywhere from the groin to the ankles, although they usually appear on the back of the calves or the inner legs. Usually accompanied by dull aches and a heavy feeling in the legs, varicose veins can also cause swollen feet and ankles, as well as severe pain. The National Institutes of Health (NIH) estimates that 60 percent of all men and women suffer from some form of vein disorder.

To understand how varicose veins are formed, it's important to first be aware of how veins are designed, as well as their purpose. This is explained in "Circulation 101" below. If a vein's one-way valves, which keep the blood flowing back to the heart, fail to work properly, the blood will back up and overfill the vein. Eventually, the blood-clogged vein will begin to bulge. Varicose veins occur in the legs because the blood coursing through the leg veins has to work against gravity to get back to the heart.

Although varicose veins seem to run in families, the exact reason for their development is not known. Contributing factors can include lack of regular exercise, standing or sitting for extended periods, heavy lifting, chronic constipation, obesity, and pregnancy. Generally, varicose veins do not cause serious health problems. In some cases, however, they can cause complications such as bleeding under the skin or blood clot formation. It is important to speak with your doctor for treatment recommendations.

There are a number of simple steps you can take to improve symptoms of varicose veins: keep your legs elevated, massage your legs, choose clothing that is not tight fitting, reduce the salt in your diet so you can decrease water retention, avoid sitting with your legs crossed, wear compression stockings, and exercise regularly. The nutrients recommended in the table below can also be helpful.

Circulation 101

The job of the circulatory system—the heart and blood vessels—is to keep blood continually traveling through the body. Basically, the heart pumps fresh nutrient-rich, oxygenated blood through the arteries to various parts of the body. When the blood makes the return trip to the heart, it does so through the veins. On this return trip, the blood is no longer powered by the pumping heart—instead, the muscles surrounding the veins expand and contract, squeezing the veins and pushing the blood along. The veins themselves are designed with one-way valves that keep the blood flowing in the right direction.

SUPPLEMENTS TO TREAT VARICOSE VEINS

Supplements	Dosage	Considerations
Coenzyme Q_{10}*	100 to 300 mg a day	If you are on blood-thinning medications, speak to your healthcare provider before using CoQ_{10}. Since some medications can cause a deficiency of this nutrient, speak to your healthcare provider to determine if you might need a larger dose.

EPA/DHA (fish oil)*	2,000 mg once a day	Choose a source that contains vitamin E to prevent oxidation.
Ginkgo biloba*	60 to 120 mg twice a day	Do not use with blood-thinning medications or supplements.
Gotu kola*	200 to 400 mg once a day	Do not take gotu kola if you have liver disease. Stop using gotu kola at least two weeks before a scheduled surgery.
Grape seed extract*	100 to 200 mg once a day	Do not use with blood-thinning medications or supplements.
Horse chestnut*	300 to 600 mg once a day	Avoid this supplement if you are allergic to latex. Also avoid if you are taking a blood-thinning medication or supplement. Horse chestnut can interact with some medications, so speak to your healthcare provider to learn if any drugs you're taking might make it wise to avoid this supplement.
OPCs*	50 to 100 mg once a day as pine bark extract, such as pycnogenol	OPCs can interact with some medications, so speak to your healthcare provider to learn if any drugs you're taking might make it wise to avoid this supplement.
Vitamin C	500 mg twice a day	Do not take high doses if you are prone to kidney stones or gout. High doses can also cause diarrhea.
Vitamin E*	400 IU once a day	Take mixed tocopherols, the more active type of vitamin E. Consult your healthcare provider first if you are taking a blood thinner.

*This supplement can have a blood-thinning action. See page 328 for more information.

WEIGHT GAIN AND OBESITY

According to the National Health and Nutrition Examination Survey (NHANES), 35 percent of men and 40.5 percent of women in the United States are obese—a condition defined as having a body mass index (BMI) equal to or greater than 30. Two-thirds of adults are considered overweight. Being obese or overweight increases your risk of over thirty-five diseases, including heart disease, insulin resistance and diabetes, memory loss, stroke, arthritis, sleep apnea, and cancer, to name just a few.

To achieve effective weight loss—and then keep the weight off—it is important to consider the cause of the weight gain. Weight gain can be rooted in many different practices and problems, including consuming more calories than you burn; getting insufficient exercise; or having an underactive thyroid, food allergies, hormonal problems, neurotransmitter imbalance, an inability to detoxify, chronic inflammation, essential fatty acid deficiency, sleep deprivation, or yeast overgrowth. Some foods, like sugar, are actually chemically addicting, making it difficult to adopt a healthier diet. That's why it's worthwhile to consult with a healthcare professional who can help you in your weight-loss efforts by determining and addressing the cause of your problem.

If you need to lose weight, it's important to select the healthy eating program that you feel is right for you. Never use the word "diet"; it will only make you hungry. Once you choose a program, begin that day. If you feel that you are going to be deprived, you may gain three pounds between now and the day you intend to start your eating plan. The program you choose should be one that you can continue throughout your life. If you start on a weight-loss program that greatly reduces your calories, you may end up gaining all the weight back. If you lose weight slowly, however, you will be more likely to keep the weight off.

Usually, people who want to lose weight try to restrict their calories on a daily basis. This type of diet is usually not successful because it is too difficult to maintain. Recent studies have shown that intermittent caloric restriction is beneficial for weight loss and is also easier to follow than daily calorie restriction. There are several versions of "intermittent fasting" diets, with the 5:2 diet being the most popular. These programs restrict caloric intake on two days of the week (usually Monday and Thursday) to 500 to 600 calories a day, and allow five days of normal eating that provides a healthy balance of proteins, fats, and carbohydrates.

As you follow your healthy eating program and experience weight loss, keep in mind that the dosage of the medications you're taking may need to be changed, and the need for some medications may decrease. Keep you healthcare provider updated regarding your progress with weight loss.

Nutritional support has been shown to improve the benefits of a 5:2 program. The nutrients in the table below will help promote weight loss, optimize the body's use of nutrients, improve insulin sensitivity, regulate blood sugar levels, and enhance overall health.

SUPPLEMENTS TO AID WEIGHT LOSS		
Supplements	Dosage	Considerations
Alpha lipoic acid	300 mg once a day	Alpha lipoic acid can interact with medication taken for diabetes and thyroid problems. Speak to your healthcare provider to see if any of the medications you take make it unwise to use this supplement.
Asian ginseng*	100 to 400 mg a day	Do not use if you are taking a blood thinner or if you have a hormonally related cancer such as breast, prostate, uterine, or ovarian.

Berberine*	200 to 400 mg twice a day of standardized extract	Do not use this supplement during pregnancy. It can cause uterine contractions.
Bitter melon	500 to 1,000 mg capsule daily, or 50 to 100 ml juice daily	Do not use if you are pregnant or breastfeeding, if you are male and trying to initiate a pregnancy, or if you are female and trying to get pregnant. If you have blood sugar problems, monitor your blood sugar on a regular basis during treatment.
Carnitine*	2,000 mg once a day as L-Carnitine	Have your healthcare provider measure your TMAO levels before starting long-term supplementation with carnitine.
Chromium	600 to 1,200 mcg once a day as chromium picolinate	Combining with the protein picolinate allows your body to absorb chromium more efficiently. However, some chromium picolinate supplements contain more chromium than necessary. Ask your healthcare provider for a recommendation on chromium consumption.
Coenzyme Q_{10}*	100 to 300 mg a day	If you are on blood-thinning medications, speak to your healthcare provider before using CoQ_{10}. Since some medications can cause a deficiency of this nutrient, speak to your healthcare provider to determine if you might need a larger dose.
EGCG (green tea extract)*	150 mg EGCG twice a day, or 2 cups of green tea a day	Green tea extract can interact with a number of drugs. Check with your healthcare provider before taking this supplement.
EPA/DHA (fish oil)*	1,000 to 2,000 mg a day	Choose a source that contains vitamin E to prevent oxidation.
Fenugreek*	5,000 mg of seed powder a day, or 1,000 mg of a hydroalcoholic extract	Avoid fenugreek if you are allergic to chickpeas, peanuts, green peas, or soybeans. Fenugreek has mild blood-thinning effects. If you have a bleeding disorder or are taking a medication or supplement that may thin your blood, do not take this herb. Fenugreek may also negatively impact thyroid function.
Ginger*	1,000 mg three times a day	Ginger can act as a blood thinner. Check with your healthcare provider or pharmacist before taking this supplement.
Green coffee bean extract	300 to 750 mg a day	Because green coffee contains caffeine, you should avoid taking this supplement if you are sensitive to caffeine.
Magnesium	400 mg a day as magnesium glycinate	Consult your healthcare provider for dosage if you have kidney disease. Discontinue use and see your doctor if you experience abdominal pain. Take a lower dose if it causes diarrhea.

Olive leaf extract*	500 mg a day containing 20 mg of oleuropein per capsule	Olive leaf extracts can interact with many prescription medications, and may increase the effects of blood thinners. Consult your healthcare provider before using olive leaf extract if you are taking any medication. Don't use if you are pregnant or breastfeeding.
Probiotics	20 billion units once a day of *Lactobacillus gasseri* and/or *Lactobacillus plantarum*	Be sure to take the probiotics specified in the dosage column, which have been found to result in weight loss. If taking an antibiotic, take the probiotics at least two hours before or two hours after using the antibiotics. Do not take them at the same time.
Vitamin C	3,000 mg a day in divided doses	Do not take high doses if you are prone to kidney stones or gout. High doses can also cause diarrhea.
Vitamin D$_3$	Have your blood levels measured by your healthcare provider, who will determine proper dosage.	

*This supplement can have a blood-thinning action. See page 328 for more information.

WOUND HEALING

Wound healing is the body's natural process of regenerating dermal and epidermal tissue—in other words, the skin—when physical injury occurs. The events that constitute the wound-healing process overlap in time, but include blood clotting, scab formation, platelet aggregation, inflammation, the formation of new capillaries and collagen, contraction of the wound edges, growth of new skin, and formation of scar tissue. This process begins at the moment of injury, and can continue for months or even longer. It can take as long as two years for the scar to fade and potentially disappear.

The ability of wounds to heal properly is determined by adequate blood supply, appropriate wound-care techniques, and control of any existing medical problems. For healthy people, wound healing usually progresses well. People who are vulnerable to problems with wound healing include the elderly, diabetics, those with congestive heart failure, and those with suppressed immune systems.

The most important aspect of wound care is constant attention to the wound, with frequent cleansing and changing of dressings. It has also been found that a supplement program which combines antioxidant nutrients can speed wound healing by 20 percent.

SUPPLEMENTS TO ENCOURAGE WOUND HEALING

Supplements	Dosage	Considerations
Arginine	1,000 to 3,000 mg once a day	Do not take if you have kidney disease, liver disease, or herpes except under a doctor's supervision. Arginine can interact with some medications. Consult with your healthcare provider before beginning this therapy.
Carnosine	1,000 to 2,000 mg once a day	Check with your doctor before starting carnosine therapy if you have diabetes, hypertension, kidney disease, or liver damage. Too much carnosine can result in hyperactivity.
Grape seed extract*	50 to 200 mg once a day	Do not use with blood-thinning medications or supplements.
Vitamin B$_5$ (pantothenic acid)	50 mg twice a day	High doses can deplete your body of other vitamins in the B complex, so take a B-complex vitamin twice a day. Stop taking B$_5$ supplements if you begin having chest pains or breathing problems.
Vitamin C	1,000 mg twice a day	Do not take high doses if you are prone to kidney stones or gout. High doses can also cause diarrhea.

*This supplement can have a blood-thinning action. See page 328 for more information.

YEAST INFECTIONS

See Candidiasis.

Conclusion

You are now aware of the many important nutrients that can help you maintain good health. If you are dealing with a health problem, you have also learned that the right nutrients can help you manage it, sometimes used alone, and sometimes used along with conventional medical treatments, such as prescription medication. A fellowship-trained specialist in anti-aging, functional, and personalized medicine can guide you in reaching your goals by encouraging the restoration of balance to your body.

The nutritional programs described in *What You Must Know About Vitamins, Minerals, Herbs, and So Much More* are designed to treat the root cause of health problems, rather than mask the symptoms. All of the suggestions offered in these pages—which are based on up-to-date research and an understanding of the physiological processes, environmental conditions, and genetic predispositions that can affect well-being—can have a major and positive impact on your health.

Yet despite all its potentially helpful information, *What You Must Know About Vitamins, Minerals, Herbs, and So Much More* can only be as useful as you, the reader, make it. It's vital that you take responsibility for what you put into your body and how you live your life.

We are in a new age of medicine, one in which you, the patient, are an active participant in your own treatment. After all, your lifestyle choices—including your diet, exercise habits, and nutritional supplement regimen—are crucial to your overall health. Yet my job as a physician is not to blame your lifestyle choices, but to assist you as you work to optimize your health. It is my hope that this book has provided a timely reference that you and your healthcare provider can use as you design a nutritional program that is uniquely suited to your needs.

Resources

In this book, I've tried to provide all the information you need to create a supplement program that will help you achieve and maintain wellness. Although you can put together and follow this regimen on your own, it is often helpful to work with a personalized medicine specialist who can customize your program to your special needs. This can be especially important if you are managing a health condition and are already taking various medications. As you've learned in this book, certain diagnostic tests can also be valuable in guiding your supplement choices. Finally, whether you develop your own regimen or rely on the guidance of a specialist, you will benefit most if you use pharmaceutical grade supplements, which meet the highest regulatory requirements. The following lists will guide you to the resources that can help you realize your goal of good health.

PERSONALIZED MEDICINE SPECIALISTS

To ensure optimal health, it is important to work with a healthcare practitioner who will take your present health status, medical history, and genetic makeup (genome) into account in formulating a personal regimen for you, and who is also knowledgeable about nutritional supplements, their benefits, and their possible side effects and interactions. Below, you will find organizations that can lead you to local professionals who specialize in natural and alternative health; nutrition; and functional, anti-aging, and personalized medicine.

American Academy of Anti-Aging Medicine (A4M)
1801 North Military Trail
Boca Raton, FL 33431
Phone: (888) 997– 0112 (toll free)
(561) 997– 0112 (outside the US)
Website: www.a4m.com

American College for Advancement in Medicine (ACAM)
380 Ice Center Lane, Suite C
Bozeman, MT 59718
Phone: (800) 532–3688
Website: www.acam.org

DIAGNOSTIC LABORATORIES

Medical testing now makes it possible to measure your amino acids, fatty acids, organic acids, vitamin levels, hormone levels, gastrointestinal function, genome, and much more. This means that your treatment can be personalized to meet your specific needs. The following laboratories can perform tests to evaluate many important aspects of your health. Before ordering any medical test, be sure to consult with your healthcare practitioner.

Cyrex Laboratories
2602 South 24th Street
Phoenix, AZ 85034
Phone: (877) 772–9739 (US)
(844) 216–4763 (Canada)
Website: www.cyrexlabs.com/

Doctor's Data
3755 Illinois Avenue
St. Charles, IL 60174
Phone: (800) 323–2784
Website: www.doctorsdata.com

Dutch Test by Precision Analytical
3138 NE Rivergate Street, Suite #301C
McMinnville, OR 97128
Phone: (503) 687–2050
Website: https://dutchtest.com/

Genova Diagnostics
63 Zillicoa Street
Asheville, NC 28801
Phone: (800) 522–4762
(828) 253–0621
Website: www.gdx.net

Great Plains Laboratory
11813 West 77th Street
Lenexa, KS 66214
Phone: (800) 288–3383

(913) 341–8949
Website: www.
greatplainslaboratory.com/

Pathways Genomics
6777 Nancy Ridge Drive
San Diego, CA 92121
Phone: (877) 505–7374
Website: www.pathway.com

Rocky Mountain Analytical
105–32 Royal Vista Drive NW
Calgary, Alberta T3R 0H9
Canada
Phone: (866) 370–5227
(403) 241–4500
Website: www.rmalab.com

SpectraCell Laboratories
10401 Town Park Drive
Houston, TX 77072
Phone: (800) 227–5227
(713) 621–3101
Website: www.spectracell.com

ZRT Laboratory
8605 SW Creekside Place
Beaverton, OR 97008
Phone: (866) 600–1636
(503) 466– 2445
Website: www.zrtlab.com

COMPOUNDING PHARMACY

Compounding is the practice of creating personalized medications to fill the gaps left by mass-produced medicine. To meet the special needs of an individual, a compounding pharmacy can provide unique dosages, innovative delivery methods, and unusual flavorings, and can also eliminate allergens and unnecessary fillers. Professional Compounding Centers of America can help you find a PCCA Member pharmacy in your area.

Professional Compounding
Centers of America (PCCA)
9901 South Wilcrest Drive
Houston, TX 77099
Phone: (800) 331–2498
(281) 933–6948
Website: www.pccarx.com

744 Third Street
London, ON N5V 5J2
Canada
Phone: (800) 668–9453
(519) 455–0690
Website: www.pccarx.ca

PHARMACEUTICAL GRADE SUPPLEMENTS

You can find many good supplement brands at health food stores. However, it is not always easy to locate pharmaceutical grade nutrients, which is what you should take to ensure that your supplements contain all of the active ingredients listed on the label, but no fillers or contaminants. The following pharmaceutical grade companies offer many quality nutritional supplements. Visit their websites for full product lists.

Biotics Research Corporation
6801 Biotics Research Drive
Rosenberg, TX 77471
Phone: (800) 231–5777
(281) 344–0909
Website: www.bioticsresearch.com

Designs for Health, Inc.
980 South Street
Suffield, CT 06078
Phone: (800) 847–8302
(860) 623–6314
Website: www.designsforhealth.com

Body Bio
45 Reese Road
Millville, NJ 08332
Phone: (888) 327–9554 (toll free)
(856) 825–8338 (outside the US)
Website: www.bodybio.com

Douglas Laboratories
112 Technology Drive
Pittsburgh, PA 15275
Phone: (800) 245–4440
Website: www.douglaslabs.com

Life Extension
5990 North Federal Highway
Fort Lauderdale, FL 33308
Phone: (800) 678–8989
Website: www.lifeextension.com

Metagenics
25 Enterprise
Aliso Viejo, CA 92656
Phone: (800) 692-9400
(949) 366–0818
Website: www.metagenics.com

Ortho Molecular Products
1991 Duncan Place
Woodstock, IL 60098
Phone: (800) 332–2351
Website: www.
orthomolecularproducts.com

Vital Nutrients
45 Kenneth Dooley Drive
Middletown, CT 06457
Phone: (888) 328–9992 (toll free)
(860) 638–3675
Website: www.vitalnutrients.net

Xymogen
6900 Kingspointe Parkway
Orlando, FL 32819
Phone: (800) 647–6100
Website: www.xymogen.com

References

The information and recommendations presented in this book are based on over a thousand scientific studies, academic papers, and books. If the references for all these sources were printed here, they would add considerable bulk to the book and make it more expensive, as well. For this reason, the publisher and I have decided to present a complete list of references, categorized by chapter and topic, on the publisher's website. This format has the added advantage of enabling us to make you aware of further important studies and papers as they become available. You can find the references under the listing of my book at www.squareonepublishers.com.

Index

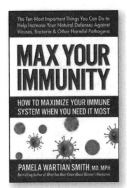
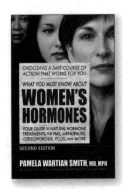

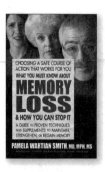

What You Must Know About Memory Loss & How You Can Stop It

A Guide to Proven Techniques and Supplements
to Maintain, Strengthen, or Regain Memory

Pamela Wartian Smith, MD, MPH

Contrary to popular belief, not all memory loss is caused by the aging process. In *What You Must Know About Memory Loss & How You Can Stop It,* Dr. Pamela Wartian Smith describes what you can do to reverse the problem and enhance your mental abilities for years to come. You'll learn about the most common causes of memory loss, including nutritional deficiencies, hormonal imbalances, toxic overload, poor blood circulation, and lack of physical and mental exercise. The author explains how each cause is involved in impaired memory and supplies a list of proven remedies.

$15.95 US • 240 pages • 6 x 9-inch paperback • ISBN 978-0-7570-0386-8

What You Must Know About Allergy Relief

How to Overcome the Allergies You Have & Find the Hidden
Allergies That Make You Sick

Earl Mindell, RPh, and Pamela Wartian Smith, MD

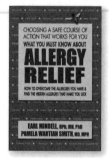

When most people have allergies, they know it. But for many others, allergies and intolerances are *hidden* culprits that lie at the heart of a number of health conditions. If you are an allergy sufferer or have a recurring health issue that you can't seem to resolve, this is the book for you. Written by a pharmacist and medical doctor, it provides important answers to common questions about allergies— what causes them, how they can affect you, and how you can overcome them. Up-to-date and easy to understand, *What You Must Know About Allergy Relief* offers the tools to identify hidden allergies and the means to relieve their symptoms.

$17.95 US • 288 pages • 6 x 9-inch paperback • ISBN 978-0-7570-0437-7

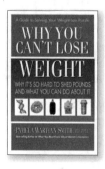

Why You Can't Lose Weight

Why It's So Hard to Shed Pounds and What You Can Do About It

Pamela Wartian Smith, MD, MPH

If you have tried to slim down without success, it may not be your fault. In this revolutionary book, Dr. Pamela Smith discusses the eighteen most common reasons why you can't lose weight, and guides you in overcoming the obstacles that stand between you and a trimmer body. It's time to learn what's really keeping you from reaching your goal. With *Why You Can't Lose Weight,* you'll discover how to shed pounds and enjoy radiant health.

$16.95 US • 256 pages • 6 x 9-inch paperback • ISBN 978-0-7570-0312-7

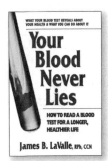

Your Blood Never Lies

How to Read a Blood Test for a Longer, Healthier Life

James B. LaValle, RPh, CCN

A standard blood test indicates how well the kidneys and liver are functioning, the potential for heart disease, and a host of other vital health markers. Unfortunately, most of us cannot decipher these results ourselves or even formulate the right questions to ask—or we couldn't, until now. In simple language, Dr. LaValle explains all of the information found on these forms, making it understandable and accessible so that you can look at the results yourself and know the significance of each marker. He even recommends the most effective treatments for dealing with problematic findings and provides the names of test markers that should be requested for a complete physical picture.

$16.95 US • 368 pages • 6 x 9-inch paperback • ISBN 978-0-7570-0350-9

Magnificent Magnesium

Your Essential Key to a Healthy Heart & More

Dennis Goodman, MD

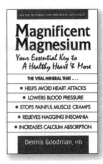

Despite the development of many "breakthrough" drugs, heart disease remains the number-one killer of Americans. In *Magnificent Magnesium,* world-renowned cardiologist Dr. Dennis Goodman shines a spotlight on magnesium, the mineral that can maximize your heart health without side effects. The author first establishes a firm foundation for understanding heart disease. Next, he examines the important role magnesium plays in life processes and explores how a deficiency of this substance can lead to many common health conditions. The author then details magnesium's astounding heart-healthy benefits, along with the additional advantages it provides for other diseases. Finally, he offers clear guidelines on how to select and use this mineral to greatest effect.

$14.95 US • 192 pages • 6 x 9-inch paperback • ISBN 978-0-7570-0391-2

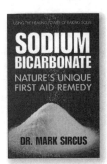

Sodium Bicarbonate

Nature's Unique First Aid Remedy

Dr. Mark Sircus

What if there were a natural health-promoting substance that was inexpensive and available at any grocery store? There is. It's called sodium bicarbonate, also known as baking soda. *Sodium Bicarbonate* begins with an overview of baking soda, chronicling its use as a home remedy. Author Mark Sircus then details how this extraordinary substance can alleviate a number of health disorders and suggests the most effective way to use sodium bicarbonate in the treatment of each condition. Let *Sodium Bicarbonate* help you look at baking soda in a whole new way.

$16.95 US • 208 pages • 6 x 9-inch paperback • ISBN 978-0-7570-0394-3

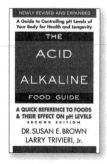

The Acid-Alkaline Food Guide, SECOND EDITION

A Quick Reference to Foods & Their Effect on pH Levels

Susan E. Brown, PhD, and Larry Trivieri, Jr.

In the last few years, researchers around the world have increasingly reported the importance of acid-alkaline balance. *The Acid-Alkaline Food Guide* was designed as an easy-to-follow guide to the most common foods that influence your body's pH level. Now in its Second Edition, this bestseller has been expanded to include many more domestic and international foods. Updated information also explores (and refutes) the myths about pH balance and diet, and guides you to supplements that can help you achieve a pH level that supports greater well-being.

$8.95 US • 224 pages • 4 x 7-inch paperback • ISBN 978-0-7570-0393-6

Glycemic Index Food Guide

For Weight Loss, Cardiovascular Health, Diabetic Management, and Maximum Energy

Dr. Shari Lieberman

By indicating how quickly a given food triggers a rise in blood sugar, the glycemic index (GI) enables you to choose foods that can help you manage a variety of conditions and improve your overall health. This easy-to-use guide teaches you about the GI and how to use it. It provides both the glycemic index and the glycemic load for hundreds of foods and beverages. Whether you want to manage your diabetes, lose weight, increase your heart health, or simply enhance your well-being, the *Glycemic Index Food Guide* is the best place to start.

$7.95 US • 160 pages • 4 x 7-inch paperback • ISBN 978-0-7570-0245-8

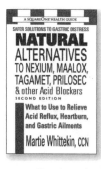

Natural Alternatives to Nexium, Maalox, Tagamet, Prilosec & Other Acid Blockers, SECOND EDITION

What to Use to Help Relieve Acid Reflux, Heartburn, and Other Gastric Ailments

Martie Whittekin, CCN

Written by Martie Whittekin, an experienced clinical nutritionist, *Natural Alternatives to Nexium* examines the underlying causes of acid reflux, heartburn, and other acid-related gastric ailments. It then provides natural alternatives to medications for both immediate and long-term relief.

$7.95 US • 272 pages • 4 x 7-inch paperback • ISBN 978-0-7570-0210-6

**For more information about our books,
visit our website at www.squareonepublishers.com**